THE CONSUMER'S GUIDE TO TREATING COMMON ILLNESSES

DR. RUTH LEVER

A FIRESIDE BOOK

PUBLISHED BY SIMON & SCHUSTER, INC.

New York · London · Toronto · Sydney · Tokyo · Singapore

FIRESIDE
Simon & Schuster Building
Rockefeller Center
1230 Avenue of the Americas
New York, New York 10020

Originally published in Great Britain by Penguin Books

FIRESIDE and colophon are registered trademarks
of Simon & Schuster Inc.

Designed by Irving Perkins and Assoc.
Manufactured in the United States of America

10 9 8 7 6 5 4 3 2 1

Library of Congress Cataloging-in-Publication Data
Lever, Ruth.
     [Guide to common illnesses]
     The consumer's guide to treating common illnesses / Ruth Lever.
        p.   cm.
     Previously published: A guide to common illnesses. Great Britain:
Penguin Books, c1990.
     "A Fireside book."
     Includes indexes.
     1. Medicine, Popular—Handbooks, manuals, etc.   I. Title.
RC81.L623   1992
616—dc20   92-18688
                                                        CIP

ISBN: 0-671-74716-9

For my husband, John,
with my love

CONTENTS

7

8   Contents

ANXIETY AND PHOBIAS   49

ARTHRITIS   56

ASTHMA   71

BACK PAIN   81

BED-WETTING (NOCTURNAL ENURESIS)   92

BREAST LUMPS   96

BRONCHITIS   107

DIVERTICULAR DISEASE   152

EAR INFECTIONS   157

ECZEMA   166

12   Contents

EPILEPSY 178

FIBROIDS 188

GALLBLADDER DISEASE 192

HAIR LOSS   203

HEMORRHOIDS (PILES)   209

HERPES SIMPLEX   213

14   Contents

MIGRAINE   298

MONONUCLEOSIS, INFECTIOUS   306

MOUTH ULCERS AND BAD BREATH (HALITOSIS)   309

NOSEBLEEDS   313

OSTEOPOROSIS   317

18   Contents

PSORIASIS   354

RHINITIS   368

RINGWORM 374

SCHIZOPHRENIA 380

SHINGLES (HERPES ZOSTER) 387

SINUSITIS 391

22   Contents

LIST OF
DIAGRAMS

THE PURPOSE AND STRUCTURE OF THIS BOOK

AS THE "RESIDENT DOCTOR" on the TVS program "Problem Page" in Britain and, now as the writer of an "Ask the Doctor" column in a weekly magazine, I have become aware that in the letters I receive asking for advice certain questions come up again and again. They include:

> *My doctor thinks I may have A and is sending me for tests. What will they entail?*

> *My doctor tells me I have B. How will it affect my life?*

> *I have just been told that I have C. What treatment will I have to undergo?*

> *My doctor has prescribed D. What is it for and what are the side effects?*

> *I have been treated by my doctor for E but nothing seems to help. Is there a complementary therapy I could try?*

> *I have F and feel it would help to talk to other sufferers. Is there an organization I can join?*

There are, of course, reasons why these questions keep cropping up. When a diagnosis is first made, it is not always easy for a patient to take in everything that is being said. Sometimes, the doctor uses language the patient doesn't understand. Sometimes he or she doesn't have time to explain everything thoroughly. Sometimes the patient's anxiety gets in the way of understanding. And, very often, so much is said that the patient can only remember a fraction of it. Unfortunately, there is also a limit to how much one can say in a few minutes on a television program or in a couple of columns in a magazine. I began to feel more and more that what was needed was a full description of a number of common illnesses that would answer all these questions in depth and that the patient could keep for reference to read again whenever necessary. And it was from that idea that this book stemmed.

Each chapter covers a common illness or group of illnesses although, in some cases, for the sake of completeness, I have mentioned one or two rarer conditions that fall within a common group. As far as infections are concerned, I have included only those which are extremely common (such as herpes simplex which affects some 20 million people in the United States) and have omitted conditions such as tuberculosis and AIDS which, although on the increase, have, thankfully, not yet reached such proportions. I have also omitted infectious diseases which are of a limited duration, such as the common cold and childhood infections.

The purpose of this book is not self-help but explanation. However, I have included a short "self-help" section in some chapters where it is appropriate.

TESTS

Having to go to the hospital or doctor's office for tests is always a little alarming and I hope that, by explaining what is likely to happen, this book will relieve some of the anxiety that patients naturally feel. Recently, however, I read an article in a magazine in which the writer commented that a friend of hers, having had some tests for cancer of the cervix, was unwilling to return to the hospital, having been unprepared "for the indignity of the procedure or the stinging pain." I was horrified by this and wrote a letter to the magazine in which I said:

It is unfortunate, of course, that she found the colposcopy uncomfortable, but the stinging pain to which you refer is only momentary (and is not experienced by all patients). . . . As to indignity . . . doctors are not there to humiliate their patients but to help them and, wherever possible, to prevent them from becoming ill or to restore them to health. There is no indignity in this. It would be a tragedy if this woman failed to return for further investigations. . . . To die from cancer which could have been cured is senseless.

It is inevitable that some tests will be uncomfortable or unpleasant. It is therefore vital to remember that they are being done for the patient's benefit in order to restore him or her to health. The diseases that can be diagnosed, treated and, in many cases, cured, are likely to be far more uncomfortable, unpleasant, and long-term than any tests.

Someone who is anxious about a test (or any procedure) should ask the doctor to explain it as he goes along. This is usually very reassuring—and may even be interesting!

RECENT ADVANCES

Most chapters have a paragraph or two on recent advances in diagnosis and treatment for that particular illness. This book was originally completed in January 1989 for the British edition, but has, as much as possible, been revised and brought up to date for this edition.

DIAGRAMS

Some diagrams may be appropriate to more than one chapter but, for reasons of space, can only be printed in one place. A list is therefore given at the beginning of the book for ease of reference.

ORGANIZATIONS

Many of the organizations listed in this book are charities, working on a very limited budget. When writing to any of them for information, please enclose a stamped addressed envelope for the reply.

THE APPENDICES

Although I have tried to avoid jargon, there are some one-word medical terms that need eight or ten words to explain them. In such cases, I have used the medical term, but an explanation appears in the glossary at the back of the book and at least once in the text. I have also tended to use medical terms where they are words that are finding their way into common usage (such as *uterus* rather than *womb*), but here again an explanation is included in the glossary.

Drugs are prescribed under their chemical or generic names. One drug may be made by a number of different companies; thus, it has several different brand names, which are sometimes used in prescriptions. I have listed all the drugs mentioned in the text, together with their various trade names, at the back of the book. If any do not appear here, it is because they are manufactured only under their chemical names. Some drugs are mentioned in several sections of the book but are detailed only once in the appendix; however, they are also listed in the index, which will direct the reader to the appropriate section of the appendix.

New drugs are being introduced all the time, while others are discontinued. It is possible, therefore, that by the time this book is published, one or two of the drugs I mention may no longer be in use and others will have taken their place.

Finally, I have also included a pronunciation guide, since some of the medical terms I have included are very long and awkward, and others, although shorter, may offer the possibility of being pronounced two or more ways.

HOW TO USE THIS BOOK

THE FIRST FEW PARAGRAPHS in each section tend to relate to the whole section and should be read before going on to any individual part of it.

Some illnesses, diagnostic techniques, and forms of treatment that are mentioned in passing in some sections may be dealt with in greater depth elsewhere, so please use the index to make sure you have found all the information relevant to any particular subject.

Before consulting the sections on complementary treatment, please read the introductory section on complementary therapies.

COMPLEMENTARY THERAPIES

I HAVE NOT ATTEMPTED to list all the therapies that may be helpful in the treatment of an illness. Complementary therapies tend to treat the whole patient, not just the part that is diseased, and therefore it is more a question of whether the patient will respond to a particular therapy rather than whether a certain illness will. Some therapies, like healing and radionics, can be helpful in an enormous range of problems, but the treatment does not vary enormously from case to case, so on the whole these are not listed. I have only mentioned an individual therapy for a particular illness where it has been possible to suggest what might be prescribed in such a case; therapies not listed may still be helpful.

Although I have mentioned specific complementary treatments (for example, herbs and homeopathic remedies), this is not a recommendation for self-treatment except as a first-aid measure. One will inevitably get the best results by going to see a therapist who has trained, usually for several years, in his specialty, rather than by trying something out from the health food shop. The exception is the Bach remedies, of which there are only thirty-eight and whose use is easily mastered.

ACUPUNCTURE

Acupuncture has been used in China for thousands of years. It is based on the theory that the body's energy or vital force (called Chi) circulates through a series of channels or meridians. Each of these channels has the name of an organ of the body (such as the Heart channel and the Liver channel) and is specifically linked with that organ. Each organ has a special function, over and above the function that is recognized in Western medicine. Thus, for example, the energy of the kidney is said to control the reproductive system and hearing.

31

The channels can be invaded by "harmful Chi," which takes the form of heat, damp, wind, cold, dryness, and poor diet. It is this invasion that causes illness by disrupting the normal flow of Chi. Along the meridians are points that can be used to control the body's energy flow and to expel harmful Chi when a needle is inserted into them.

The acupuncturist's choice of which points to use will be based on the patient's symptoms, the appearance of her tongue, and her pulse, among other diagnostic techniques.

ALEXANDER TECHNIQUE

This system of posture training can be invaluable when problems stem from or are made worse by a faulty posture.

AROMATHERAPY

The life force of a plant is said, by aromatherapists, to be captured in its essential oil. Each oil has specific properties that make it valuable in the treatment of certain diseases. The oils may be taken by mouth, inhaled, used in the bath, or massaged into the skin, depending on the individual case.

BACH FLOWER REMEDIES

These flower remedies were discovered by Dr. Edward Bach, who was an eminent physician. He felt that some of his patients did not get well as fast as they should and that this was due to their state of mind. He was convinced that flowers had properties that could affect the mind and he started to investigate these. The resulting thirty-eight remedies (and the combination "Rescue Remedy" useful for all forms of shock and fright) are exceptionally gentle and very effective. Each is appropriate for a different negative state of mind, such as anxiety, melancholy, fear, or exhaustion. They have no side effects of any kind, can be taken quite safely with any other type of medication and, what is more, can be taken as often as they are needed—every ten minutes if necessary. Four drops are put on the tongue and left for a few seconds before swallowing. They are best not taken within ten minutes of eating, drinking, or smoking. Bach remedies are available from many health food shops or by contacting the Dr. Edward Bach Healing Society, 644 Merrick Road, Lynbrook, NY 11563; 516/593-2206.

CHIROPRACTIC

This system of manipulation focuses primarily on the spine.

HEALING

There are many types of healers. Some believe their healing ability comes from God and that it is therefore a semireligious experience. Others believe that they are merely acting as a channel for a natural energy. Some move their hands above the patient; others touch the patient. Some use visualization as part of their therapy, so that the patient is taking part in his own treatment. Healing has been reported to be effective in the treatment of many kinds of disease and, even in cases where a cure is not possible, may help to improve the patient's quality of life.

HERBALISM

Although herbalists use many herbs that are also used, in a refined form, by traditional practitioners, the theory on which their use is based is somewhat different. For a start, herbalists believe that the whole plant is more effective in treatment than any one of its component parts. And, for the most part, they use herbs not to treat an individual symptom as such but rather to raise the level of health of the patient, clean toxins out of the body, restore normal function to the diseased part, and leave the body to heal itself, which it is then in a position to do.

HOMEOPATHY

Homeopathy is based on the premise of "like cures like." A substance that will produce a certain set of symptoms in a healthy person will, if given to someone who has developed those symptoms as a result of a disease, cure him. Homeopathic remedies are used in enormous dilution and thus produce few side effects, while being extremely powerful.

There are over two thousand remedies, each of which has its own "symptom picture." The task of the homeopath is to match, as closely as possible, the patient's personality and habits, as well as his symptoms, to a particular remedy.

HYPNOTHERAPY

Hypnotherapy is a form of deep relaxation that can be used in the treatment of any illness that has a psychosomatic component (that is, anything that can be brought on or made worse by mental factors such as stress or anxiety).

NATUROPATHY

This is mainly based on a healthy way of life and much of the advice given by a naturopath concerns diet. I have therefore tended to include such ideas in the "self-help" sections, as most of them are quite safe to follow on one's own. However, naturopaths sometimes recommend fasts and these should never be undertaken without the advice and guidance of a qualified therapist.

NUTRITION THERAPY

Much of what we eat today is deficient in vitamins and minerals. Not only have a lot of vegetables been grown in mineral-deficient soil but the food itself has been harvested long before it reaches the supermarket shelves, so its vitamins have started to break down. Some types of cooking and processing destroy vitamins still further, but "junk" foods increase our needs for these vital nutrients. It is scarcely surprising, therefore, that many nutrition therapists maintain that everyone nowadays needs to take vitamin and mineral supplements. A number of symptoms can be laid very firmly at the door of nutrient deficiencies and can be treated very successfully with nutritional supplements. I have tended to avoid giving dosages for supplements in the text, since these can vary enormously depending on the individual patient. However, the following is a suitable daily intake for the average adult: 7500 i.u. of vitamin A; 400 i.u. of vitamin D; 100 i.u. of vitamin E; 1000 mg of vitamin C; 25 mg each of vitamins B_1 (thiamine) and B_2

(riboflavin), and 50 mg each of vitamins B_3 (nicotinic acid), B_5 (pantothenic acid), and B_6 (pyridoxine); 5 mcg of vitamin B_{12} and 50 mcg each of folic acid and biotin; 25 mg each of choline, inositol, and PABA; 150 mg of calcium; 75 mg of magnesium; 10 mg each of iron and zinc; 2.5 mg of manganese; 25 mcg of selenium and 20 mcg of chromium. Several multivitamin/multimineral preparations contain quantities similar to these. Those that do not contain copper are preferable, since most people get adequate amounts of copper from their drinking water.

OSTEOPATHY

This is a form of manipulation by fully trained medical doctors that seeks to restore normal function to the joints and muscles of the body.

RADIONICS

A form of absent healing, radionics uses a piece of the patient's hair as a "witness" to link patient and practitioner. A well-known doctor once remarked that the most extraordinary thing about radionics is that it works. How it works no one knows—even the practitioners have no single theory. However, it has been reported to be useful in a wide range of illnesses and, like healing, may help to improve the patient's quality of life even when a cure is not possible.

Addresses of organizations holding lists of qualified complementary practitioners may be found at the back of the book.

REFLEXOLOGY

Reflexology is a system of foot or hand massage based on the theory that the entire body is reflected in the sole of the foot or the palm of the hand. Thus, massage of a particular point will affect the organ with which it is linked. Not only is the treatment very soothing and relaxing but it has been reported to be effective for a wide range of ailments.

FURTHER READING

Barlow, W. *The Alexander Technique*. Arrow, 1979, London, and Warner Books, 1980, New York.

Bayly, Doreen. *Reflexology Today*. Thorsons, 1984, Wellingborough, UK, and Thorsons, 1984, New York.

Brown, Barbara. *Stress and the Art of Biofeedback*. Bantam, 1978, New York.

Buchman, D. *Herbal Medicine*. Rider, 1983, London.

Byers, Dwight C. *Better Health with Foot Reflexology*. Ingham Publishing, 1983, Saint Petersburg, Florida.

Cade, C. Maxwell, and Nona Coxhead. *The Awakened Mind*. Element Books, 1986, United Kingdom.

Carroll, D. *The Complete Book of Natural Medicine*. Summit Books, 1980, New York.

Chaitow, Leon. *Osteopathy*. Thorsons, 1982, Wellingborough, UK, and Thorsons, 1985, New York.

Chancellor, P. *Handbook of Bach Flower Remedies*. C. W. Daniel, 1985, Saffron Walden, UK, and Keats, 1980.

Clark, Linda. *Handbook of Natural Remedies for Common Ailments*. Pocket Books, 1976, New York.

Connelly, Dianne. *Traditional Acupuncture: The Law of the Five Elements*. Center for Traditional Acupuncture Inc., 1979.

Coulter, Catherine R. *Portraits of Homeopathic Medicines: Psychophysical Analyses of Selected Constitutional Types*. Wehawken Book Co., 1986.

Coulter, Harris L. *Homeopathic Science and Modern Medicine*. North Atlantic Books, 1981.

Dintenfass, J. *Chiropractic: A Modern Way to Health*. Harcourt Brace Jovanovich, 1971, New York.

Fulder, Stephen. *The Handbook of Complementary Medicine*. Coronet Books, Hodder & Stoughton, 1984, United Kingdom.

Gelb, Michael. *Body Learning*. Aurum Press, 1985, London, and Delilah Books, 1981, New York.

Goldstein, J. *The Experience of Insight*. Wildwood House, 1981, London, and Shambhala Publications, 1983, New York.

Gordon, Richard. *Your Healing Hands*. Wingbow Press, 1978, Berkeley, CA.

Green, Elmer, and Alyce Green. *Beyond Biofeedback*. Dell Publishing Company, 1977, New York.

Griggs, Barbara. *Home Herbal*. Pan, 1983, London.

Grossman, Richard. *The Other Medicines*. Doubleday, 1985, New York, and Pan, 1986, London.

Hoffman, D. *Holistic Herbal*. Findhorn Press, 1984, Forres, UK.

Hyne Jones, T. W. *Dictionary of the Bach Flower Remedies*. C. W. Daniel, 1985, Saffron Walden, UK.

Inglis, Brian, and Ruth West. *The Alternative Health Guide.* Michael Joseph, 1983, London.

Iyengar, B. K. S. *Light on Yoga.* Allen and Unwin, 1985, London, and Schocken, 1977, New York.

Jarvis, D. C. *Folk Medicine.* Pan, 1961, London, and Fawcett, 1985.

Kaptchuk, Ted. *Chinese Medicine, The Web That Has No Weaver.* Rider, 1986, London, and Congdon and Weed, 1984, New York.

Krieger, Dolores. *Therapeutic Touch.* Prentice Hall, 1979, Englewood Cliffs, NJ.

Lankton, Stephen R. (ed.) *Elements and Dimensions of an Ericksonian Approach.* Brunner-Mazel, 1985, New York.

Leibold, G. *Practical Hydrotherapy.* Thorsons, 1980, Wellingborough, UK.

LeShan, Lawrence. *How to Meditate.* Thorsons, 1985, Wellingborough, UK., and Bantam, 1975, New York.

Lidell, Lucy. *The Book of Massage.* Ebury Press, 1984, London, and Simon & Schuster, 1984, New York.

Lidell, Lucy. *The Book of Yoga.* Ebury Press, 1983, London, and Simon & Schuster, 1983, New York.

Lindlahr, H. *Philosophy of Natural Therapeutics.* Maidstone Osteopathic Clinic, 1975, Maidstone, UK.

Lindlahr, H. *Practise of Natural Therapeutics.* Maidstone Osteopathic Clinic, 1985, Maidstone, UK.

MacManaway, Bruce, and Johanna Turcan. *Healing.* Thorsons, 1985, Wellingborough, UK, and New York.

Newman Turner, Roger. *Naturopathic Medicine.* Thorsons, 1984, Wellingborough, UK.

Ohashi, Wataru. *Do-It-Yourself Shiatsu.* Allen and Unwin, 1979, London, and E. P. Dutton, 1976, New York.

Panos, M., and J. Heimlich. *Homeopathic Medicine at Home.* Corgi, Transworld Publishers, 1984, London, and Tarcher, 1981, Los Angeles.

Poteliakhoff, Max, and M. Carruthers. *Real Health: Ill Effects of Stress and Their Prevention.* Davis-Poynter, 1981, London.

Powell, Eric. *The Natural Home Physician.* C. W. Daniel, 1975, Saffron Walden, UK.

Rolf, Ida. *Rolfing, The Integration of Human Structures.* Harper & Row, 1977, New York.

Ryman, Daniele. *The Aromatherapy Handbook.* Century Hutchinson, 1984, London.

Scofield, A. G. *Chiropractic.* Thorsons, 1982, Wellingborough, UK.

Stanway, Andrew. *Alternative Medicine.* Macdonald and Janes, 1979, London, and Penguin, 1986, London, and Penguin, 1982, New York.

Stoddard, Alan. *The Back: Relief from Pain.* Dunitz, 1979, London.

Tappan, Frances M. *Healing Massage Techniques—A Study of Eastern and Western Methods.* Prentice Hall, 1978, Reston, VA.

Thie, John F. *Touch for Health, A Practical Guide to Natural Health.* De Vorss and Co., 1979, Princeton, NJ.

Tisserand, R. *The Art of Aromatherapy.* C. W. Daniel, 1985, Saffron Walden, UK.

Valentine, T., and C. Valentine. *Applied Kinesiology.* Thorsons, 1985, Wellingborough, UK, and Thorsons, 1985, New York.

Vithoulkas, G. *Homeopathy, Medicine of the New Man.* Thorsons, 1985, Wellingborough, UK, and Arco, 1979, New York.

Wright, B. *Natural Healing with Herbal Combinations.* Green Press, 1984, Burwash, Suffolk, UK.

ACNE

INCIDENCE, CAUSE, AND DESCRIPTION

Acne is a skin condition that probably affects 80 percent of all adolescents to a greater or lesser degree. It usually begins around the time of puberty, affecting both boys and girls, and, in most cases, has cleared up by the early twenties. Boys are more likely to be severely affected, about 5 percent continuing to have problems into their thirties, compared with 1 percent of girls. Similarly, only one girl in two hundred is likely to suffer from severe acne whereas with boys the proportion is about one in twenty-five.

Various factors are known to cause acne, such as contact with mineral or vegetable oils or crude petroleum (occupational acne), and, sometimes, the contraceptive Pill or the use of steroids. However, in the vast majority of cases it seems to be caused by androgens, sex hormones that are secreted for the first time at puberty.

Although androgens are the male sex hormones, they are also produced in small amounts by girls. Among other effects, they stimulate the production of facial and body hair, which is kept soft by an oily substance called sebum. This is secreted by tiny sebaceous glands in the skin, which enlarge and become more active in response to these hormones. Acne occurs when the sebaceous glands become overactive and the exit from the gland is blocked by a deposition of keratin—the hard substance that forms an important part of the hair and nails and that helps to toughen skin. Sebum is therefore produced at a faster rate than it can leave the gland which, as a result, swells up. Normally harmless bacteria called *Propionibacterium acnes* tend to colonize in the swollen gland, where they feed on the sebum. Inflammation occurs and pimples and pus-filled spots (pustules) may develop. In severe cases, the glands may burst into the skin, producing cysts.

The first signs of acne are often whiteheads and blackheads. They are both caused by blocked sebaceous glands, the difference being that blackheads (whose color comes from melanin, the pigment present in

39

the skin and the hair) can be squeezed out or can work their way out of the duct, whereas whiteheads can't. In many cases, the condition doesn't progress any further and, after a few months or years, the skin becomes clear again. In more serious cases, in which pustules or cysts develop, scarring may occur as these heal.

The commonest site for acne is the face. Sometimes it may be months or even years before the condition spreads to the chest, back, shoulders, or neck, but occasionally the chest may be the only area involved. Repeated pressure or friction on the skin may make the condition worse—for example, violin players may find that the area under the chin is most severely affected.

TRADITIONAL TREATMENT

Over 90 percent of patients with acne respond to treatment. However, this often needs to be prolonged over months or even years. Two main forms are available: topical (applied directly to the skin) or systemic (taken internally).

Topical Treatment
Benzoyl peroxide is an exfoliating agent—that is, it helps the top layer of the skin to peel off—and it also prevents bacteria from multiplying. It is available as a gel, cream, or lotion, sometimes in combination with sulphur, which is also an exfoliating agent. It needs to be used for a considerable time and may, at first, produce redness and dryness of the skin, which will diminish after a while.

Tretinoin (or retinoic acid) is sometimes used alternately with benzoyl peroxide (one at night and the other in the morning) or it may be used alone. It is a derivative of vitamin A, which plays an important role in the maintenance of healthy skin, and it reduces the abnormal production of keratin at the mouth of the sebaceous glands. It is therefore very useful for the treatment of whiteheads and blackheads but is less effective in more advanced forms of acne. It can cause irritation and redness, especially if the skin is exposed to strong sunlight. Both benzoyl peroxide and tretinoin need to be used for a minimum of six months and it may take several weeks before any improvement is noticed.

Topical antibiotics are sometimes used in the treatment of acne, although some doctors avoid them because patients may become allergic to them.

In severe cases when cysts form, steroids injected into them may help them to resolve.

Systemic Treatment

The most popular treatment for acne is the antibiotic tetracycline. Used together with topical benzoyl peroxide, it is very effective. However, it is not well absorbed if taken with food, so the patient has to remember to take it between meals. Antacids, iron supplements, and milk can also interfere with its absorption. It must be taken for a minimum of three months and often much longer, although some improvement is usually obvious after about two months. Other antibiotics are sometimes used and may be helpful when tetracycline has failed. These include trimethoprim-sulfamethoxazole, minocycline, doxycycline, and erythromycin.

Although the initial changes of acne are brought about by androgens, nothing can be done about this in boys, since these are the hormones that transform them into men. However, in girls, whose development depends on the female hormones estrogen and progesterone, antiandrogen treatment can be used. In the United States, this is most commonly accomplished with oral contraceptives containing mestranol or ethinylestradiol. These drugs can be used to treat patients with acne and who need birth control.

The most recent innovation in the treatment of acne is isotretinoin (13-cis-retinoic acid) which, like the topical tretinoin, is a derivative of vitamin A. Its main effect is to reduce the production of sebum while stimulating the shedding of old skin cells. Because it can have serious side effects it is available only to those patients with severe acne who are referred to dermatologists familiar with using it. It commonly causes a dryness of the lips and soreness at the corners of the mouth, a dry rash on the face, nosebleeds, and conjunctivitis. Older patients may develop arthritis. It can also affect the liver and the levels of fat in the blood, so blood tests are taken every six weeks during treatment in order to monitor this. Any abnormalities would mean that the patient would be taken off the medication immediately. Normally, however, treatment is continued for about four months. Facial acne improves in between 80 and 90 percent of patients, while acne on the back and chest improves in about 60 percent. The effect of one course may last up to six years. Because isotretinoin can cause malformations in an unborn child, sexually active women must use adequate contraception throughout the course of treatment and for two months afterward.

RECENT ADVANCES

An Italian chemist has developed a method of getting rid of acne scars that is said to be effective in 80 percent of cases. It is available from qualified beauty therapists under the trade name AS-43 Suntronic treatment. A pad soaked in a liquid that contains protein is put over the affected area and a very small electric current is passed through it, stimulating the skin to repair itself. The treatment is marketed by the Mediform Clinic, 22 Harcourt House, 19 Cavendish Square, London. It is also widely available in Europe but not in the United States.

One day it may be possible to vaccinate youngsters against acne. Scientists at the Medical Academy in Krakow, Poland, prepared a vaccine from the bacteria proprionibacterium, which is known to colonize the sebaceous glands of patients with acne. This vaccine was then used in a double-blind trial involving 320 adolescents. In the group given the vaccine, definite improvements were noticed in the skin.

COMPLEMENTARY TREATMENT

Acupuncture
Points are used to relieve the stagnation of Chi in the channels of the face, said to be the cause of acne.

Aromatherapy
Chamomile, lavender, juniper, and bergamot are among the oils that may be helpful.

Herbalism
Herbs are used to reduce toxicity, which is believed to be associated with any chronic skin condition, and to restore the function of the skin to normal. Among those that may be prescribed are dandelion root and burdock root. Echinacea and poke root are used for their antiinflam-

matory properties; red clover, which is also used, may have estrogenic action.

Homeopathy
Kali brom. may help patients who have pustules and blind boils, especially on the face, neck, and upper part of the back. For those with oily skin, blackheads, and pimples, selenium may be prescribed. For patients whose pustules are painful and discharge yellow pus, hepar sulph. may be appropriate.

Nutrition
Supplements of B complex (particularly B_6), C, and E, and of the mineral zinc may be recommended since these are very important for the health of the skin, as is vitamin A, which may be added to the list for patients who are not already taking isotretinoin. Eating foods that are rich in sulphur such as onions and garlic may be helpful. Patients are likely to be advised to avoid sugar, cigarettes, and fried and fatty foods.

SELF-HELP

Ultraviolet light or sunlight may sometimes improve acne, but its effect is only temporary.

Excessive washing is not helpful.

ANOREXIA AND BULIMIA

THESE TWO POTENTIALLY life-threatening eating disorders mainly affect young women and are thought to be caused by psychological factors. It is only in the past few years that bulimia has been recognized as a separate disease entity, although both conditions can occur together.

ANOREXIA NERVOSA

Definition, Incidence, Causes, and Symptoms

The word *anorexia* is used by doctors, without the *nervosa* suffix, to describe loss of appetite due to any cause. However, *anorexia nervosa* is defined as a disease in which the patient, who has an intense wish to be thin and an overwhelming fear of fatness, starves herself so that she weighs less than 75 percent of the standard weight for her height and build.

Surveys have shown that anorexia nervosa affects between 1 and 2 percent of school-age girls and female university students. However, it is thought that many more have less severe degrees of the disease. Ninety-five percent of cases begin in late adolescence, usually between the ages of sixteen and seventeen. The condition is rare over the age of thirty and affects twenty females for every male.

Various theories have been put forward as to its cause. Some specialists see it as an attempt by young women to escape back into childhood, away from the problems of adolescence. Others suggest that it occurs mainly in girls who do not feel in control of their lives and that starvation is their way of trying to gain control over themselves and the people around them. One symptom of the disease is an absence of periods (amenorrhea), but in about 20 percent of cases this occurs before there is any dramatic weight loss, which has led some authorities to suggest that, in such cases, the condition may be caused by a hormonal imbalance.

Anorexia nervosa is more common among the daughters of professional people and seems to affect girls in certain occupations, such as nursing or ballet, more frequently than others. It is also far more common in those cultures where thinness is equated with beauty than in those where there is less stress on weight-watching. Often the patients have been slightly overweight in the past. Having decided to lose weight, their dietary controls become more and more strict until they eat hardly anything. Carbohydrates, in particular, are avoided. In addition, the patient does exercises, takes purgatives, and may make herself vomit after eating. Her fear of being fat does not diminish as she continues to lose weight and she is unable to see how thin she has become or to recognize the fact that she has problems. She has no sex drive, her skin may become mottled and her body may be covered by a fine soft hair (lanugo), and she is likely to have a low body temperature, a low heart rate, and a low blood pressure.

The disease may take the form of one prolonged episode or may fluctuate, with the patient seeming to get better for a while and then relapsing again.

Traditional Treatment

Some patients may be treated at home but, in most cases, especially if the patient is severely malnourished, she will need admission to the hospital. If she refuses to go and it seems that her life is in danger, she can be made to enter the hospital under a psychiatric court order.

Treatment consists mainly of a high-calorie diet together with psychotherapy. Usually the patient is told upon admission to the hospital that she will have limited privileges but can earn them by putting on weight. She will be watched carefully to ensure that she does not take purgatives and does not make herself vomit. Support and counseling are offered and, in some cases, antidepressants may be helpful.

Prognosis

The outlook for patients with anorexia nervosa is variable. The longer they have been ill and the more severe their weight loss, the poorer are their chances for a complete recovery. Patients who purge themselves or make themselves vomit, who suffer from bulimia, who have problems in their relationships with others, or whose illness began at a relatively late age are also less likely to do well. Follow-up studies of patients, done between four and ten years after the onset of the disease, have shown that about 2 percent had died from starvation, 16 percent were still seriously underweight, and 19 percent were moderately underweight; 29 percent still had no periods and in 17 percent the periods were irregular; 36 percent were still using purgatives. Recently an American study has suggested that anorexic women are more likely than others to develop osteoporosis at an early age. One of the most life-threatening complications is cardiac dysrhythmia, which can result from low potassium levels caused by poor intake of food and vomiting. In the long term, between 2 and 5 percent of patients with chronic anorexia nervosa may commit suicide.

Complementary Treatment

Aromatherapy
Bergamot, clary sage, or rose may be helpful.

Herbalism
Several herbs are appetite stimulants and condurango may be especially helpful in the treatment of anorexia nervosa.

Homeopathy
Remedies that may be helpful include natrum mur., silica (especially for pale, cold patients with sweaty hands and feet), and arg. nit. (particularly when anorexia is associated with phobias).

Hypnotherapy
Hypnosis may be of limited use in anorexia. It can be used to discover the cause of the patient's anxieties and to help her to overcome them by expressing them in another, less harmful, way. However, it is only possible to hypnotize a willing patient, so the many anorexics who refuse to believe that there is anything wrong with them would not be suited to this therapy.

Nutrition

Anorexia may be associated with a raised level of zinc in the body. If tests show that this is the case, it can be corrected by taking supplements of other minerals such as copper, iron, calcium, and manganese. However, these supplements should be prescribed by a qualified nutrition therapist as it is essential to get the balance correct.

BULIMIA NERVOSA

Symptoms, Incidence, and Complications

This condition may occur together with anorexia nervosa or as a separate entity. The patient is preoccupied with food and indulges in episodes of bingeing after which she makes herself vomit. She has a fear of not being able to stop eating and uses drugs such as laxatives, diuretics, appetite suppressants, or thyroid extracts to control her weight.

Bulimia affects a slightly higher age group than anorexia, the average age of onset being eighteen. In the United States, between 5 and 30 percent of girls in high schools, colleges, and universities are said to be suffering from it to a greater or lesser degree. Like anorexia, it is far more common in females than in males.

Patients are often depressed and may at times become suicidal. They may indulge in antisocial behavior, such as stealing, and may become addicted to alcohol or to drugs.

There are many physical problems that may result from persistent bingeing and vomiting, including inflammation of the esophagus (gullet), distension of the stomach, pancreatitis, poor kidney function, swelling of the salivary glands, and rotting of the teeth (due to repeated contact with acid from the stomach). The loss of acid from the stomach causes an imbalance in the body chemistry and this, in turn, may result in abnormal heart rhythms and muscle spasm or paralysis. Complete loss of periods is rare, but they are usually irregular.

Traditional Treatment

Because bulimia has only recently been recognized as a disease in itself, doctors are, as yet, unsure about the best treatment and the likely outcome. However, a form of psychotherapy in which the patient keeps a diary of what she eats and tries to identify and avoid anything in her life that seems to act as a stimulus to bingeing seems to be having good results.

Recent Advances

Research in the United States has suggested that, in some cases, bulimia may be associated with a hormonal problem. It seems that cholecystokinin, the enzyme that produces a feeling of satisfaction after a meal, is secreted in abnormally small amounts in patients with bulimia, which may account for their bingeing in an attempt to feel satisfied. It is not clear, however, whether the low cholecystokinin level is the cause of bulimia or results from it, but either way it seems likely that it perpetuates the disorder. Tricyclic antidepressants that boost the secretion of cholecystokinin can be a very effective treatment.

ORGANIZATIONS

American Anorexia/Bulimia Association
133 Cedar Lane
Teaneck, NJ 07666
201/836-1800
(Publishes a newsletter five times a year.)

Anorexia Nervosa and Related Eating Disorders
P.O. Box 5102
Eugene, OR 97405
503/344-1144
(Publishes a monthly newsletter and educational material.)

National Association of Anorexia Nervosa and Associated Disorders
Box 7
Highland Park, IL 60035
312/831-3438
(Publishes a quarterly newsletter.)

ANXIETY AND PHOBIAS

ANXIETY

Definition and Incidence

Everyone feels anxious from time to time, but the medical condition known as anxiety is one in which the patient constantly feels anxious, has physical symptoms related to the anxiety, and may from time to time have sudden panic attacks during which the symptoms worsen considerably. Often a patient feels anxious and apprehensive without having any clear idea what is causing these symptoms—this is known as free-floating anxiety.

Anxiety affects some 5 percent of the adult population, women twice as often as men. It usually begins between the ages of fifteen and forty and, in most cases, is mild. Hospital admission is rarely necessary. However, the condition may be a long-term one and there is a danger that patients may become dependent on tranquilizers or on alcohol.

Symptoms

Physical symptoms of anxiety may be due to muscle tension, to over-breathing, or to excessive activity of the sympathetic nervous system. This part of the nervous system, which is not under voluntary control, governs the way in which the body reacts to a threatening situation. The bodily changes that are temporarily brought on by fear (such as diarrhea, pain in the chest, dry mouth, dizziness, and a wish to urinate) may continue to trouble the patient suffering from anxiety over a long period of time. Other symptoms include excessive sweating, sleeplessness, unpleasant dreams, palpitations, breathlessness, indigestion, impotence or loss of the sex drive, ringing in the ears, blurred

49

vision, restlessness, and inability to concentrate. Panic attacks in which there is a sudden feeling of terror and impending doom may be associated with overbreathing, or hyperventilation. Rapid breathing in and out expels more carbon dioxide from the lungs than is normal and this upsets the balance of oxygen to carbon dioxide in the bloodstream, which has the result of making the blood more alkaline—a condition known as respiratory alkalosis. This, in turn, produces other chemical changes in the blood that cause various symptoms such as dizziness, tingling (especially in the arms and legs), and spasm of the muscles in the hands and feet. A patient who develops these symptoms, particularly if associated with palpitations or chest pain, may think that he is having a heart attack, which will increase his anxiety still further.

Tests

Occasionally, a patient may develop the physical symptoms of anxiety without the mental symptoms and may have to go through numerous tests of the digestive system, heart, lungs, and so on before the diagnosis of anxiety is made. However, in most cases, the diagnosis is clear. For a patient who hyperventilates, there is a simple test that is most useful in demonstrating to both patient and doctor that it is anxiety that is causing the unpleasant symptoms. The patient is asked to overbreathe deliberately for two to three minutes. As he does so, he will develop the tingling, chest pain, dizziness, and so on of which he has been complaining. He is then given a paper bag and asked to breathe in and out of that. By doing this, he rebreathes the carbon dioxide that he has just breathed out. This brings the level of the blood gases back to normal and the symptoms subside. Not only does this reassure the patient but it also offers him a way in which he can control his attacks in the future.

Traditional Treatment

As well as the "paper-bag" technique, patients who suffer from hyperventilation can be offered training in how to breathe slowly and in relaxation techniques.

Psychotherapy takes several forms. The simplest form—supportive psychotherapy—may help to minimize the symptoms of an anxious patient until the condition clears up of its own accord (which, in many cases, it does). Recurring attacks, however, may warrant behavior therapy (in which the patient's behavior patterns are changed in order to help her cope with her condition) or even psychoanalysis (in which the root cause of the problem is investigated). However, psychoanalysis is very lengthy and expensive, and not all patients are suited to this form of treatment.

Tranquilizers such as diazepam, chlordiazepoxide, oxazepam, temazepam, and lorazepam may greatly reduce symptoms of anxiety and, taken at night, may give the patient a good night's sleep. However, they cannot be taken for more than three or four weeks without the risk that the patient will become tolerant of them (needing a higher dose for the same effect) and addicted to them. Side effects include drowsiness, confusion, and unsteadiness. Patients who have been on such tranquilizers for a long time and suddenly stop taking them are likely to develop withdrawal symptoms such as insomnia, anxiety, trembling, and muscle twitching. Patients who suddenly stop taking a high dose may even have convulsions. It is important, therefore, when stopping tranquilizers after a prolonged period to come off them gradually over the course of several weeks.

Because of the problems associated with tranquilizers, some doctors prefer to treat patients suffering from anxiety with beta blockers (described in the section on high blood pressure). The effect of these is to reduce overaction of the sympathetic nervous system and thus to relieve the symptoms that this produces.

PHOBIAS

Definition and Symptoms

A phobia is an irrational intense fear of a specific object, activity, or situation. The patient is aware that the fear is irrational and tries to fight against it, but this only brings on extreme anxiety and, in the end, the attempt is given up.

The condition usually appears before the age of forty and affects two or three times as many women as men. Probably some 20 percent of the population are affected by what are known as simple phobias—fear of dogs, cats, spiders, and so on—but few of these are disabling. These types of phobia often begin in childhood. Agoraphobia—a fear of leaving one's home—affects between 3 and 7 percent of the population and usually begins in early adult life. It may be very disabling and may result in the patient becoming housebound.

Closely related to the phobias are the obsessions. These are irrational actions that the patient feels compelled to carry through. Failure to do so brings on anxiety. For example, a woman living alone may feel herself compelled to lock up all her kitchen knives every night in case someone should break in and stab her. Or a patient may be unable to leave her house without checking five or six times that she has turned the stove off or locked the front door. A hand-washing obsession is not uncommon, with the patient constantly feeling that his hands are dirty and, as a result, washing them twenty or thirty times a day. Obsessional phobias, in which the patient is constantly afraid that he may do something terrible against his will, may also occur.

Traditional Treatment

Desensitization therapy consists of asking the patient to imagine the thing of which he is afraid and, as the fear develops, teaching him how to relax and reduce his anxiety. Very gradually, over a period of weeks or months, he imagines more and more intense situations until finally he can cope with the object of his phobia.

Flooding treatment is based on the fact that if an animal cannot escape from the thing of which it is frightened, it loses its fear. The patient is asked to imagine situations that produce a considerable amount of fear until, ultimately, the fear is exhausted. Implosion is a variation on this, in which the situation imagined is exaggerated so as to be the worst possible. Although successful, there is little evidence that these forms of treatment are any better than desensitization.

The best treatment for agoraphobia is programmed practice, in which the patient is taken outside her house and exposed to situations that produce a limited amount of anxiety. She is taught how to cope with this and, practicing for at least an hour each day, gradually becomes able to deal with situations that she could not face previously.

Obsessional phobias are sometimes helped by drug treatment. The drugs used include chlorpromazine, trifluoperazine, imipramine, and desipramine. Chlorpromazine and trifluoperazine, although useful, have a wide range of side effects, not least of which are trembling, restlessness, and abnormal body movements. However, not all patients are affected and, for those who are, adjusting the dose can usually minimize the problem. Imipramine and desipramine may cause dry mouth, drowsiness, blurred vision, constipation, and excessive sweating, all of which usually decrease as treatment continues.

COMPLEMENTARY TREATMENT

Acupuncture
In the Chinese theory of energy flow around the body, the heart is said to be the seat of the mind and the spirit. Thus, disturbances of the mind such as anxiety are seen as being due to a dysfunction of the heart. This may be due to a deficiency of Chi or to the presence of phlegm and heat. In the first case, points will be chosen to stimulate the Chi of the heart and, in the second, to eliminate phlegm and heat. In both cases, points will also be used to strengthen and pacify the spirit.

Aromatherapy
Lavender, geranium, and marjoram are among the oils that may be recommended for patients with anxiety.

Bach Flower Remedies
Agrimony is for the person who is calm and cheerful on the outside but anxious on the inside and who tries to keep active as a way of coping with the anxiety.

Aspen will help someone who is anxious for no apparent reason and whose fears may be associated with death or with sleep; he may also suffer from faintness, headaches, and trembling. Red chestnut is useful for the sort of person who can always find something to worry about and who tends to worry about other people's problems and the problems of the world.

Cherry plum is for the treatment of severe anxiety where the patient is suicidal or worries that he is going insane. It may also be helpful in the treatment of obsessions.

Mimulus is used to treat specific fear such as fear of animals, the dark, or being alone. Rock rose is for sudden fear and is useful in the treatment of panic attacks and as a sedative after nightmares.

White chestnut treats what the medical profession calls *rumination*—the constant thinking over minor worries and building them up into major anxieties. Patients may also complain of insomnia, depression, and guilt.

Rescue remedy is a combination of cherry plum, clematis (which revives faintness), impatiens (for stress and nervous tension), rock rose, and star of Bethlehem (for shock, grief, and distress) and is a wonderful emergency treatment for all manner of experiences, ranging from anxiety before going to the dentist to shock following a car accident.

Herbalism

A number of herbs act as relaxants and tranquilizers and may be useful in the treatment of anxiety. These include scullcap, valerian, vervain, and lemon balm.

Homeopathy

Calc. carb. may be prescribed for someone who readily becomes anxious and discouraged, who is apprehensive, forgetful, or confused, and who may have palpitations. Phosphorus may be appropriate for the oversensitive patient who constantly needs reassurance and ignatia for the person who overreacts to situations and tends to exaggerate her problems. For the patient who is greatly lacking in confidence and covers up by being irritable and touchy, lycopodium may be helpful. Severe anxiety associated with restlessness may be treated with arsenicum alb. Phobias may respond to arg. nit. or gelsemium.

Hypnotherapy

This can be extremely helpful in the treatment of patients with anxiety and phobias. Hypnosis itself is a form of deep relaxation that can have a considerable calming effect. When in a hypnotic trance, the patient is given suggestions that he will feel more relaxed and is taught how to hypnotize himself to reinforce this training. In the treatment of phobias, hypnosis may be combined with the desensitization techniques described above and, in addition, with analytical techniques that may enable the patient to discover the cause of his phobia and thereby to overcome it.

Nutrition
Magnesium is a natural tranquilizer and may be recommended.

ORGANIZATIONS

National Institute of Mental Health
5600 Fishers Lane
Rockville, MD 20857
301/443-3673

ARTHRITIS

DEFINITION

Literally *arthritis* means inflammation (-itis) of a joint (arthr-), but in some arthritic conditions inflammation does not play a large part. The term is used to include any condition in which one or more joints become painful, stiff, or limited in function for a prolonged period of time, and encompasses gout and joint infections as well as rheumatoid arthritis and osteoarthritis (the two commonest forms). Some patients suffering from psoriasis develop arthritis and the condition may also occur as part of a generalized reaction to an infection, as in the case of Reiter's syndrome, which predominantly affects men and in which other symptoms may include a discharge from the urethra and conjunctivitis.

Because there are so many facets to arthritis, and because some of its forms are quite uncommon, this section will be restricted to osteoarthritis, rheumatoid arthritis, and gout. Millions of people in the United States have various joint complaints, the majority of which represent osteoarthritis. Psoriatic arthritis is mentioned in the section on psoriasis.

RHEUMATOID ARTHRITIS

Although rheumatoid arthritis (RA) primarily attacks the joints, it also affects other parts of the body. It is thought to be an autoimmune disease—that is, one in which the body is attacked by its own immune system. Why this should happen is not known, although there are theories that it may be precipitated by a viral infection. Whatever the cause, it is of comparatively recent origin since archeologists have found that, although a number of ancient skeletons show evidence of having suffered from gout and septic arthritis (infection of a joint by bacteria), there is no convincing evidence of rheumatoid arthritis occurring before about 1800.

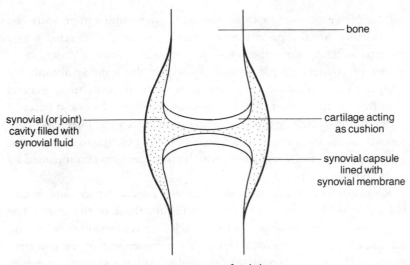

The structure of a joint

Nowadays, RA is a common disease, affecting between 2 and 4 percent of the population and usually starting between the ages of thirty and fifty. Among young adults, it is six times more common in women than in men, but in older patients the sexes are more equally represented.

Affected joints become inflamed and swollen, causing pain and, sometimes, deformity, and the lining of the joint cavity (synovium) becomes thickened. The disease may also affect the heart, lungs, eyes, and nervous system.

Symptoms and Course

The main symptom of rheumatoid arthritis is usually increasing stiffness and pain in the small joints, of which those of the hands are often the most severely affected. In about 10 percent of cases the patient has a single attack and then recovers completely, and in about 25 percent the disease remains relatively mild with long symptom-free periods elapsing between attacks, but in 65 percent the symptoms are moderate to severe, with a flare-up every few months.

RA may start in a number of different ways. The patient may, for a time, simply be aware that her joints are stiff when she wakes in the morning. Gradually the stiffness worsens and more joints become involved. However, in some cases, the onset can be much more acute and a previously healthy patient may, literally overnight, develop severe arthritis affecting a number of joints. Another mode of onset, commoner in younger people, is that in which the joint symptoms are comparatively minor but the patient is quite ill with more general symptoms such as fever, weight loss, and anemia. In one quarter of patients, the disease begins in a single joint, often the knee, and later spreads. In the early stages of RA many patients complain of tiredness, loss of appetite, and weight loss, which are sometimes accompanied by fever and sweating.

Rheumatoid arthritis usually affects the hands, wrists, and knees, but can involve almost any joints, including those of the spine. The hands may become deformed as the muscles waste, the joints swell, and the muscle tendons contract and pull the bones out of their normal position. Typically, the fingers are pulled sideways, away from the thumb (this is known as ulnar deviation). The fibrous sheaths in which the tendons are encased may also swell, causing pain when the fingers are moved; sometimes the tendons themselves rupture, so that the patient can no longer move her fingers. The skin of the hands may become very thin and fragile, and prone to infection or ulceration.

The bones in the feet may become displaced, giving the patient the sensation of walking on pebbles. Deformity of the toes may occur and this may result in ulceration, because the tips of the toes, which are not normally weight-bearing, now have pressure put on them during walking.

About 30 percent of patients, usually those whose arthritis is more severe, develop small nodules under the skin. These tend to occur near joints and over areas that are subject to pressure, being commonest just below the elbow. They are not tender, but may persist for months or years. Two thirds of all patients have a moderate degree of anemia, which may be made worse if aspirin is used to treat their arthritis.

About 10 percent of patients recover completely from RA. In 40 percent the condition persists but causes no disability. Another 40 percent suffer from a moderate degree of disability and 10 percent become severely disabled. When the disease starts slowly at an advanced age it usually remains relatively mild.

Younger women who suffer from rheumatoid arthritis often find that the condition improves when they become pregnant and recent research has shown that the contraceptive Pill seems to have a protective effect against the disease, but some studies do not show such a connection. Hopefully, future research will provide more information.

Diagnosis

The diagnosis of rheumatoid arthritis is often made from the symptoms and an examination. However, it is sometimes necessary to differentiate it from other forms of arthritis. Eighty percent of patients have what is known as rheumatoid factor (RF) in their blood, but this test is not specific, RF being found in other diseases as well. Anemia is often present and needs to be diagnosed so that it can be treated. X-rays are very helpful in establishing the diagnosis of RA.

Traditional Treatment

In recent years, many new drugs have been developed for the treatment of arthritis, most of them falling into the NSAID (nonsteroidal anti-inflammatory drug) category.

NSAIDs

These include drugs such as ibuprofen, indomethacin, and naproxen. They are very effective in many cases, but can cause unpleasant side effects, usually affecting the stomach and intestines. Occasionally a patient has to stop taking the medication because of symptoms such as indigestion, nausea, and abdominal pain. A recent study looked at a group of patients who had been taking NSAIDs long term and discovered that over 70 percent of them had inflammation of the small intestine. Specialists are unsure whether the use of NSAIDs can actually cause an ulcer to form in the stomach or duodenum, but have no doubt that they can delay healing once an ulcer has occurred. Some doctors, therefore, are very cautious about giving these drugs to patients who have a history of ulceration. Elderly people, in particular, need to be watched closely since they are more likely to suffer from complications if they develop ulcers than those in a younger age group. In some cases, where the patient seems at risk of developing an ulcer but where an NSAID is essential, additional antiulcer medication may be prescribed as a preventive measure.

Patients who take anticoagulants may have to reduce their dosage if they start to take NSAIDs as well, since the latter can interfere with blood clotting. They can also induce water retention, which may make them unsuitable for patients with certain heart conditions. And some preparations may need to be avoided by asthmatic patients as they tend to increase the irritability of the lungs.

Aspirin

This is an effective painkiller and antiinflammatory drug but, like NSAIDs, it may upset the stomach and may cause bleeding from the stomach or intestines.

Gold

Gold is given by injection as the compound sodium aurothioglucose or by mouth as auranofin, and tends to be used only if aspirin and NSAIDs have been unsuccessful. It takes between six and twelve weeks to work and provides relief in 40–60 percent of cases. Sometimes this relief is only partial, but in other cases a total remission occurs. However, the results after a single course may be only temporary and up to 50 percent of patients develop side effects. The commonest of these is a rash which, although usually mild, may occasionally cause severe peeling of the skin. Mouth ulcers can also occur. Much less common is suppression of the bone marrow, with a consequent reduction in the number of blood cells and platelets (vital for the process of clotting) in the blood. Monthly blood tests are essential and, since gold may also damage the kidneys, the urine is regularly checked for the presence of protein.

Other "Second-Line" Drugs

One of these is penicillamine which, like gold, may take twelve weeks or more to work. Its success rate and side effects are also similar to those of gold and monthly blood tests and urine tests must be done.

Drugs that suppress the immune system, such as azathioprine, may be used (usually together with steroids) if gold and penicillamine have failed.

Methotrexate is a drug that prevents the rapid turnover of cells and, as such, is used successfully in the treatment of both cancer and psoriasis. However, in the past ten years it has also been used to good

effect by rheumatologists. Short-term side effects include gastrointestinal upsets, hair loss, and soreness of the mouth.

Steroids
These are normally kept for cases in which the patient is suffering from
a more generalized illness and in which other parts of the body, such
as the heart, blood vessels, or spleen, have been affected. In younger
patients they are used only if all other forms of treatment have failed.
However, they are sometimes prescribed in less severe cases when one
or two joints are particularly troublesome; in such cases they are not
taken by mouth but are injected directly into the joint. Usually this
relieves pain and stiffness for a week or two only, but for some patients
the effect is long-lasting. Unfortunately, steroids don't prevent the
disease from continuing to destroy the joint.

Surgery
In some patients, the disease continues to progress despite treatment,
and surgery may become necessary to restore function to the joints or
to relieve pain. A commonly used operation, particularly for the fingers
and knees, is synovectomy in which the lining of the joint capsule (the
synovium) is removed. This regrows within three or four weeks, but
the operation seems to delay the rheumatoid process, sometimes for
several years.

Other operations include repair of ruptured tendons, which may
restore movement to the fingers, and fusion of joints, which will relieve
pain, although movement will be prevented. Nowadays, operations to
replace joints (arthroplasty) are quite common and may give good
results.

Recent Developments

Recently the interest of traditional practitioners has been caught by the
use of evening primrose oil (EPO) and fish oils in the treatment of
arthritis. Both these oils contain essential fatty acids that are converted
by the body into substances important for the control of inflammation.
Research at Albany Medical College has shown clinical and biochemical
benefit in rheumatoid arthritis patients who supplemented their diets
with fish oils; the effects were more pronounced with higher doses used

for longer periods of time. Another study at the Harvard Medical School also suggested an antiinflammatory effect of fish oil supplementation.*

Complementary Treatment

Acupuncture
According to Chinese acupuncture theory, arthritis is caused by a blockage to the flow of energy, or Chi, around the body. If Chi cannot flow normally, the body cannot function properly. In chronic arthritis the blockage is said to be due to cold and damp. In acute forms, when the joints are red and swollen, it is said to be due to heat and wind. In either case, the aim of treatment is to rid the body of the causative factors and to restore the flow of Chi to normal.

Aromatherapy
Pain and inflammation may be reduced by use of a number of essential oils. Commonly used are juniper, thyme, rosemary, and chamomile.

Herbalism
Like traditional medicine, herbal medicine treats RA by reducing inflammation and pain, but also aims to rid the body of those toxins that have accumulated and are preventing recovery. Among the many herbs that may be prescribed, dandelion root and burdock root are used to cleanse toxic conditions, while white willow is a painkiller, containing salicylates—chemical relatives of the traditional drug, aspirin.

Homeopathy
Because RA can present in a multitude of ways, there are many remedies that may be appropriate for its treatment. Bryonia, for example, may be prescribed if the pain is worse upon movement and at night, but it is better for rest and cold. Rhus tox. may be given if the pain is worse for rest, cold, and damp, but it is better for heat and continued movement. If the patient complains of pain moving from joint to joint,

* Cleland, L. G., et al. "Clinical and Biochemical Effects of Dietary Fish Oil Supplements in Rheumatoid Arthritis," *Journal of Rheumatology* 15:10, 1988.

which is better when the joint is exposed to the air, pulsatilla may be needed.

Nutrition
In some cases, arthritis seems to be an allergic process that can either be brought on or made worse by certain foodstuffs or drinks, notably wheat, sugar, salt, coffee, tea, dairy products, or citrus fruit. A nutritionist may recommend an exclusion diet to see whether avoiding any of these results in a lessening of symptoms.

Some patients with arthritis have low levels of copper in their blood, whereas others seem to have an excess. The former group may benefit from taking a multimineral tablet containing copper or from wearing a copper bracelet. (Advocates of this approach claim that molecules of copper can actually be absorbed through the skin into the bloodstream.) However, an assessment of the patient's copper status will be made before such treatment is recommended, since additional copper may make the symptoms worse for someone whose levels are already high. For such a patient, supplements of vitamins A, C, and E, together with the mineral zinc, will help to reduce copper to within normal limits.

Supplements of vitamins A, C, D, and B_5 may be helpful in some cases, as may dolomite, a tablet containing calcium and magnesium.

Some patients with RA will respond to the amino acid histidine, taken together with vitamin C.

Self-Help and Paramedical Assistance

A vegetarian diet containing no refined carbohydrates may sometimes be recommended by a naturopath.

Some years ago it was found that an extract from the New Zealand green-lipped mussel could be very effective in the treatment of rheumatoid arthritis, although it must not be taken by anyone who is allergic to shellfish. This substance is available from health food shops under various trade names.

It is very important for a patient with rheumatoid arthritis to keep mobile and, to this end, special exercises may be taught by a physiotherapist. However, when joint pain is severe, bed rest for a short period may be helpful. It is also important to maintain a good posture—patients should sleep on a firm mattress with only a small pillow and should sit on chairs that have firm seats and straight backs.

Heat can reduce pain and spasm, and paraffin baths are especially good for relieving pain in the hands and wrists. Using a splint at night, especially for the wrists, helps to rest the joints and to prevent deformities from occurring.

Special adaptations to the home may be essential. These include faucet handles that are easy to turn on and off, a raised toilet seat, and rails to assist walking and to enable the patient to get in and out of the bath or shower.

Patients whose hands are affected by arthritis may find it very difficult to open child-proof medicine bottles. Ask your pharmacist for easy-open bottles.

OSTEOARTHRITIS

Osteoarthritis is usually said to be a disease of wear and tear. It affects less than 1 percent of people age twenty but over 80 percent of those age seventy. The cartilage that cushions the articulating surfaces of the bones becomes soft and splits and then gradually wears away. The bone underneath the cartilage gets thicker and new bone is formed around the edges of the joint. Gradually the joint becomes stiff and painful. Osteoarthritis usually develops in middle-age women and may involve one joint or several. It tends to run in families and, in the majority of cases, is a mild disease.

Symptoms and Course

The joints most frequently affected by osteoarthritis are the knee, hip, spine (particularly in the neck and lower back), the fingers, elbows, thumbs, ankles, and big toes. The shoulders and wrists are seldom involved. Osteoarthritis of the knee is more likely to affect women than men, but for the hip the position is reversed. Joints that have been damaged are particularly susceptible and may become osteoarthritic within ten years of the original injury.

Osteoarthritis affects only the joints and is not a systemic (generalized) disease. Another way in which it differs from rheumatoid arthritis is that hand function does not become impaired since it is the finger joints nearest the nails that are likely to be involved, whereas in RA it is the second finger joints and the knuckles. However, characteristic bony swellings, known as Heberden's nodes, may form on the affected finger joints and these may be painful.

The symptoms of osteoarthritis are pain, limitation of movement, and stiffness. Most cases progress slowly and only a small proportion of patients develop any major disability. The pain is usually worse upon exercise, but is often mild and aching in character. The stiffness is worse after rest, but wears off after a few minutes of movement; the severe morning stiffness associated with rheumatoid arthritis does not occur.

The joints may look quite normal, but sometimes they are enlarged and, in such cases, may be tender. Often only one joint is affected.

When it affects the hip, osteoarthritis causes pain, generally in the groin or the buttock, but occasionally in the thigh. It is usually worse when the patient stands or walks and may keep him awake at night when the muscles relax. The hip may become distorted, partly due to muscle spasm around the joint and, as a result, the gait may be affected. The leg may become shortened and this, in turn, may put a strain on the spine.

Osteoarthritis of the spine (spondylosis) is widespread among the general population in the United States. Sometimes no symptoms occur but patients may complain of pain, which is due to a nerve being trapped between the affected bones. Occasionally, a nerve in the chest may become trapped, producing a pain that may be mistaken for angina.

Most people over the age of forty have some degree of osteoarthritis, which can be demonstrated on X-ray. But symptoms occur only in about 10–20 percent, of whom two thirds are women, although the disease probably affects the two sexes equally. By the age of eighty, some 85 percent of the population are affected, but may often be symptom-free despite quite considerable joint deformities. However, injury may cause sudden severe pain in a joint that was previously symptomless. Symptoms are likely to be made worse by obesity and are also more likely to occur during menopause or when the patient is suffering from another disease, such as chronic depression or thyroid deficiency.

Diagnosis

This is made by X-ray, which shows the joint spaces to be smaller than normal, with extra lips of bone growing around the edges of the joint surfaces.

Traditional Treatment

NSAIDs
Although these can be useful in an acute flare-up of osteoarthritis, some specialists think that they may, if used long term, make the condition worse. Many patients need only simple painkillers such as aspirin or acetaminophen to control their pain.

Steroids
As with RA, a steroid injection into an acutely painful joint may give temporary or long-lasting relief from pain.

Surgery
Sometimes if the joint becomes swollen it is necessary to insert a needle and draw out the fluid.

Synovectomy can be combined with a clearing out of debris from the joint—fragments of cartilage or bone that have broken off. This is particularly useful for the treatment of the knee joint.

Another operation used is osteotomy in which the bone below the affected joint is divided and then allowed to heal again. How this works is unknown, but it may dramatically relieve pain and the effect may last for several years. However, the result is unpredictable and not all patients respond well.

Fusion of a joint (arthrodesis) is the best way to relieve severe pain, especially in young people, but inevitably causes some disability.

Complementary Treatment

Those therapies listed in the section on rheumatoid arthritis may also be beneficial to sufferers from osteoarthritis. Since most complementary prescriptions are based on the patient's symptoms and appearance rather than on the orthodox diagnosis, many of the same treatments may be appropriate for all forms of arthritis. In addition, osteopathic or chiropractic manipulation may be useful for patients with osteoarthritis, helping them to retain maximal possible movement in the joints and to maintain good posture. However, manipulative therapies are not usually suitable for those whose joints are inflamed as a result of rheumatoid arthritis.

Self-Help

It is important for patients to avoid long periods of immobility. Swimming is an ideal form of activity to keep the joints mobile.

Overweight patients may find it helpful to lose weight, thus relieving their joints of some extra stress.

GOUT

Cause

Gout is a condition in which an excessive amount of the waste product uric acid circulates in the blood. Because it is impossible for all this acid to be held in solution, it is deposited in the body tissues in the form of urate crystals. It is the immune system's attack on the crystals that produces the symptoms of gout.

The cartoonist's picture of a person with gout is that of an elderly man who drinks excessively, but this is not necessarily the case. Five percent of patients are women and the condition can occur in young people, although it is rare under the age of forty. Also, the patient does not have to be a heavy drinker. However, in those who are prone to gout anything that causes the body to manufacture uric acid—and this includes red meat and liver as well as alcohol—may precipitate an attack. The condition may run in families and, for some reason, is rare in Scots and in patients suffering from rheumatoid arthritis.

Course of the Disease

Gout usually affects the hands and feet, especially the big toes, and sometimes the wrists, ankles, knees, elbows, and shoulders. The first attack tends to involve only a single joint (the big toe in 50 percent of cases), but later others may be affected. The joint suddenly becomes very painful and swollen and is usually red and impossible to move. Attacks seem to occur more often in the springtime and may be accompanied by a slight fever. The first episode subsides gradually over a period of a few days to a few weeks, but there are likely to be recurrences. These may occur at intervals of a few months or of several years. Repeated attacks will damage the joints involved, so that full function will not be regained when the inflammation has died down. As well as dietary indiscretions, attacks may be brought on by stress or trauma, surgical operations, and some antibiotics. The rapid turnover of skin cells that occurs in psoriasis also raises the level of uric acid in the blood, so patients suffering from both conditions may find that a flare-up of the rash brings on an attack of gout.

As well as being deposited in the joints, urate crystals are also laid down in the soft tissues (particularly those of the ear lobes, hands, and feet) of some 25 percent of patients. Here, after a number of years, they form hard little lumps, known as *tophi,* that are relatively painless but may cause progressive stiffness and aching and, ultimately, deformities. If they become large, they may ulcerate through the skin. Sometimes urates are deposited in the kidneys where they may form stones or, if they are laid down within the body of the kidney, may interfere with its function and cause the blood pressure to rise.

Diagnosis

Blood tests usually show a raised level of uric acid, although occasionally this may be normal. There may also be increased amounts of uric acid in the urine during an attack. X-rays may show rounded erosions, caused by the crystals, near the edges of affected joints. The true diagnosis of gout involves demonstrating urate crystals in joint fluid.

Traditional Treatment

Colchicine
This drug is so specific for gout that if the patient takes it and gets better this is considered to confirm the diagnosis. It usually relieves the

pain within 24–48 hours, but it is unpleasant to take and often causes diarrhea, nausea, vomiting, and cramps.

NSAIDs
These may be useful in an acute attack.

Steroids
Injected into a joint, hydrocortisone usually relieves pain within 24–36 hours.

Allopurinol
This is used in cases of chronic gout to lower the level of uric acid in the blood. Because there is a risk that initially it may increase the number of acute attacks, it is often given together with colchicine for the first six months. It works by preventing the formation of uric acid from its precursor, xanthine, which is a more soluble substance.

Uricosuric Drugs
These work by increasing the concentration of uric acid that is excreted in the urine. The patient needs to take them regularly and to drink plenty so that the uric acid can be flushed out. They should not be taken by people with kidney stones since they may precipitate an attack of renal colic; allopurinol is usually used instead. Other side effects include stomach upsets and rashes.

Uricosuric drugs include probenecid and salicylates (the aspirin family of drugs). However, aspirin itself should not be taken by patients with chronic gout since it can cause retention of uric acid.

Complementary Treatment

Acupuncture
Gout is treated in a similar way to an acute attack of rheumatoid arthritis.

Aromatherapy
Juniper, benzoin, chamomile, rosemary, and basil are among the essences that may be used.

Herbalism

Celery seed and nettle are specific herbs that have been reported to increase the body's excretion of uric acid. Other herbs are also used to reduce pain and inflammation. Colchicum autumnale is related to the refined product, colchicine, used by traditional practitioners.

Homeopathy

A wide range of remedies is available. These include calc. carb. for patients who develop gout whenever the weather changes, nux vomica for a first attack coming on after drinking a lot of wine, and ledum for pain situated in the ball of the big toe that is worse with heat but is associated with little swelling. Homeopaths, too, use colchicum when the big toe and heel are very painful, red, and tender, the pain moves from one joint to another, and the patient is irritable and feels weak.

ORGANIZATIONS

Arthritis Foundation
1314 Spring Street, NW
Atlanta, GA 30309
404/872-7111
(Publishes *Arthritis Today* bimonthly.)

ASTHMA

INCIDENCE AND CAUSE

Asthma affects between 3 and 6 percent of the general population in the United States, with most new cases occurring in children under five. Fortunately, many of them grow out of the condition, with as many as 25 percent free of symptoms after adolescence. New cases continue to develop after childhood and half of all newly diagnosed asthmatics over age forty are cigarette smokers with prior histories of emphysema or chronic bronchitis; still many have never smoked (true adult-onset asthma). In young children asthma is about twice as common in boys as in girls, whereas this trend gradually disappears or starts to reverse in adults. Usually the attacks are intermittent, but some patients have persistent symptoms.

Inhaled air enters the windpipe (trachea), which divides to form the two main bronchi. These, in turn, divide many times, forming the bronchi leading to the even narrower bronchioles that finally end in little sacs, called alveoli. In the alveoli, the air is separated from the bloodstream by only a single layer of cells. Oxygen diffuses through this layer to enter the blood and is carried to the body tissues, while the waste product, carbon dioxide, diffuses out into the alveoli and is exhaled. All but the smallest bronchioles have in their walls a layer of muscle that constricts and relaxes in response to certain stimuli to regulate the breathing. However, in an asthma attack, this muscle contracts dramatically, narrowing the air passages. The patient finds breathing is difficult (typically, it is harder to breathe out than to breathe in) and wheezing can be heard as the air is forced down the narrowed tubes. As the attack continues, the lining of the tubes may become inflamed and swollen and mucus is secreted, which narrows the passages still further. An asthmatic attack in a very young child may be more severe than in an older child in whom the bronchioles are proportionately larger.

In children, it is often an allergy (usually to grass pollen, house dust

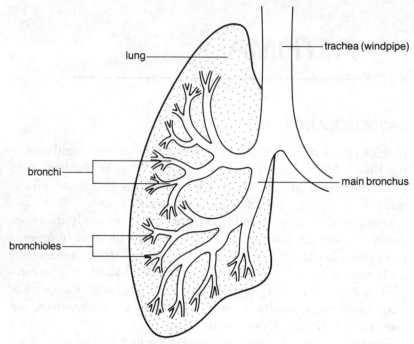

The lungs: bronchi and bronchioles

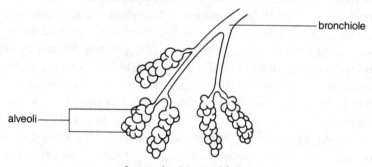

A terminal bronchiole

mite, or to animals) that triggers an attack of asthma. Grass pollen allergy is also responsible for the symptoms of hay fever and some patients may suffer from this too. The house dust mite is a minute creature that is found everywhere and thrives in house dust. It has no harmful features apart from the fact that certain people are allergic to it. Eradicating it can be very difficult, if not impossible. Asthmatic patients may also suffer from another disease associated with allergy—eczema. This may appear during the same period as the asthma or one condition may be superseded by the other. One third of patients have relatives who have suffered from asthma, and many come from families where there is a history of hay fever or eczema.

However, not all asthma attacks are due to an allergy. Some 40 percent are precipitated by an infection—a heavy cold or a chest infection—and others may be brought on by an emotional upset.

Annual asthma mortality in the United States in people ages five to thirty-four is 0.4 per 100,000. After age thirty-four asthma deaths are more likely to occur in older patients whose chronic asthma is complicated by chronic bronchitis.

SYMPTOMS

In acute asthma the attack may come on quite suddenly, often during the night, in which case the patient wakes up feeling breathless. Or it may be preceded by a head cold or a dry, hacking cough. The main symptoms are a tight feeling in the chest and difficulty in breathing out. The breathing becomes wheezy and the patient may cough, without bringing anything very much up from the chest. As the attack progresses, the breathing becomes rapid and shallow, and the patient looks pale and anxious and avoids the effort of speaking. In a severe attack the breathing becomes irregular and the wheeze may be less noticeable as less air goes in and out of the lungs. The patient becomes increasingly restless and the relative lack of oxygen in the blood may turn his lips blue. His pulse may race, but only if the attack has been brought on by an infection will he have a fever. An attack may last for minutes or hours, or rarely, for days. Sometimes the patient will vomit and, following this, his breathing may become easier.

Effort of any kind makes the symptoms worse, as does anxiety, so that a vicious circle may arise as the patient becomes more and more anxious over his inability to breathe normally. He is usually most comfortable sitting, leaning forward, with his arms resting on something that is at the same level as his shoulders, since this is the position in which breathing is easiest. A number of extra muscles (the so-called accessory muscles of respiration) are brought into play at the top of the rib cage, around the base of the neck, in order to keep the chest moving, and upon breathing in, the spaces between the ribs may appear to be sucked in. A patient suffering from chronic asthma often has a distended barrel-shaped chest with very little movement visible upon respiration. After a prolonged attack the patient will be very tired, his chest and abdomen may be sore, due to the overuse of muscles, and he is likely to cough up a great deal of mucus including wormlike "casts"—the plugs of mucus that have formed in the small bronchioles.

Normally there are no symptoms between attacks, but adult patients who suffer from chronic asthma may become breathless upon slight exertion, may wheeze frequently, may have a cough that is particularly troublesome during the night, and may bring up sputum first thing in the morning. The cough may persist for months, especially during the winter. Superimposed on these symptoms, acute attacks of asthma can be brought on by a chest infection and these patients often suffer from chronic bronchitis in addition to asthma. Some children who have acute asthma may also have a recurrent dry cough that is usually worse in the evening or early morning. Sometimes this is their only symptom and they do not proceed to the full-blown asthma attack.

STATUS ASTHMATICUS

This is a condition in which an attack continues for many hours or days and is not relieved by the patient's usual medications. It is a life-threatening condition and usually requires hospital treatment.

Because the attack progresses without any relief, mucus accumulates in the smallest of the bronchioles and may block them completely, adding to the patient's breathing difficulties. If a whole section of the lung becomes plugged, it may collapse and pneumonia may develop. Finally, the amount of oxygen being taken in may become so small that the patient can die from suffocation.

TESTS

Between attacks, the asthmatic patient may appear perfectly normal. However, tests of lung function may become abnormal after exercise. A child who is suspected of having asthma may be told to run around for a few minutes before being asked to blow into a machine, known as a spirometer, which will measure the capacity of his lungs. The two measurements that are generally used are the FEV1 and the FVC. The FEV1 is the forced expiratory volume in one second—the patient is asked to take a very deep breath, hold it, and then breathe out forcibly as hard as he can into the spirometer tube. The amount of air that he forces out during the first second is measured by the machine. The FVC is the forced vital capacity—the total amount of air that the patient can force out of his lungs after taking the largest possible breath in. On the whole, spirometers are used by hospital doctors and some GPs, but most GPs have smaller, portable machines called peak flow meters. Such a machine measures the peak expiratory flow or PEF—the maximum rate at which the air can flow from the lungs—a measurement comparable to the FEV1. Here again, the patient is asked to breathe forcibly into the machine, which he holds in his hand, after filling his lungs as deeply as he can.

People who are in the throes of an acute asthma attack, those who suffer from chronic asthma, and most asthmatic patients who have just exercised will have levels of FEV1, FVC, and PEF that are lower than normal. If, however, they are given a drug to relieve the constriction in the lungs (a bronchodilator), the FEV1 usually rises fairly quickly.

Other investigations that may be done are chest X-ray, which will show up any areas of lung infection or collapse, skin tests to check for allergies, which may be precipitating attacks and, in status asthmaticus, blood gases. This last test shows the levels of oxygen and carbon dioxide in the arterial blood, which reflects the balance of gases in the lungs. It serves as a guide to the severity of the attack and monitors the efficacy of the treatment being given. The blood is usually taken from the femoral artery (in the groin) or from the radial artery in the wrist.

TRADITIONAL TREATMENT

Nowadays it is possible to give drugs that will prevent asthma attacks from happening as well as drugs to relieve and cut short attacks when they do occur.

Cromolyn sodium is a commonly used drug with practically no side effects whose action is to inhibit the release from the tissues of histamine and other chemicals involved in the development of an allergic reaction. Its action is entirely preventive and it has no effect once these substances have begun to act and an asthma attack is under way. It has to be taken regularly up to four times a day and is usually prescribed only for patients who have frequent asthmatic attacks, but it may also be used for those in whom asthma is brought on by exercise, in which case it should be taken ten to fifteen minutes before the activity begins. Cromolyn sodium seems to be particularly effective for children.

Bronchodilators are given once an attack has started, to relieve the spasm in the lungs. They may be divided into two main groups, the xanthine drugs, such as theophylline and aminophylline, and the beta adrenergic drugs, such as isoetharine, albuterol, and terbutaline. The xanthine drugs, although effective, may have considerable side effects such as irritability, hyperactivity, abdominal pain, an increased heart rate, and vomiting of blood. However, if a small dose is taken first and then, if necessary, followed by gradually increasing doses, the side effects are usually minimal. A long-acting form of theophylline is said to be particularly helpful in controlling attacks that occur during the night, but may cause nausea, headache, and digestive problems. Among the beta adrenergic drugs, terbutaline seems to have a longer-lasting action, so these too may be useful for patients who have nocturnal asthma.

Steroids are also effective against asthma, but because of the dangers of long-term side effects they are usually prescribed for limited periods, except in the case of patients whose asthma is incompletely controlled by any other drugs. Many doctors feel that too many asthmatics die because they are not given steroids or are given them too late. Used regularly to prevent attacks from occurring, they have few side effects and are usually stopped slowly after about a year of treatment.

Many of the drugs mentioned here can be given either by mouth or through an inhaler, the latter method often being preferred since it is likely to have fewer side effects. There are various forms of inhalers and even quite young children (over the age of four) can usually manage to use one of them successfully.

If a patient fails to respond to basic treatment in an asthma attack, hospital admission may be necessary. The treatment of status asthmaticus includes the administration of oxygen, intravenous steroids, and a bronchodilator, either inhaled or in the form of aminophylline given intravenously. The patient is likely to be considerably dehydrated (because rapid, shallow breathing results in the loss of a great deal of moisture from the lungs) so he will need plenty of fluids and, if he is unable to drink due to the severity of the attack, a drip will be set up. If the attack has been brought on by an infection, antibiotics will also be necessary. In a very severe case, the patient may need to have his breathing assisted by a mechanical respirator for a short period.

Most asthmatic patients are kept under review by a hospital specialist, although those whose attacks are mild and infrequent are usually looked after by their GPs. In either case, regular checkups are important.

In some cases, where the attacks are shown to be brought on by an allergy to grass pollen or to the house dust mite, desensitizing injections may be effective.

RECENT ADVANCES

Measuring the lung function of small babies has always been difficult, but now an inflatable jacket has been developed in Australia that makes this possible.

Some asthmatic patients may be suffering from an allergic condition without realizing it. A professor of allergy at the University of Virginia has found that patients who have both asthma and athlete's foot are likely to be allergic to the ringworm fungus that is causing their foot condition. When the athlete's foot is treated, the patient's need for asthma medication is reduced.

An experiment carried out at St. Thomas's Hospital in London showed that when men increased the amount of salt in their diet, their bronchi and bronchioles became more sensitive and more likely to go into spasm. However, the same effect was not demonstrated in women. These results suggest that men who suffer from asthma might be well advised to reduce their salt intake.

At the University of Natal in Durban, South Africa, doctors have found that when asthmatic children lie down it is more difficult for them to breathe and that they are likely to cough and wheeze less during the night if they sleep propped up. This applies particularly to children ages two to three.

Methotrexate is a drug that has been used for some time in the treatment of cancer because of its ability to kill abnormal cells. It is also used successfully in severe cases of psoriasis and has been found useful in the treatment of arthritis. Now researchers in the United States have found that giving it once a week to fourteen patients with severe asthma allowed them to reduce their dose of steroids. The only side effects seemed to be transient nausea and, in one patient, a rash. Other studies will be needed to confirm these results.

COMPLEMENTARY TREATMENT

Acupuncture
Asthma is divided into three types—the cold type (acute asthma), the hot type (acute asthma associated with an acute chest infection), and the deficiency type (chronic asthma).

For the cold type, points will be chosen that have the effect of warming and strengthening the lungs, expelling the cold and clearing phlegm. For the hot type, the aim of treatment is to cool the heat and clear phlegm. For chronic asthma, in which there is said to be a deficiency of energy or Chi in the lungs, points will be chosen that will strengthen the lungs and their Chi. In all three types, points are also used that produce relaxation of the bronchi.

Alexander Technique
Improving the patient's posture may have the added benefit of helping him to breathe more easily.

Aromatherapy
A large number of essential oils may be used including eucalyptus, hyssop, lavender, aniseed, cajuput, lemon, and thyme.

Herbalism
Among the herbs used to treat asthma are ephedra (which relaxes the bronchi), coltsfoot (which soothes the irritated airways and is an expectorant, helping the patient to cough up mucus), grindelia (an expectorant and antispasmodic), lobelia (which has expectorant and antiinflammatory properties), and skunk cabbage, thyme, bloodroot, and sundew (all of which are expectorants).

Homeopathy

The patient may be given one of a large number of remedies appropriate for different types of asthma. Ipecac may be helpful for patients whose attack is associated with a rattling in the throat, sweating, anxiety, nausea, and a feeling of chill. Patients who require arsenicum are often elderly and are usually worse after midnight and worse for lying down or for movement. Kali carb. is useful if the patient is worse for movement, especially walking, and suffers from dizziness and diarrhea. Lobelia may be prescribed if the attack is associated with nausea, vomiting, giddiness, and a feeling of heaviness in the chest and abdomen. If the attack follows an upset stomach or a period of great mental exertion, nux vomica may be appropriate, but if it follows exposure to wind or to cold, the patient may require aconite. Sambucus is especially useful for children who develop an acute attack during the night.

Hypnotherapy

Very often a mild asthma attack may be made worse by the patient's anxiety, which causes additional spasm in the bronchi. Under hypnosis, a patient can be taught how to relax when the first symptoms of breathlessness arise. Once this has been learned and used on a few occasions, he will begin to feel confident in his ability to control an asthma attack and this will reinforce the power of the technique. For some patients, it may be possible, by using self-hypnosis, to prevent an attack from developing altogether. Often additional techniques are taught that are used in conjunction with self-hypnosis, such as one in which the patient visualizes his bronchi relaxing and performs some action (such as unclenching clenched fists) to mirror this and "cause it to happen."

Manipulation

Patients who have had asthma for many years may develop a curvature of the spine and a pigeon chest. Manipulation can improve the mobility of the spine and loosen the rib cage so that breathing becomes easier and deeper.

Nutrition

The lining (mucosa) of the bronchi and bronchioles needs vitamin A in order to stay healthy. A supplement of this may be recommended, together with vitamin C, which helps to inactivate any inhaled substances that may spark off an asthma attack.

SELF-HELP

Measures should be taken to reduce the house dust mite population—feather pillows and quilts should be replaced by others with synthetic filling and a plastic cover should be put over the mattress. Reducing humidity, in which the mites thrive, is also important. A powder called Acarosun, available from the Fisons Drug Company, 755 Jefferson Road, Rochester, NY 14623, is sprinkled onto carpeting, binds the excrement of the dust mite, then is vacuumed away (the excrement is supposedly the allergenic property).

Some children seem to be allergic to milk, so exclusion of milk from the diet may be helpful. However, a calcium supplement, in the form of dolomite, will need to be taken regularly. In some cases goat's milk can be substituted. Fish, eggs, nuts, and berry fruits may also bring on attacks, especially in the very young. Some children are allergic to animals and will have to be denied the pleasure of keeping a pet.

Garlic is effective in reducing mucus and may be taken in capsule form.

Because steroid inhalers may promote the growth of monilial infections (thrush—see separate section) in the mouth, patients should brush their teeth after using such preparations in order to minimize the risk of this occurring.

Patients, especially children, who wish to undertake some form of exercise should opt for something such as swimming or walking rather than a sport that necessitates sudden bursts of activity and that may more readily bring on an attack of asthma.

ORGANIZATIONS

Asthma and Allergy Foundation of America
1717 Massachusetts Avenue
Suite 305
Washington, DC 20036
202/265-0265
(Publishes *Advance,* a bimonthly newspaper, and educational materials.)

BACK PAIN

INCIDENCE

The incidence of back pain is estimated to be 60–80 percent of the population in the industrialized world. Approximately 75 million Americans complain of back pain, and for every 1000 workers there are 1400 lost workdays because of back pain. This, however, is only the tip of the iceberg—it is estimated that for every one of these patients there are another eighteen who do not seek medical advice. Fortunately, nearly half of all those affected are better within a week and over 90 percent have recovered within two months. The majority of sufferers are women, but in many cases the problem is related to the patient's occupation: 64 percent of all those who are involved in heavy work will suffer at some time from back pain, and each year one sixth of all nurses will be affected to some extent.

TYPES OF PAIN

Back pain is not a single entity—it can have many different causes— and so the types of pain that patients may experience can differ quite considerably.

Pain can be sharp or aching, constant or intermittent, localized or diffuse, and may be relieved by a variety of postures. If a nerve is irritated, as well as a relatively sharp pain at the site of irritation, a dull ache may be felt further along the length of that nerve. So, for example, a prolapsed ("slipped") disc which is pressing on the nerve that runs down the leg and into the foot may cause an ache in the toes. This is known as referred pain.

CAUSES OF BACK PAIN

There are many causes of back pain. However, the commonest single cause is a prolapsed intervertebral disc, which accounts for 20 percent

81

of cases. A further 15 percent are caused by a number of uncommon conditions, while the remaining 65 percent are labeled "non-specific"—in other words, the patient's symptoms and the findings upon examination do not point to any particular physical cause.

Specific causes of back pain, apart from a prolapsed disc, include fractures of the vertebrae, dysfunction of the joints, arthritis, inflammation, ligament problems, and osteoporosis. Muscle spasm can cause considerable pain and often exacerbates that due to another cause. Occasionally, pain originating in the abdomen may be felt in the back—for example, in patients suffering from pancreatitis (inflammation of the pancreas). Rarely, back pain may be caused by an infection or a growth in the bone itself.

Fractures of the vertebrae (the bones making up the spine) are usually the result of injury. However, a child or adolescent who takes part in a lot of sports may sustain a spontaneous stress fracture in one of the lower lumbar vertebrae, and elderly people may develop crush fractures as the result of osteoporosis (see section on osteoporosis).

PROLAPSED INTERVERTEBRAL DISC (SLIPPED DISC)

The disc that cushions adjacent vertebrae is made up of two parts—the tough outer annulus fibrosus and the jellylike inner nucleus pulposus. With age, the disc degenerates. It is possible that this occurs unevenly, setting up stresses in the annulus fibrosus, making it more likely to tear. If it does tear, the nucleus pulposus flows out, producing symptoms by stretching the annulus fibrosus and pressing on the adjacent nerves.

Usually the patient is young or middle-age and the first attack strikes suddenly when, after twisting, bending, or coughing, she suddenly finds herself in severe pain and unable to move. There is often a history of injury to the back at some time in the past. However, sometimes the pain comes on in a less spectacular manner, increasing gradually over the course of a day. The patient may also be aware of pain running down into her buttock, thigh, or leg, and, occasionally, may just have pain in the leg with very little in the back. Normally only one side is affected and the patient may assume a lopsided posture in an attempt to relieve the pain.

Prolapsed discs seem to occur most frequently in those parts of the

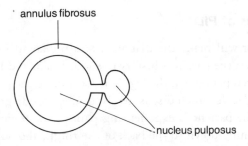

annulus fibrosus

nucleus pulposus

A prolapsed disc

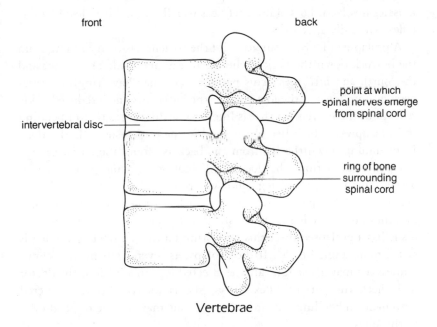

front

back

point at which
spinal nerves emerge
from spinal cord

intervertebral disc

ring of bone
surrounding
spinal cord

Vertebrae

spine that are the most mobile. Thus, they are commonest in the lumbar spine (lower back), fairly common in the cervical spine (neck), and quite rare in the thoracic spine (chest region). It is customary to refer to a disc by the numbers of the vertebrae between which it lies. Thus, the disc lying between the fourth and fifth lumbar vertebrae is known as L4/L5, while that between the fifth lumbar and the first sacral (near the pelvis) vertebrae is L5/S1. It is L5/S1 that is found to have prolapsed in the majority of cases of PID.

Diagnosis of PID

The doctor will make the diagnosis of a prolapsed intervertebral disc primarily on the patient's history of sudden pain and locking, together with referred pain down the leg. The location of the pain will allow the doctor to decide which disc is involved. She will diagnose a prolapse of L4/L5 if the patient is experiencing pain in the region of the hip and groin, running down to the back of the thigh, the outer surface of the lower leg, the back of the foot, and the first or second and third toes. Tingling, soreness, or numbness may be associated with the pain and the patient may find it difficult to point her toes due to weakness of the muscles involved. Loss of knee reflex is usually L3/L4 disc; loss of ankle reflex is usually L5/S1 disc.

A prolapse of L5/S1 is suggested if the patient has pain running from the buttock down the back of the leg to the underside of the foot and the fourth and fifth toes. This patient, too, may have tingling, soreness, or numbness in the lower leg or the outer toes and a reduced ankle reflex, but the movement that is likely to be difficult is that of bending the foot upward. Inability to lift the big toe up is usually L4/L5 disc. Pain running down the leg from the back is often called sciatica.

Upon examination, the doctor will look for specific points of tenderness in the back and leg, and will probably try the "straight leg raising test." The patient sits on the couch with her legs stretched out in front of her. The leg in which she feels the pain is slowly raised and, if she has a prolapsed disc, this will bring on the pain before the leg is raised to an angle of 45°. If the prolapse is severe, raising the symptomless leg may also aggravate the affected leg. In addition, the doctor will check the patient's flexibility—she is likely to have restricted movement in bending forward, although she may be able to bend fully to the sides.

An X-ray is seldom taken since there is usually nothing to be seen until the patient has had her problem for several years, at which point there may be evidence that the space occupied by the disc between the vertebrae is narrowed. However, if surgery is proposed, a myelogram, in which a radio-opaque dye is injected into the spinal canal, may be done to show up distortion of the affected disc. The MRI (magnetic resonance imaging) shows this as well and is noninvasive.

SPONDYLOSIS

This severe form of osteoarthritis affects the spine and is associated with degenerated intervertebral discs. Spondylosis affects older patients, who complain of pain, stiffness, and limited movement that is relieved by rest. The pain occurs in either the neck or the lower back and may radiate to the arms or the legs. Often the patient will have periods when the pain suddenly gets worse and movement becomes more difficult.

An X-ray will show the characteristic appearance of an arthritic spine. However, many older people have these changes without suffering from any symptoms and it is not known why this condition should cause pain only in some and not in others.

SPONDYLOLISTHESIS

This is a condition in which one vertebra becomes displaced and slips forward, causing pain that is relieved by stooping. It is responsible for 15 percent of cases of back pain that occur in people under the age of twenty and may in some cases be due to a slight deformity in the vertebra itself, although in others it is caused by injury. In the elderly, L4 may slip forward on L5 as a result of osteoarthritis. Diagnosis can be made on an X-ray.

RHEUMATOID SPONDYLITIS (RHEUMATOID ARTHRITIS OF THE SPINE)

This is comparatively rare. It often begins in the sacroiliac joints situated between the lower part of the spine, or sacrum, and the pelvic bones. The patient complains of a continuous ache and stiffness in the back or the buttocks and thigh, often accompanied by other symptoms of rheumatoid arthritis (see section on rheumatoid arthritis). The pain is often worse after resting and is eased by exercise, and it commonly occurs at night or in the early hours of the morning. It is frequently aggravated by changes in the weather.

ANKYLOSING SPONDYLITIS

This form of arthritis mainly affects young men, although it sometimes attacks women and may begin at any age before fifty. It affects 1–2 percent of the population and is the commonest of the so-called seronegative arthritides (in other words, arthritis where the diagnostic rheumatoid factor, found in the blood of patients with rheumatoid arthritis, is absent). It is thought to be a reactive arthritis, triggered off in a genetically susceptible individual by a particular stress such as an infection.

It causes recurrent episodes of stiffness together with low back pain, which may be aching in character and may radiate down the legs. Unlike the one-sided pain from a slipped disc, that of ankylosing spondylitis is usually symmetrical. One third of patients also develop arthritis changes in the shoulders, hips, knees, and ankles, and one quarter suffer from recurrent inflammation of the eyes. Other symptoms may include fever, fatigue, weight loss, chest pain, pain in the sole of the foot and the Achilles tendon, and a skin rash.

It used to be thought that ankylosing spondylitis was always a progressive disease in which the bones of the spine gradually fused and the patient was left with a rigid "poker back," often in a stooped and deformed position. However, in very few cases does the spine fuse completely and modern treatment can control the symptoms in the majority of patients.

In early cases, the diagnosis usually has to be made from the history, since it may be some time before the classical picture of blurring of the sacroiliac joints and calcification of the ligaments of the spine are visible on X-ray. Morning stiffness that is relieved by exercise suggests this diagnosis, as does a finding of tenderness over the sacroiliac joints. A blood test for HLA-B27 (an antigen) also suggests the diagnosis.

SPINAL STENOSIS

In this condition, the spinal canal and the canals through which the spinal nerves leave the vertebral column are narrowed as the result of osteoarthritis, a prolapsed disc, previous surgery, spondylolisthesis, or a disease of the bone itself. Pain is felt in the back and the buttock, is eased by bending over, and is made worse by standing up straight or walking downhill. It may be accompanied by referred pain, numbness, tingling, or weakness in the affected part, all of which may be brought on by walking and may be relieved by sitting down.

NONSPECIFIC BACK PAIN

In the majority of cases of back pain no particular cause can be found. One specialist believes that many of these patients are suffering from spinal stenosis, which may be hard to diagnose. However, the MRI may diagnose this. In some cases, the pain may be due to ligament strain or muscle spasm caused by awkward movement or incorrect use of the back when lifting. The episodes may be recurrent but usually settle within two weeks. The pain may radiate to the buttocks and thighs, often gets worse with prolonged walking, sitting, or standing, and is usually most severe in the evenings.

TRADITIONAL TREATMENT

This varies according to the diagnosis that has been made. In all cases painkillers are helpful. Nonsteroidal antiinflammatory drugs (NSAIDs) such as indomethacin and flurbiprofen are effective in rheumatoid spondylitis and in ankylosing spondylitis.

It is customary to recommend a period of bed rest on a firm mattress until the acute symptoms have disappeared, but a study carried out in the United States in 1986 showed that two days in bed was as effective as seven and in some ways better, since prolonged bed rest allowed the back muscles to become weak, adding to the patient's problem. Spinal support, in the form of a corset, may be used following bed rest and may be particularly helpful as a long-term treatment in patients with spondylosis and spondylolisthesis.

Manipulation and stretching the spine with traction may be used, especially for patients with a diagnosis of a prolapsed disc. In some cases injections into the spinal joints or the spinal canal of steroid and local anesthetic can be effective. Physiotherapy in which the patient is taught exercises to strengthen the back muscles will often help not only to relieve the pain but also to prevent further episodes.

Patients suffering from spinal stenosis can be helped by physiotherapy, exercises, and posture training, and over half find relief from the use of transcutaneous electrode nerve stimulation (TENS). A gadget is strapped to the skin in the affected area and delivers a tiny electrical stimulus to the nerve in such a way as to anesthetize it.

In many cases of prolapsed disc, the basic treatment of bed rest and painkillers, possibly with some traction, will suffice. However, when attacks occur frequently and are both prolonged and severe, doctors may consider surgery to be appropriate. Because the results of surgery cannot be guaranteed, caution must be exercised when offering operative treatment and it is usually only suggested for certain patients.

The most commonly performed operation is partial removal of the prolapsed disc, or laminectomy. This reduces pain in up to 96 percent of patients, but the relief is total in only 15 percent. Such an operation may have to be performed as an emergency if a disc has prolapsed in such a way that it is pressing on the nerves that run to the bladder, resulting in paralysis of the muscles of the bladder wall and consequent retention of urine. Extensive weakness of the leg muscles is also a clear indication for surgery.

A more recently introduced form of treatment is chemonucleolysis in which the disc is dissolved by injecting into it an enzyme called chymopapain. A general anesthetic is not necessary, the procedure being performed under local anesthetic and sedation. It is done in the operating room, and the surgeon checks the position of his needle by using X-rays, which means that this technique cannot be used for pregnant women. After the treatment, the patient is kept in bed for forty-eight hours, during which time her back pain may be severe and she may need powerful painkillers. She is then allowed up, wearing a corset, which she continues to wear for four weeks.

One percent of patients have a severe allergic reaction to chymopapain and, although this is easily dealt with, the treatment involves the use of adrenaline. This makes chemonucleolysis inadvisable for people who have recently had a heart attack or who have liver or kidney disease. A second injection of chymopapain increases the risk of such a reaction to 12 percent, so this form of treatment is very rarely offered a second time.

Since the discs dry up of their own accord with age, chemonucleolysis is inappropriate for older patients. It is also unsuitable for adolescents who may still be growing. The ideal patient is between twenty and forty, has three or more attacks of back pain a year lasting over a month each time, with leg pain that is eased by bed rest. A myelogram or scan will be done before treatment and it is important that the location of the patient's symptoms correspond exactly to the disc that is seen to be prolapsed. In this way, the surgeon will have no doubt that he is treating the correct disc. Because it is vital that the enzyme is injected into the center of the nucleus pulposus, and because it is sometimes difficult to do this with an L5/S1 disc, patients with a prolapse at this level are more likely to be offered surgery.

If all these conditions are adhered to, and if chemonucleolysis is offered only to patients who are perfectly suitable, it is said to have an 80 percent success rate. However, 10 percent of those treated may need surgery at a later date and 2 percent may have severe backache for up to a year following the procedure. In the United States, some surgeons no longer offer this form of treatment since they consider the long-term results to be inferior to those of laminectomy.

RECENT ADVANCES

A new method of treatment has been introduced for prolapsed discs that looks as though it will be very effective for selected patients. One English surgeon has reported that he has used it on fourteen patients; in thirteen cases it was highly successful and only one patient still needed a laminectomy. Known as nucleotomy, the technique consists of inserting a special needle into the center of the prolapsed disc and using it to cut through the disc material and suck out the debris. As a result of this procedure, the pressure inside the disc is relieved and the prolapsed section can fall back into the space that has been cleared. Done under local anesthetic, and aided by X-rays, nucleotomy takes only an hour and the patient can go home the same day. Relief of pain is almost immediate in successful cases. However, because not all patients are suitable for this operation, laminectomy is likely to remain the standard procedure for the treatment of a prolapsed disc.

COMPLEMENTARY TREATMENT

Acupuncture
Back pain is associated with stagnation of the flow of energy or Chi in the affected area. This may be due to blockage of the channels by wind, cold, and damp. Treatment consists of using points to warm the chan-

nels, to dispel the wind, cold, and damp, and to restore the normal flow of Chi. Specific points can also be used to relieve pain.

Alexander Technique
This is a system of posture training whose aim is to relieve the body of all unnatural tensions. Back pain is always associated with muscle spasm and abnormal posture, so Alexander training can be very effective, helping not only to relieve the pain but to prevent its recurrence.

Aromatherapy
Ginger, juniper, marjoram, sage, geranium, and lavender are among the essential oils that may be used in treating back pain.

Chiropractic
A chiropractor offers manipulative treatment for musculoskeletal disorders, especially where these are related to spinal problems. Some forms of back pain may respond very well because manipulation improves the flexibility of the spinal joints and muscles, even if it is incapable of curing the degenerative process causing the trouble. Treatment also aims to improve the strength of the muscles that support the spine.

A chiropractor will examine the patient's back in the same way as a doctor and will take X-rays. The manipulation used is localized on the exact area in which the problem lies and is accompanied by massage, exercises, and advice on posture. Several sessions of treatment may be necessary, depending on the individual patient.

Herbalism
Herbs may be used to reduce muscle spasm, such as yarrow, cramp bark, or lobelia, or to reduce inflammation and relieve pain, such as white willow (which contains aspirinlike compounds) and vervain. Lady's slipper has all these actions.

Homeopathy
Of the many remedies that may be suitable for patients with back pain, rhus tox. is one of the most commonly used. It is often prescribed when the pain has resulted from straining and is associated with stiffness upon first moving; the pain is usually better for heat, firm support, and

continued movement. Other remedies include bryonia, which may be indicated when the pain is severe, shooting in quality, and travels from the lower back down to the ankles; the patient tends to feel cold and to walk stooped over. Arnica is useful when the pain is due to injury, especially if there is a lot of bruising. Sulphur may help patients with chronic sciatica that is worse for warmth, especially if it is on the left side. Patients whose low back pain is dull, severe, and usually worse in bed and in the morning may be helped by nux vomica.

Osteopathy
Osteopathic manipulation is different from that used by chiropractors but equally effective, especially in the treatment of prolapsed discs. Chronic or recurrent back pain that is associated with a previous injury or that is worst for rest and better for exercise is also likely to respond well, as is pain due to strain or muscle tension. Several sessions of treatment may be necessary.

ORGANIZATIONS

The Back Pain Association, 31-3, Park Rd., Teddington, Middlesex, England TWII OAB (tel. 081/977-5474), is involved in fund-raising for research into the causes and treatment of back pain and offers leaflets on ways of preventing back pain from occurring. There is no similar group in the United States, but the Arthritis Foundation (see page 70) may be of some help.

BED-WETTING (NOCTURNAL ENURESIS)

INCIDENCE AND CAUSES

This is a very common problem among children, but in the great majority of cases the cause is unknown. In about 5 percent of cases, there is some underlying physical disorder such as a urinary tract infection, diabetes, chronic constipation, or epilepsy, but these children almost always have other symptoms so that diagnosis is made easier.

The age at which children "should" be dry is difficult to assess, but most doctors will not start treating for bed-wetting before the age of five or six. On average about one child in five wets the bed more than once a week at the age of three, one in ten at the age of five, and one in thirty-five at the age of fourteen. Bed-wetting is commoner in boys than in girls and commoner in children who are emotionally deprived, such as those living in institutions. Some 10 percent of bed-wetters will also have trouble controlling their bladders during the day.

In 70 percent of cases, bed-wetting runs in the family, with the mother, father, or a brother or sister having been affected. It is customary to divide patients into two groups—those who have never been dry (primary enuresis) and those who were dry but have started to wet again (secondary enuresis). Primary enuresis is commoner than secondary, but since both types are treated in the same way, the distinction is purely academic.

Sometimes when a child who is dry starts to wet again, it is at a time when something important is happening in his life, such as starting school or the birth of a new brother or sister. However, this does not necessarily mean that the child is worried or upset by the event and some specialists deny that bed-wetting is associated with stress. Often when a child goes on vacation or stays with relatives he will suddenly become dry again, but the reason for this is unclear.

TESTS

Before any treatment is offered, the urine will be checked to rule out any infection and, if necessary, a few basic tests of balance, coordination, and sensation will be done to see whether there might be anything wrong with the nervous system. If an underlying organic disease is suspected, this will be investigated and treated.

TRADITIONAL TREATMENT

There are many methods that have been used to treat bed-wetting, some more successful than others. In the first place, the child needs to understand that the mechanism that controls the bladder is very complex and that bladder control is something that has to be learned in the same way that he must learn to swim or ride a bicycle. Keeping a star chart (with a gold star for every night that he is dry) and praising or rewarding him as he gains better control can be very productive. Admonishing or punishing him when he is wet, on the other hand, can be very counterproductive and parents should try not to express their annoyance or anger to the child on the occasions when the bed is wet.

Waking up the child at night is sometimes helpful, but the time at which he is roused should be varied or he will just tend to wet at that particular time. Fluids before bedtime should not be restricted because it is important that the bladder learns to cope with normal amounts of urine. If less is given, it just gets used to holding less.

Drug treatment is available in the form of the tricyclic antidepressant imipramine or the antispasmodic propantheline, both of which seem to have the effect of relaxing the bladder muscle so that it does not contract abnormally. This has a 50 percent success rate, but unfortunately up to 70 percent of those helped relapse again later. However, it is useful in the short term, for example, if the child is going on a vacation.

The most effective treatment the doctor can offer is the enuresis alarm. This consists of a urine-sensitive pad that is put (depending on the model) either on the bed or inside the pajamas with an alarm wired up to it that is placed by the bedside or attached to the pajama top. As soon as the pad becomes wet, the alarm goes off, causing the child to jump. This results in automatic contraction of the muscles at the base of the bladder and the flow of urine stops. While the alarm is still sounding, it is necessary for a parent to come into the room and wake the child so that he can turn the alarm off himself. Eventually, a reflex will develop in which the sensation of starting to wet will cause the child to jump and wake up. The alarm has an 80 percent success rate after about three months of treatment, with only a 13 percent relapse rate. Some children who do not respond right away may do so with a different type of alarm—some respond better to bells, others to buzzers. If the parent wakes the child each morning by pressing the test button on the device, this will also help him to associate the sound of the alarm with waking up. The child should keep a record chart to show the nights on which he stays dry. But, in the early stages, encouraging signs are smaller wet patches in the bed and wetting later at night. Nylon sheets, pants, and pajamas should be avoided, as should comforters, since these tend to make the user sweat, and sweating can dampen the pad and lead to false alarms. After two weeks of consecutive dry nights, in order to reduce the risk of relapse, the child should be given more to drink in the hour before bedtime and continue to use the alarm until he has had another two weeks of dry nights.

RECENT ADVANCES

It is thought that some children who wet the bed do so because of a deficiency of antidiuretic hormone or ADH, which results in the production of abnormally large amounts of urine. ADH controls water secretion by the kidney and, if inadequate amounts of the hormone are produced, the bladder fills up faster than normal. Based on this theory, a synthetic form of ADH, desmopressin, has been produced as a nasal spray. One puff into each nostril at night should be enough to control bed-wetting in some children.

COMPLEMENTARY TREATMENT

Acupuncture
As in the case of incontinence (see separate section), bed-wetting is said to be due to a lack of Chi in the kidney and treatment uses specific

points that will strengthen the kidney and restore its energy flow to normal.

Aromatherapy
Cypress or pine may be recommended.

Herbalism
St. John's wort, which is used to treat anxiety states, may also be very helpful in the treatment of bed-wetting where the problem seems to result from stress. Horsetail and cornsilk act by making the lining of the bladder less irritable. Other herbal remedies may also be prescribed.

Homeopathy
For a child who wets the bed quite early in the night, belladonna may be helpful, whereas one who passes large amounts later on and is anxious and irritable may benefit from lycopodium. Gelsemium may be prescribed if the child is of a nervous disposition and wets himself during the day as well as at night.

Hypnotherapy
Children over the age of about six may often benefit from treatment by hypnosis. Some pediatricians treat them in groups, while others see them individually. The aim of treatment is to convince the child that his bladder can expand to hold more urine than it now manages to cope with at night and to enable him, if it really does become full, to wake and go to the toilet, rather than wetting the bed. It also reduces the anxieties that the child may have about his inability to stop wetting.

ORGANIZATIONS

Society for Pediatric Urology
c/o Dr. Dixon Walker
Box J-247
J. Willis Miller Health Center
University of Florida
Gainesville, FL 32610
904/392-2501

BREAST LUMPS

THERE ARE A NUMBER of conditions that can produce lumps in the breast, but most of them are fairly rare. The only common causes are fibroadenosis, fibroadenomas, and cancer. Any woman who finds a lump in her breast tends to think that it must be cancer, but only one in every ten breast lumps turns out to be malignant.

FIBROADENOSIS (CHRONIC MASTITIS)

This condition, in which the breasts are lumpy and tender, is ten times commoner than cancer of the breast. The tenderness and lumps are most noticeable just before a period and are often confined to the upper outer quadrant of the breast and the segment that stretches up into the armpit. Also known as chronic mastitis, fibroadenosis occurs between the ages of fifteen and fifty and is thought by some specialists to affect most women to a certain extent.

The hormonal changes that occur at the time of ovulation each month act on the lining of the womb and on the breast to prepare them for pregnancy. The breast tissue enlarges, but if pregnancy does not occur it subsides again until the next ovulation. Because this happens every month, the breast may become increasingly lumpy and cysts may form. The condition is more common in women who have never had babies and in those who have not breast-fed, and it may become less of a nuisance after a woman has fed her first baby. Although symptoms may be particularly severe around the time of the menopause, the condition tends to disappear after this, since the monthly hormonal changes are no longer occurring.

It is usual for one breast to be more severely affected than the other and the pain may be made worse by moving the arm. The glands under the arm may be tender as well. Sometimes the lumpiness of the breast may be the first sign to appear or there may be a discharge from the nipple, which may be blood-stained, yellow, green, or brown. Occa-

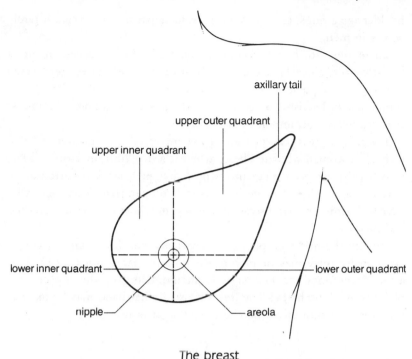

upper outer quadrant

upper inner quadrant

axillary tail

lower inner quadrant

lower outer quadrant

nipple

areola

The breast

sionally, the first sign is a smooth, spherical swelling, which may be quite large.

FIBROADENOMA

This is a very mobile lump with well-defined margins which tends to slip away from the examining fingers. Also known as a "breast mouse," it occurs primarily in women between the ages of fifteen and thirty-five and usually grows to a size of 1–3 cm in diameter. Rarely, there may be more than one in the same breast.

CANCER

Breast cancer is the most prevalent form of malignant disease in the Western world. In the United States, it accounts for about one third of all cases of cancer, affecting one in every ten to eleven women. It is second only to lung cancer as a cause of cancer death. It tends to occur in older age groups, especially after the menopause. Breast cancer rarely occurs in men.

There seems to be an environmental factor in the development of breast cancer, since Japanese women in the United States are affected much more frequently than those who live in Japan. Similarly, it is commoner in Danish women than in their near neighbors, the Finns. It is relatively uncommon in Africa and Asia.

The risk of breast cancer seems to be increased, to a greater or lesser extent, in women who are obese, who eat a diet high in saturated fat, who have never been pregnant, whose first pregnancy occurred at an advanced age, whose first period was at a comparatively early age, who have had benign breast disease previously, or whose mother or sister has had breast cancer.

Usually the first sign of breast cancer is a painless lump, although occasionally there may be pain or discomfort that is pricking in character. Sometimes the first sign is an indrawing of the nipple or a blood-stained discharge. The lump is usually hard and may be fixed to the overlying skin or to the chest, so that it is immobile.

PHYLLOIDES TUMOR

This relatively rare variant of the fibroadenoma occurs mainly in women over the age of forty. It feels tender, warm, and cystic, grows quite rapidly, and can become very large. The skin over the tumor may become thin and the veins on the surface of the breast may dilate. Very rarely, it may break through the skin, forming an ulcerating mass. Unlike cancer, it rarely attaches itself to the skin or to deeper structures, but remains mobile. Occasionally there may be a clear discharge from the nipple.

INTRADUCT PAPILLOMA

This is an uncommon little growth that occurs within the milk ducts of the breast, just under the nipple. It affects women between the ages of twenty and fifty, being rare under the age of twenty-five and commonest in the over-thirty-fives. The first sign is usually a blood-stained discharge, sometimes with a lump detectable under the areola (the dark skin around the nipple). Occasionally there may be more than one papilloma present.

FAT NECROSIS

Necrosis means death of the tissue involved. Fat necrosis in the breast occurs after injury, and bruising may be visible, although occasionally the woman may not remember having hurt herself. The patient is usually an overweight middle-aged woman. A painful lump is often the first sign, although pain may be absent. The lump may then become smaller and, being attached to the skin, may pull it inward, producing a dimple.

BREAST ABSCESS

This is a fairly rare condition that most often occurs in women who are breast-feeding. The cause is commonly a cracked nipple, through which bacteria have entered the milk ducts. This is why breast care and hygiene are so important for nursing mothers. The breast becomes red, hot, swollen, and very painful, and if incorrectly treated the abscess may become chronic.

MONDOR'S DISEASE

In this uncommon condition, the veins that run across and under the breast become thrombosed (that is, the blood within them clots). The cause is unknown, although it may occur after injury. The affected veins may be felt as long cordlike strands, some 3 mm across, in the outer part of the breast, often extending up into the armpit or down toward the abdomen. They are usually tender at first and may remain noticeable for up to a year.

RETENTION CYST

This is similar to a sebaceous cyst anywhere else on the body and occurs in the areola around the nipple.

PAPILLOMA OF THE NIPPLE

This is a small benign growth that arises from the areola or the nipple. It may grow to the size of a cherry and is always attached to the breast by a thin stalk.

TESTING OF BREAST LUMPS

Some breast lumps—such as papilloma of the nipple and Mondor's disease—are easy to diagnose, but others will need further testing in order to differentiate the benign tumors from cancer. Very often a doctor can make a diagnosis of fibroadenosis just from examination of the breast, but sometimes when there is an obvious lump mammography and biopsy may be suggested.

A cyst is a fluid-filled swelling that may occur without there being any other indication of breast disease. However, it is most frequently associated with fibroadenosis. It is often easy to diagnose. If the doctor holds a flashlight pressed to one side of the breast lump and the light shines through it, this is a clear indication that there is fluid in the lump. This technique is called transillumination. A further test is to insert a needle into the lump and extract all the fluid possible; if the fluid is clear and if the lump has completely vanished by the end of the procedure, this will confirm the diagnosis of a simple cyst. However, if the fluid is blood-stained or if a lump can still be felt, further tests are necessary, although in many cases the condition will be found to be benign.

Mammography is a fairly simple procedure in which the breast is squeezed between two X-ray plates and either one or two pictures are taken. Cancer may show up as a darker patch on the X-ray. However, benign tumors may also look dark and so, if any abnormality is seen, a biopsy is usually performed as well.

TRADITIONAL TREATMENT

Most benign tumors will not recur if removed, but it is not uncommon for cysts to recur in a breast with fibroadenosis. Forty percent of all phylloides tumors grow again unless they are removed with a wide margin of normal breast tissue so that, if the tumor is very big, a mastectomy may have to be performed. In the case of multiple intra-duct papillomas, it may be necessary to remove all the major milk ducts leading from the breast to the nipple, which means that breast-feeding will no longer be possible.

Mondor's disease needs no treatment and will subside of its own accord in time. Fibroadenosis usually needs no treatment, if there is no obvious lump, but if the patient complains of persistent pain, hormone treatment may be given for four to six months. Among the agents commonly used are danazol and bromocriptine.

A breast abscess that has only just started to form will often subside if the patient is treated with antibiotics. However, for those whose abscesses are beginning to "ripen" and for those who do not show a fairly immediate response to antibiotics, drainage is necessary. This is done under general anesthetic. The abscess is cut open and the pus is cleaned out. The wound is packed with a dressing that will prevent the resulting hole from closing over. Healing thus occurs from the base of the wound, and this helps to guard against a recurrence of the infection. The dressings are changed daily, less and less being packed into the wound as it becomes smaller.

The treatment of cancer depends very much on how advanced the tumor is and on who is treating the patient, since different surgeons have their own preferences. However, nowadays, many specialists are happy just to remove the lump with a wide margin of normal tissue ("lumpectomy") rather than to remove the entire breast. In most cases lumpectomy is combined with radiotherapy. Recent studies suggest that life expectancy following this form of treatment is as good as it is after mastectomy. Usually, a radioactive implant is inserted into the breast during the operation and is removed forty-eight hours later. Then a course of radiotherapy is given in the outpatients' department. Because the first "port of call" for a cancer that is spreading is the lymph glands in the armpit, it is usual to "sample" (just a few are taken) these to see if the cancer has spread there, which may change the treatment protocol, whatever type of operation is being performed.

Mastectomy may be of three kinds. In the simple mastectomy just the breast tissue (plus the lymph glands) are removed. In a radical mastectomy the muscle on which the breast lies is taken in addition. In an extended radical mastectomy, the lymph glands that run down the front of the chest are also removed. These more mutilating types of operation are less commonly performed nowadays than in the past.

Some forms of breast cancer are hormone-dependent—in other words, they thrive on estrogen. In such cases a drug that suppresses estrogen may be given or, in a premenopausal patient, the ovaries may be surgically removed. In postmenopausal women, the antiestrogen drug tamoxifen, which has a minimum of side effects, is commonly used. It has been shown that treatment with tamoxifen is as effective as surgery for breast cancer occurring in women over the age of seventy—a fortunate finding, since many elderly patients tolerate operations badly. Hormone therapy may also be valuable when cancer that seemed to have been cleared recurs; radiotherapy, too, can be useful in such cases. Chemotherapy (the use of drugs that kill cancer cells) is also effective, particularly in nonhormone-dependent tumors or when the cancer has spread to other parts of the body.

In the few men who develop breast cancer, a radical mastectomy is performed and this usually necessitates a skin graft to cover the wound. If the tumor is hormone-dependent, removal of the testes (orchiectomy) may be required.

Two percent of breast cancers occur in pregnant women. In the first half of pregnancy, the treatment is the same as for nonpregnant women and, if radiotherapy or chemotherapy is used, the pregnancy may have to be terminated, since both of these can cause severe deformities in the unborn child. If, however, the patient is nearing the end of her pregnancy, it may be feasible to induce labor and deliver the baby before beginning treatment. In some cases, it may be possible to wait a few weeks before starting treatment in order to allow the fetus to become a little more mature before it is delivered.

Patients are followed up at regular intervals following an operation for cancer of the breast so that any recurrence may be treated immediately.

Breast cancer is classified according to stages, stage one including all those cases in which the cancer appears to be confined solely to the breast itself, without any evidence of spread. *At least 80 percent of patients who are treated at this stage are still alive five years later, but for more advanced growths, the outlook is less good. This is why it is so important for a woman to see her GP immediately when she discovers a lump in her breast, just in case it turns out to be malignant.*

RECENT ADVANCES

Trials of lumpectomy plus radiotherapy have shown how successful the treatment is. Doctors at the University of Kansas Medical Center treated 110 cases of breast cancer in this way and found only two recurrences during the following four years, while doctors at the Albert Einstein College of Medicine in New York observed a recurrence rate of 14 percent within five years, when they followed up 201 patients.

Some would like to introduce a nationwide screening program in which all women over the age of fifty will be offered mammography. The age limit has been chosen for two reasons. One is that breast cancer is commoner in older women and the other is that, before the menopause, the density of the breast tissue reduces the reliability of the test. The American Cancer Society recommends a baseline mammogram before the age of forty. It has been estimated that some 10 percent of women who have mammograms will have to be recalled for reassessment and further tests, although only a small proportion of these will be found to have cancer.

However, some younger women are at higher risk of developing breast cancer than others, because the disease seems to run in the family. A Family Cancer Clinic has been set up by the Royal Free and University College Hospitals in London to offer screening to any woman over the age of thirty whose mother or sister developed breast cancer before she was fifty.

There has been some debate in the medical press as to how effective mammography is as a screening process, but in a New York survey of 62,000 women over a period of eighteen years it was found that in those who were offered mammography the death rate from cancer of the breast fell by one third. Similarly, both Holland and Sweden reported a 30 percent drop in mortality following the introduction of mammography.

A technique developed at the Royal Marsden Hospital in London is able to show whether or not an abnormality that has shown up on a mammogram is malignant, without a biopsy being necessary. The new technique records blood flow within the breast and shows it on a screen. Normal breast tissue and benign tumors appear blueish, while cancers, which always have an increased blood flow, appear red. Cancers as small as half a centimeter across can be picked up and the intensity of the color shown can guide specialists as to the kind of treatment required.

The need for biopsies may also be reduced by a technique now being used in a few centers across the world. This is needle aspiration. A tiny needle is inserted into the lump and a small section of the tissue is removed and examined under a microscope.

Other methods of screening that will pick out women who are particularly at risk of developing breast cancer are constantly being sought. At the Christie Hospital in Manchester, doctors took tiny pieces of skin from women whose mothers and grandmothers had had breast cancer. Then, in the laboratory, they grew some of the cells (the fibroblasts) contained in the skin samples and found that, in half of the cases, they took on the character of cancer cells and became invasive. The women are now being followed up to see whether those whose tests were abnormal are those who develop cancer.

In another study at the University of California School of Medicine, breast fluid was drawn off through the nipple from 3194 women. The cells contained in the fluid were abnormal in 420 cases, and researchers were able to follow up 335 of these. Subsequently 19 of these women developed breast cancer, compared with 6 in a similar-size group who had had normal results.

At the Royal Liverpool Hospital, surgeons found viruslike particles in the white blood cells of thirty-one out of thirty-two patients with early breast cancer, but only in three out of twenty-seven healthy women. The particles were also seen in the breast, in the macrophage cells that, like the white cells, are part of the body's defense against foreign tissues such as bacteria, viruses, and cancer. Further research is going to be necessary to determine whether the virus itself is causing the cancer or whether it just reduces the effectiveness of the white cells and macrophages, making them less able to fight cancer when it arises. If it turns out that the virus is a causative factor, it may be possible at some time in the future to develop a vaccine against it.

At Rockefeller University in New York, it was found that patients with breast cancer had 50 percent more 16-alpha hydroxy estrone in their blood than healthy women. This estrone is a breakdown product from estrogen and it is thought that it becomes bound to the nuclei of the cells making up the breast tissue, stimulating them and increasing the risk of abnormal growth. It has been found that women who have a high dietary intake of saturated fat have higher blood levels of 16-alpha hydroxy estrone, whereas those who have low intakes and who regularly eat fatty fish or take fish oil supplements tend to have low levels.

In Toronto, two groups of women considered to be at risk of developing breast cancer were observed over a period of five years. One group followed a low-fat diet and only one member developed cancer, while the others ate a normal diet and produced six cases over the five years. Very recently results of another study have seemed to show that women who drink heavily have a greater risk of developing breast cancer than occasional drinkers.

It has also been suggested that taking the contraceptive Pill may have some effect on the breast and increase the risk of developing cancer. But although a recent study carried out at Oxford University confirmed the findings of the Imperial Cancer Research Fund epidemiology unit that women who took the Pill for four or more years before having their first full-term pregnancy had more than double the risk of those who had not, several other studies, including a much larger one in the United States, showed no such risk. And since new, low-dose Pills are being introduced constantly, none of these studies has really been able to determine the true effects of the modern Pill.

Tests that can assess the severity of a cancer are also important since they can ensure that appropriate treatment is given. Normally, the lymph glands under the arm are removed, but not totally, in all operations for breast cancer, since there is no way of knowing whether or not the tumor cells have spread there. However, doctors working for the Imperial Cancer Research Fund have discovered a method of detecting spread, which may eventually mean that it will be possible to pick out those women in whom spread has not occurred and avoid having to do this extra piece of surgery. The test makes use of an antibody that sticks to tumor cells. This is attached to a mildly radioactive substance and injected into the patient. A special camera is then used to detect the antibodies—if they are clustered in the glands, this is a clear indication that the glands should be removed.

COMPLEMENTARY TREATMENT

The use of complementary therapies in the treatment of cancer is described in the section on cervical cancer.

ORGANIZATIONS

See also the section on cervical cancer.

Y-ME Breast Cancer Support Program
c/o Sharon Greer
18220 Harword Avenue
Homewood, IL 60430
312/799-8338
(Publishes the *Y-ME Newsletter*.)

Breast Cancer Advisory Center
P.O. Box 224
Kensington, MD 20895

BRONCHITIS

THE WORD *bronchitis* simply means inflammation of the air passages of the lungs—the bronchi and bronchioles. (See the diagram showing the structure of the lungs on pg. 72.) Bronchitis can be acute or chronic.

ACUTE BRONCHITIS

Acute bronchitis is caused by an infection, probably 90 percent of cases being due to viruses and 10 percent to bacteria. It usually begins with a hacking cough and after 24–48 hours the patient begins to bring up phlegm, which is white, yellow, or green. Children tend to swallow phlegm rather than spit it out and the irritation this causes to the stomach lining may cause vomiting.

In many cases the patient is feverish and often a wheeze can be heard as he breathes in and out, forcing air through bronchial tubes that have become narrowed by inflammation and excessive mucus secretion. The cells that form the lining of the bronchi possess microscopic fingerlike projections called cilia, whose function is to sweep mucus upward out of the respiratory tract. These cilia are paralyzed by cigarette smoke, so smokers may take much longer to recover from an attack of acute bronchitis than nonsmokers. If infected mucus settles low down in the respiratory tract, it may cause pneumonia. Among nonsmokers, this is more likely to occur in the very young and the very old.

It is not uncommon for children to develop acute bronchitis, those suffering from measles or whooping cough being particularly susceptible. Viral bronchitis, which often attacks children under the age of five, tends to occur in localized outbreaks. Although infants may appear to be seriously ill with bronchitis, the infection is very seldom fatal. However, after recovering from the condition many children will continue to have a dry cough for several weeks.

107

CHRONIC BRONCHITIS

This is altogether a more serious illness than acute bronchitis. Traditionally, it is defined as a condition in which the patient coughs, bringing up phlegm, on most days during a period of three consecutive months for more than two successive years. In other words, the condition is long-term and recurrent.

The most important causative factor is cigarette smoking. Whereas only 5 nonsmokers in every 100,000 will die each year from chronic bronchitis, 49 who smoke under twenty-five cigarettes a day and 106 who smoke more than this will die each year. Stopping smoking, even quite late in the disease, may make a difference to the patient's life expectancy, the average death rate from bronchitis of ex-smokers being 38 per 100,000.

Chronic bronchitis is commoner in older people and in men. Exposure to air pollution is also a factor in its development. In Britain it affects one middle-aged man in ten and causes the loss of 30 million working days a year. It is often known as "the British disease," since its severe forms are very much more common in Britain than elsewhere, possibly because it is exacerbated by the climate. Deaths from bronchitis are commoner in winter and in urban areas, and are more likely to occur among unskilled and semiskilled workers than among the professional classes. This is probably because the former tend to smoke more heavily than the latter and are more likely to be exposed to atmospheric pollution in their place of work.

Chronic bronchitis usually begins between the ages of thirty and sixty. The symptoms may come on very gradually or may follow an attack of acute bronchitis or pneumonia. To begin with, persistent phlegm, requiring frequent clearing of the throat, may be the only symptom. This phlegm is produced by overactivity of the mucus-secreting glands that are found in the lining of the air passages. As more and more is produced, the patient starts to cough some up each morning when he wakes. Eventually the cough may continue throughout the day. At first the phlegm is clear, although it may contain black specks that are particles of carbon left in the lungs from smoking. The cough is likely to become worse toward the end of the day, particularly if the patient has been exposed to dust or cigarette smoke, or has been in crowds or has drunk alcohol. There may also be a feeling of discomfort in the sinuses, across the cheekbones and forehead, together with a dripping of mucus from the sinuses down the back of the throat, making it sore. Coughing may come in fits, particularly at night or upon waking in the morning, and may be started off by taking a deep breath.

Acute chest infections in patients suffering from chronic bronchitis (acute on chronic bronchitis) are not uncommon, particularly in advanced cases. In healthy lungs there are no infective organisms present in the air passages, but the excessive mucus produced in chronic bronchitis makes it easier for viruses and bacteria to live there. Viral infections increase the mucus secretion still further and encourage bacterial growth. If a bacterial infection takes hold, the mucus thickens and may become yellow or green and the air passages become acutely inflamed. This may cause permanent damage to the lungs, especially if it is not possible to eradicate the bacteria from the phlegm completely, in which case repeated episodes of infection are likely to occur. The final picture of a patient with severe chronic bronchitis is one in which any form of exertion is impossible since it causes bouts of coughing, wheezing, and breathlessness.

For those patients who give up smoking early in the course of the disease and who manage to avoid recurrent chest infections, the outlook is good. However, the poorer the lung function becomes, the more likely the patient is to die from respiratory failure or from heart failure.

EMPHYSEMA

This condition often occurs in conjunction with chronic bronchitis and may be responsible for much of the breathlessness experienced by patients. In emphysema, damage to the air passages results in dilation or destruction of the alveoli—the tiny air sacs through which oxygen diffuses into the blood and carbon dioxide diffuses out into the lungs. The normal elasticity that aids breathing out is lost, the lungs become overinflated, and the patient is constantly breathless.

PULMONARY HEART DISEASE

The word *pulmonary* is used to describe anything related to the lungs, such as their blood supply (pulmonary circulation) or tests of how they are working (pulmonary function tests). Pulmonary heart disease may occur as a result of poor air flow from the lungs into the blood. If inadequate amounts of air get through to the alveoli because of narrowing of the air passages, insufficient oxygen enters the bloodstream, which remains overloaded with carbon dioxide. As a result, the blood vessels that carry the blood to and from the lungs constrict. This occurs as an automatic reaction, which may be reversed in the early stages if the condition of the lungs improves. However, if there is no improvement, pulmonary hypertension may eventually occur, in which the blood pressure in these vessels is a great deal higher than it should be. This, in turn, puts strain on the right side of the heart whose function is to pump blood through the pulmonary circulation, and it may cease to function effectively.

TESTS

Tests are usually unnecessary in acute bronchitis since the diagnosis is easily made upon examination. However, tests may be needed for patients with chronic bronchitis, not only to confirm the diagnosis but to ascertain the extent of the lung damage that has occurred.

A chest X-ray taken early in the course of the disease is likely to be normal, as are X-rays of the sinuses. A culture of the sputum may show bacteria growing there. Lung-function tests (described in the section on asthma) may also be normal at first.

Occasionally the doctor may suspect that there is a more sinister cause for the patient's chronic cough and in such cases may suggest bronchoscopy or bronchography. In the former, a small tube with a tiny inbuilt camera is passed into the patient's lungs under anesthetic. Through this the specialist can see whether there are any localized problems such as a foreign body that has been inhaled, tuberculosis, or a tumor. In bronchography, the air passages of each lung in turn are filled with a substance that will show up on X-ray. A film can then be taken that will demonstrate any abnormalities. In chronic bronchitis, it may show the wide mouths of the many overactive mucous glands together with narrowing of the smaller airways.

At a later stage in the disease, a chest X-ray may show enlargement of the right side of the heart, indicating a degree of pulmonary heart disease. This may also show up on an electrocardiogram. Results of the lung-function tests will begin to deteriorate and a blood count may show an excess of red cells. Production of these cells, whose function is to carry oxygen in the bloodstream, is stimulated by a continuing lack of oxygen in the blood. Increased numbers are also to be found in the blood of people who spend their lives at very high altitudes where the atmosphere is thin, and in smokers.

TRADITIONAL TREATMENT

Acute Bronchitis
Although 90 percent of cases are viral and therefore will not respond to antibiotics, it is customary to prescribe these in all cases. There are two reasons for this. First, it is not always easy to determine which cases are viral and which are not; second, tissue that has already been damaged by a virus is susceptible to superimposed bacterial infection.

Chronic Bronchitis
The most important form of treatment is to persuade the patient to stop smoking, since this, more than anything else, will help to prevent the rapid deterioration of his health. Other preventive measures include vaccination against influenza every winter and avoidance of dusty and smoky atmospheres and fog. Overweight patients should attempt to diet, since obesity puts further strain on the heart. Physiotherapy to help the patient clear his lungs of mucus is also beneficial.

Antibiotics are given when acute bacterial infections occur and some patients may need regular small doses throughout the winter months in order to prevent acute attacks. Some patients find bronchodilators helpful; these reduce spasm in the bronchi and are usually prescribed in the form of inhalers. If right-sided heart failure occurs, this will need to be treated, usually with diuretics (as in hypertension). If the heartbeat becomes erratic, the patient may need digoxin.

In severe cases, oxygen given over a period of at least fifteen hours in every twenty-four may help to relieve the patient's symptoms. Some patients with severe breathlessness may be helped by the use of steroids, usually in an inhalable form.

COMPLEMENTARY TREATMENT

Acupuncture

Acute bronchitis is said to be due to invasion by wind and cold or by wind and heat, which obstruct the flow of energy, or Chi, in the lungs. Specific points will be used to eliminate phlegm, wind, and either cold or heat, and to restore the flow of Chi to normal. Because the lung is intimately related, in the Chinese system of energy flow, with the spleen and kidney, treatment for chronic bronchitis will include the use of points to strengthen these organs.

Acupuncture can also help patients to give up smoking.

Alexander Technique

Correct posture may help the patient with chronic bronchitis to breathe more easily.

Aromatherapy

Thyme may be useful in acute bronchitis, and niaouli, origanum, rosemary, sandalwood, and sage in chronic bronchitis. Other oils such as cajuput, eucalyptus, hyssop, and pine may be effective in either type.

Herbalism

This may be helpful in both acute and chronic bronchitis. A variety of herbs may be used. Coltsfoot relaxes the bronchial tubes, acts as an expectorant (helping the patient to cough up phlegm), and soothes the inflamed airways. Hyssop in acute bronchitis encourages sweating, thus lowering the fever, reduces the inflammation, and also is an expectorant. Other expectorants include aniseed and elecampane (both of which are particularly useful in chronic bronchitis), garlic, and thyme.

Homeopathy

The remedy needed by an individual patient will depend on his symptoms. In the early stages of acute bronchitis, when he is restless and feverish and has a dry, painful cough, aconite may be appropriate, whereas a spasmodic cough with rattling of mucus in the chest and an inclination to vomit may indicate a need for ipecac. Phosphorus may improve the condition of a patient who has tightness across the chest, wheezing, and hoarseness, and who is worse for talking and fresh air. Antimony tart. is particularly useful for children and old people who have a lot of loose phlegm in the chest and rattling wheezy breathing, but who cough up very little and are afraid of suffocating during a coughing fit.

Hypnotherapy
By helping patients to give up smoking, hypnosis may be a valuable adjunct to the treatment of chronic bronchitis. However, since it works only by strengthening the patient's resolve and reducing or preventing withdrawal symptoms, it cannot make someone give up if he doesn't really want to.

Manipulation
Both chiropractic and osteopathy may help the patient to increase the air space in his chest cavity and thus to use his lungs more effectively.

Nutrition
Vitamins A, B complex, C, and E and the minerals selenium and zinc strengthen the immune system and help the body to fight against infections. Supplements may be recommended to prevent recurrent attacks of acute or acute on chronic bronchitis. Vitamins A and C also help to maintain healthy lung tissue. A nutrition therapist may suggest that a patient avoids dairy produce, which encourages the formation of mucus.

CERVICAL CANCER

INCIDENCE AND RISK FACTORS

Cancer of the cervix, or neck of the womb, primarily affects women between the ages of thirty and fifty, although it can occur both earlier and later than this. It is commonest in married women and in the lower socioeconomic classes, and seems to be more likely to occur in those who started having sexual intercourse at an early age and who had their first pregnancy while they were still very young. An increased frequency in women who have had a large number of sexual partners and who have been infected with genital herpes or with genital warts suggests that infection must, in some way, play a part in the development of this type of cancer. For a reason yet to be explained adequately, some racial groups are far less prone to develop cervical cancer than others—it is quite rare in Jewish and Muslim women but comparatively common in Puerto Ricans.

In the United States, cervical cancer is the commonest gynecologic cancer in women ages fifteen to thirty-four. However, it does not cause as many deaths as cancer of the ovary, which is far less easy to diagnose at an early stage.

PAP SMEARS

Because cervical cancer can be detected at a very early stage in its development using the Pap smear, it is possible to cure it in very many cases. The American Cancer Society recommends three annual smears starting at age eighteen or with the beginning of sexual activity, then every one to three years at the patient's or doctor's discretion. Some preventive medicine experts feel that women over the age of sixty-five can stop screening. Most young women will have smears more frequently than this, since they are usually performed at family planning and during ante- and postnatal care. Unfortunately, the bulk of cases of cervical cancer occur in older women, who may have completed their family and are no longer receiving such care. It is important that these women arrange to see their gynecologists in order to continue to have regular smears.

Not only does the smear show up abnormal cells but it will also indicate if there is any infection present on the cervix, such as thrush. The majority of patients who are recalled after having a smear have either an infection that needs treating or dysplasia—a condition in which the cervical cells show some abnormality although they are not frankly malignant.

STAGES OF CERVICAL CANCER

Cervical cancer is broken down into stages according to how advanced it is, the earliest being CIN, or cervical intraepithelial neoplasia. CIN I includes all patients with mild dysplasia. Eighty-five percent of cases of CIN I disappear of their own accord, but because the remaining 15 percent can progress it is vital that all patients continue to be followed up until they are told that they are clear. CIN II is moderate dysplasia, and CIN III includes severe dysplasia and carcinoma in situ (cancer that has not started to invade the surrounding tissue). The three CIN stages make up stage 0.

Stages I to IV comprise invasive cancer, which is no longer confined to the layer of cells on the surface of the cervix in which it arises. In stage I, the cancer is still confined to the cervix itself. Later stages are defined by how far the cancer has spread to adjacent organs such as the rectum or bladder or, via the blood and lymphatic system, to distant parts of the body.

SYMPTOMS

Stages 0 and Ia (in which the cancer has only just begun to invade the cervix) produce no symptoms, but can be picked up by a Pap smear. Once the cancer has started to invade the cervix and other local tissues, vaginal bleeding may occur after intercourse or between the periods and may also affect postmenopausal women. If the condition is allowed to progress, the patient may develop a foul-smelling watery discharge that may be blood-stained.

A more advanced cancer may obstruct the ureters that lead from the kidneys to the bladder, interrupting the normal flow of urine and causing kidney failure. Pain in the back and pain and swelling of the legs may also occur. Involvement of the bladder may produce pain upon passing water and blood-stained urine. Spread to the rectum (back passage) may cause bleeding, pain upon defecation, or diarrhea.

TESTS

A Pap smear is a quick and easy procedure. It may be slightly uncomfortable for a matter of seconds, but this is a small price to pay for a test that can detect cancer at an early enough stage to allow it to be cured.

If an abnormality is found, the patient may be referred for colposcopy. This takes slightly longer than a smear and is usually done in the outpatients' department. The patient lies on her back with her legs apart and a metal instrument is inserted into the vagina so that the doctor can see the cervix. The smear is repeated and a swab is taken to check for infections. The cervix is swabbed with a saline solution and a special microscope is used to inspect it. The saline will cause the blood vessels on the cervix to stand out so that any abnormalities can be seen. Then the cervix is swabbed with dilute acetic acid, which may sting briefly. This shows up abnormal areas of cells as white patches. Finally a swab of iodine is used, which will show normal areas as brown and abnormal areas as white or yellow. A little instrument is inserted into the cervical canal, so that the doctor can also inspect the cells that line it. If any abnormal areas are seen either on the surface of the cervix or in the canal, a biopsy is taken. A tiny piece of tissue, no larger than a grain of rice, is pinched out and any resulting bleeding is stopped by holding a silver nitrate stick against the area for a few minutes. This is not a painful procedure so no anesthetic is needed.

Depending on the findings of the biopsy and the symptoms of which the patient is complaining, other investigations that may be performed include proctoscopy (inspection of the rectum using a little metal instrument), cystoscopy (inspection of the bladder under general anesthetic, using a fine telescope), X-ray of the kidneys (intravenous pyelogram), and other X-rays.

TRADITIONAL TREATMENT

Patients with CIN can often be treated in an outpatient unit without needing admission to the hospital. Techniques used include electrocautery, electrocoagulation diathermy, laser, and cryocautery. In other words, the abnormal tissue can be destroyed either by burning or freezing. Diathermy is a painful procedure and therefore has to be done under a general anesthetic. All these methods cure the condition in over 90 percent of patients. However, follow-up is vital to ensure that those few who do not respond are given further treatment.

If the cancer cells seem to be extending up the cervical canal, a cone biopsy is performed. This is done under general anesthetic and entails a few days in the hospital. A cone of tissue is removed from the cervix, reaching up the canal. This procedure helps confirm the diagnosis and in many cases will also cure the condition by removing all the cancerous tissue. The commonest complication is bleeding. This may occur within twelve hours of the operation, in which case a return to surgery may be necessary, or it may happen a week or so after the operation, when it is often associated with infection and the patient may need to be treated with antibiotics. The bleeding may be heavy, but is usually easily controlled. Occasionally, the cervix is damaged so that either it becomes scarred (causing pain at period times and retention of blood in the womb) or it becomes lax (causing miscarriage). In the latter case, a special stitch can be inserted into the cervix once the patient knows she is pregnant to prevent it from opening until the pregnancy has reached full term.

Patients who have had a cone biopsy or treatment with a laser must avoid using tampons and refrain from having sexual intercourse for a month afterward.

Patients who continue to have abnormal cells on smears taken after a cone biopsy, or who have other gynecological problems such as fibroids, may be offered a hysterectomy even though their cancer is at a very early stage.

Where the cancer has started to invade the cervix but has progressed no further, surgery may be performed. This usually takes the form of a radical, or Wertheim's, hysterectomy in which the entire womb, the tubes, the upper third of the vagina, and the local lymph glands are removed. Some specialists also remove the ovaries, but others consider this unnecessary, especially in younger women.

More advanced cases are treated with radiotherapy. However, some physicians treat all patients with invasive cancer with this method whether the cancer is at stage I, II, III, or IV. Usually a radioactive implant is inserted into the womb and external radiotherapy is given in addition. Both surgery and radiotherapy have their drawbacks. Surgery, which is only suitable for certain patients, may be followed by bleeding, infection, and bladder problems. The shortening of the vagina may be a disadvantage in young sexually active women. Radiotherapy, however, may cause sickness and diarrhea at the time of treatment and, later on, shrinking of the vagina (causing sexual difficulties), bladder problems, and constipation or diarrhea. Vaginal shrinkage can be minimized by giving the patient an estrogen cream to use once radiotherapy has been completed.

Surgery may sometimes be appropriate when the cancer has invaded the bladder or the rectum but seems to involve no other structures. The rectum can be removed and the healthy end of the large intestine can be brought out to the abdominal surface as a colostomy. If the bladder is removed, the urine flow has to be diverted. This is done by removing a piece of large intestine and forming it into a sac. The ureters, which carry the urine from the kidneys, are inserted into this sac and an exit is formed in the abdominal wall through which the urine can be passed.

PROGNOSIS

Doctors usually assess the results of treatment for cancer in terms of five-year survival—in other words, how many patients are still alive five years after the original diagnosis was made. For stage I cancer of the cervix, this is around 90 percent. Since recurrence, if it occurs, is likely to do so within eighteen months of treatment, one can, in this instance, talk about a 90 percent cure rate. Stage II has about a 75 percent five-year survival rate. For stage III, it is around 40 percent. Even in stage IV, the most advanced form, 10 percent of patients will still be alive in five years. The results for patients treated with surgery and those having radiotherapy are much the same.

RECENT ADVANCES

In 1987, scientists at the Department of Veterinary Pathology at Glasgow University who were investigating tumors caused by the papilloma virus in cows found that they could cure them by injecting them with a preparation made from the same tumors. The virus concerned is identical with the virus that causes genital warts in humans and that is thought to be associated with the development of cervical cancer. Antogenous vaccines are being developed to treat human papilloma virus infections that cause various types of warts. This research suggests that one day it may be possible to produce a vaccine against some forms of cervical cancer.

In 1988 doctors at the Whittington and Royal Northern Hospitals in London found that smokers were more vulnerable to viral infections of the cervix than others. Smoking seemed to reduce the normal immune response of the cells of the cervix, so that viruses were not readily destroyed. The doctors also found nicotine (known to be a carcinogen) in the cervical secretions. It seems likely, therefore, that smokers have a greater risk of developing cervical cancer than nonsmokers. A study at the University of Utah School of Medicine also found an increased risk of cervical cancer among smokers and from passive smoking as well.

COMPLEMENTARY TREATMENT

Because traditional treatment of cancer of the cervix is nowadays so effective, it would be extremely foolhardy to rely solely on complementary treatment for this complaint. However, the complementary therapies can be invaluable as an adjunct to traditional treatment, since their action is to stimulate the patient's immune system, which allows the body to play a greater role in fighting the disease. Naturopaths may recommend a diet consisting mainly of uncooked organically grown fruit and vegetables. Nutritionists are likely to suggest large doses of vitamins and minerals. Vitamins B, C, E, and folic acid strengthen the immune system, as does zinc. Vitamins C and E, zinc, manganese, and selenium help to defend the body against damage caused by carcinogens, and vitamins C and A detoxify carcinogens, preventing them from causing harm.

Herbal medicine, homeopathy, acupuncture, radionics, and healing can all play a role in strengthening the patient's resistance and raising her level of health.

Visualization is a technique that has been pioneered in the United States by a psychologist, in which the patient pictures her cancer slowly being overcome by her medication and her body getting stronger. It has proved the truth of the old adage of "mind over matter," since it seems to be remarkably effective in many cases.

ORGANIZATIONS

American Cancer Society
261 Madison Avenue
New York, NY 10016
212/599-3600

Cancer Connection
H & R Block Building
4410 Main Street
Kansas City, MO 64111
816/932-8453

Foundation for Alternative Cancer Therapies
Box 1242
Old Chelsea Station
New York, NY 10113
212/741-2790

International Association of Cancer Victors and Friends
7740 W. Manchester Ave.
No. 110
Playa Del Rey, CA 90293
310/822-5032

National Coalition for Cancer Survivorship
323 Eighth Street, SW
Albuquerque, NM 87102
505/764-9956

FURTHER READING

Cancer and Its Nutritional Therapies by Dr. Richard A. Passwater (published in the United States by Keats/Pivot but available in the United

Kingdom) is a straightforward and informative overview of how optimum nutrition is being used to treat malignancy.

Getting Well Again is by Carl and Stephanie Simonton and James L. Creighton, all of whom have pioneered the use of self-help techniques, including visualization, in the treatment of patients with cancer. Published by Bantam, it explains the techniques that they have used and contains many interesting case histories.

Love, Medicine, and Miracles, by Bernie Siegel, is published by Harper & Row.

CONSTIPATION

DEFINITION AND CAUSES

Constipation may be defined as a condition in which the patient moves his bowels less than three times a week or in which he passes small or hard stools or needs to strain. It is extremely common and may be a symptom of a number of diseases (one textbook lists thirty-two causes of constipation). The commonest cause is poor bowel habits. These may arise in children as a result of problems with toilet training or may occur later in life for a variety of reasons. Most frequent, perhaps, is a change in daily routine. For example, someone who normally defecates (moves his bowels) after breakfast each day changes jobs and has to catch an earlier train. He no longer has time to go to the toilet after breakfast and by the time he reaches work the urge to defecate has passed. Similarly, children may become constipated when they go to school because they do not want to use the school toilets. Sometimes a child may find a stool painful to pass and after that be unwilling to defecate in case it should hurt. Often constipation runs in families.

Another common cause of constipation is a poor diet—either inadequate in itself (for example, in the case of someone on a strict reducing diet or a patient with anorexia nervosa) or else a diet lacking in roughage. Inadequate fluid intake, or excess fluid loss such as occurs during a fever, also results in the formation of hard stools.

Constipation is frequently a symptom of irritable bowel syndrome and diverticular disease and may be the first symptom of cancer of the bowel. It can also occur in diabetes, myxedema (hypothyroidism), Parkinson's disease, multiple sclerosis, and depression. Certain drugs may cause constipation—such as opiates (morphine, heroin, codeine), aluminum salts (present in many antacids), iron, methotrexate (used in the treatment of various malignant conditions and also in psoriasis and arthritis), and aspirin—as may the toxic mineral lead.

Pregnant women frequently become constipated. This is probably partly due to the pressure of the womb on the bowel and partly to the iron supplements that they take. Sudden changes in diet or physical activity will often cause transient constipation.

Babies not infrequently go a day or two without passing a stool, but as long as the stools remain soft and the baby seems well there is usually nothing to worry about. However, one condition that starts in childhood is Hirschsprung's disease, in which the nerves leading to the lower part of the large bowel are abnormal. As a result, that part of the bowel remains constricted, making it difficult for stools to pass through, and the normal bowel above it may become distended. It is an uncommon disease, affecting fewer than one in 5000 babies, but it tends to run in families.

TESTS

It is usual to examine children who have been constipated since birth and adults who suddenly become constipated because in these cases there may be an underlying physical problem. However, because constipation is so common in older children, they are not usually tested extensively unless they fail to respond to basic treatment.

Initially the doctor will examine the patient's abdomen for any masses, inspect the anal area for any painful conditions that may be making defecation difficult (such as a split, or fissure, in the skin, or prolapsed hemorrhoids), and examine the rectum with a finger to see whether it is full of stool or empty. In patients whose constipation is due to faulty habits, the rectum is usually clogged up with stool.

If considered necessary, blood tests may be taken to check the patient's thyroid function, a urine test to check for diabetes, and a stool specimen to check for intestinal bleeding. If the diagnosis is still in doubt, the patient may need a sigmoidoscopy (inspection of the bowel with a flexible telescope) or a barium enema (X-ray of the bowel). If the cause of the constipation has still not been found, more sophisticated hospital tests may be required. A biopsy of the rectum will indicate whether or not there is a neurological cause for the constipation (that is, whether it is due to a malfunction of the nervous system as in Hirschsprung's disease), and tests that measure the pressures within the bowel will help to assess bowel function.

TRADITIONAL TREATMENT

In cases where there is an underlying physical cause for constipation, this must be treated. Sometimes surgery will be necessary to remove an abnormal segment of bowel, for example, in patients suffering from cancer of the bowel or babies with Hirschsprung's disease.

However, for those patients whose constipation is due to faulty habits, the treatment consists in changing those habits and, if necessary, giving a gentle laxative. The diet should be changed to include plenty of fresh fruit and vegetables and the amount of red meat (which slows down intestinal activity) should be reduced. Time should be allowed to move the bowels—those people who know that they usually need to go straight after breakfast should make sure that they have time to do so without missing their train or being late for school. Children must be reassured that it is quite acceptable to ask to go to the toilet when the need arises. However, straining to pass a stool when one does not feel the desire to do so may be damaging and should be avoided.

In severe cases, enemas may be necessary, or even manual removal of the stools under anesthetic, in order to clear very hard stools and allow other treatments to start working. Patients may also find suppositories (which are inserted in the rectum) helpful and there are enemas that patients can be taught to give themselves.

Normally, however, a change of diet and habits and a gentle laxative is enough. If the use of a laxative can be avoided, so much the better. If one is used, the patient should not buy it over the counter without advice, but should first consult his doctor. The best type is a hydrophilic agent—one that absorbs water in the bowel and therefore softens the stool and makes it bulky and easy to pass. These include agar and various proprietary bulking agents. Although bran is also a hydrophilic agent, it is best avoided, because in large quantities it has been known to cause blockage of the bowel. Also it is less pleasant to take than some of the other preparations. All of these may cause flatulence, but this is usually avoided by starting with a small dose and working upward until the constipation is relieved.

For those patients who fail to respond to a hydrophilic agent, lactulose may be helpful. This is a synthetic sugarlike substance that, when broken down in the bowel, draws water into the stool, making it softer and bulkier. However, it, too, may cause flatulence and also diarrhea.

As a last resort, other laxatives include docusate sodium (which softens the stools), anthracine derivatives (such as senna and cascara), or inorganic salts (such as magnesium sulphate, Epsom salts). However, these laxatives irritate the bowel and may cause diarrhea, colic, dehydration, and an imbalance in the body's chemicals.

Many doctors now advise that the old favorites castor oil and mineral oil should never be used. Castor oil can cause a severe loss of water and minerals from the body and mineral oil can produce irritation around the anus and, more important, can cause pneumonia if it "goes down the wrong way" and gets into the windpipe. There is also a suspicion that it may encourage the development of cancer if taken long term.

LAXATIVE ABUSE

Before the current interest in healthy eating, it was common for people (especially the elderly) to dose themselves regularly with laxatives. Patients suffering from anorexia nervosa may also surreptitiously take laxatives as part of their attempt to lose weight.

People who have taken laxatives over a long period of time may develop diarrhea, abdominal discomfort, and bloating, together with tiredness and lethargy. Sometimes they may become dehydrated and their body chemistry may be severely disturbed, resulting in heart or kidney problems. It is therefore very important that laxatives should only be taken over a short period unless absolutely necessary. Patients who need laxatives long term should only take hydrophilic agents, which are unlikely to cause problems.

For those patients who have become "hooked" on a laxative, it may be very hard to come off. When they do finally manage to stop taking it, the large bowel may no longer work because it has become so used to having its work done for it by stimulants. In such a case, an operation to remove the nonfunctioning section of bowel may be necessary.

COMPLEMENTARY TREATMENT

Aromatherapy
An abdominal massage with fennel or rosemary may be recommended.

Herbalism

Many orthodox laxatives are derived from herbs, such as senna and cascara. Although herbalists feel that the whole herb is likely to be more effective than an extract from it, as well as having fewer side effects, their policy when prescribing laxatives is much the same as that of a traditional practitioner. In other words, where necessary, strong laxatives may be given for a short period of time but gentle bulk laxatives such as linseed and psyllium are preferred.

Homeopathy

A patient whose stools are quite soft but who has to strain to pass them may benefit from alumina. For one who has overused laxatives in the past and who, although he frequently desires to go, manages only to pass a small amount each time, nux vomica may be helpful. Opium is used for patients who have no desire to defecate and who, when they do go, pass small, hard, dry pellets. If the passage of small, hard, dry stools is associated with great effort, pain, and burning, especially if the patient also has piles or a distended abdomen, sulphur may be prescribed. If constipation is linked with a great deal of flatulence, lycopodium may be suitable. Other remedies may also be appropriate in individual cases.

Nutrition

Figs, licorice, prunes, raw spinach, strawberries, and honey all have gentle laxative properties. A high-fiber diet will be recommended, consisting of plenty of fruit, vegetables, and whole-grain products, and a minimum of refined carbohydrates. Unsalted peanut kernels (eaten with their brown fiber coating) are a pleasant way of taking additional fiber.

Vitamin C has a laxative action in high doses and a deficiency of vitamin B_5 (pantothenic acid) may cause constipation, so supplements may be prescribed.

DEPRESSION

DEFINITION

It is only in the 1900s that psychiatry has become a medical specialty in its own right and that diseases such as depression have been recognized as having a physical basis. Older textbooks say that depression can be divided into two main groups—endogenous (arising "from within") or reactive (resulting from a particular stress or event)—whose symptoms differ from each other. However, in many cases, the symptoms of both endogenous and reactive depression can be found together and most specialists now agree that symptoms vary only according to the severity of the attack and not according to its cause.

What has been called reactive depression is now also called minor depression or depressive neurosis, while endogenous depression is also known as major depression or depressive psychosis. Neurosis and psychosis are two commonly used terms in the field of mental illness. Both may be defined simply as types of mental disorder, the difference between them being that psychotic patients lose touch with reality to a greater or lesser extent, suffering, for example, from delusions or hallucinations, whereas neurotic patients retain contact with reality and have some insight into their condition.

The other end of the scale from depressive psychosis is mania, a state in which there is a very marked elevation of mood and the patient becomes overactive, uninhibited and, even in the face of disaster, inappropriately high-spirited. Manic patients may go out on spending sprees or behave extravagantly in other ways. In manic depressive psychosis, which in some cases may be an inherited condition, patients tend to swing between depression and mania. Patients who never experience mania are said to have *unipolar* depression, whereas manic depressive psychosis is described as *bipolar*.

Depression is very common. About 12 percent of all men and eighteen percent of all women will suffer from major depression at some time during their lives. Many more suffer from minor degrees, perhaps as many as one out of every four individuals. Ninety percent of all cases are unipolar and tend to start in early middle age. Only 10 percent suffer from manic depressive psychosis, which tends to begin in the teens, twenties, or thirties. Some patients will only ever suffer from one attack, but others have recurrences. Suicide causes about 15 percent of all deaths in unintended mood disorders.

Most patients recover fully from their first attack of depression but may later relapse. Eventually 43 percent of all cases develop persistent symptoms and, of these patients, up to a third may spend long periods in the hospital.

No one knows exactly what causes depression, although it would appear to be a malfunction of certain chemicals, known as neurotransmitters, which are responsible for carrying electrical impulses between the millions of cells that make up the brain. It is these electrical impulses that are translated into thoughts and actions by the body. Some of the drugs used in the treatment of depression are known to affect the neurotransmitters in various ways.

In 1988 doctors interested in the effect of diet on depression reported the results of vitamin assays that had been carried out over the course of twelve years on patients admitted to the psychiatric unit at Northwick Park Hospital in Middlesex, Great Britain. They found that those with depression tended to have a deficiency of riboflavin (B_2), pyridoxine (B_6), and folic acid. In some cases the depression seemed to stem from the deficiency whereas in others the deficiency seemed to result from the reduction in appetite that occurred as part of the illness.

SYMPTOMS

In most cases the overwhelming symptom is a feeling of depression, which may be described in physical terms—for example, as a great weight pressing down on the shoulders. The world seems gray and the patient becomes incapable of feeling any normal emotion.

In severe cases, patients may develop inappropriate feelings of guilt, may believe that they are being persecuted, or may become convinced that they are suffering from some appalling physical disease. They feel unworthy and reproach themselves for all that they have done in the past. They are absent-minded, are unable to concentrate or to remember things, and they tend to speak slowly and monotonously. They become very pessimistic and may have recurrent thoughts about suicide or death. A psychotic patient may hear voices telling her how unworthy she is and urging her to kill herself.

Physical symptoms of depression include sleep problems (commonly waking early in the morning or sleeping too much), an increase or decrease in appetite and subsequent gain or loss of weight, constipation, loss of interest in sex, fatigue, and lack of energy. Sometimes, however, anxiety is a major symptom, in which case the patient may be agitated and restless. Some patients, while quite willing to speak to a doctor or to relatives about their physical symptoms, are loath to mention the associated mental symptoms and occasionally physical symptoms may occur without any associated change in mood.

TRADITIONAL TREATMENT

There are three methods of traditional treatment that can be used separately or together. Psychotherapy is of most value in the treatment of less severe forms of depression. Drug treatment can be useful in severe depression and mania, as well as in less serious cases. Finally, physical treatment—electroconvulsive therapy (ECT)—is reserved for the most severe cases.

Depending on the severity of the symptoms, patients may need to be admitted to the hospital or may be treatable as an outpatient by the family physician or psychiatrist.

Psychotherapy

Supportive psychotherapy, consisting of sympathy, reassurance, and explanation about the illness, may be all that some patients need. Cognitive psychotherapy is a more active treatment based on the fact that depressed patients tend to develop negative attitudes very readily. The patient is shown how to overcome these attitudes that are likely to prolong the depression. She is helped to look objectively at her ideas and feelings about herself and the world around her and to assess whether she is seeing things in their true light. She is also encouraged to start doing things that she used to do before she became ill. This treatment requires about one hour a week for an indefinite time period.

Drugs

Antidepressant drugs can be broken down into three main groups—tricyclics or heterocyclics and related drugs, monoamine oxidase inhibitors (MAOIs), and other, newer drugs. None of these drugs is a tranquilizer, like Valium, and none is addictive. It is important that at the start of treatment both patient and doctor persevere with the chosen drug for several weeks even if it seems to be ineffective. Sometimes the patient may start to sleep better (a good sign that the drug is working) some weeks before she begins to feel any improvement in herself. Once an antidepressant has started to work, it usually needs to be taken for several months and it is recommended that a patient with moderate or severe depression should continue to take her medication for at least four months after she has fully recovered in order to avoid risking a relapse. Someone who has recurrent depression may need to take drugs for several years. When treatment is completed, the antidepressant must be halted gradually since stopping suddenly may also precipitate a relapse.

TRICYCLICS (HETEROCYCLICS)

The tricyclic drugs include imipramine and amitriptyline (the two most commonly used), nortriptyline, doxepin, and trazodone. Although very effective, particularly in cases where the patient has noticeable physical symptoms, they do have drawbacks. Not only may they take two weeks before they start to work, but the full effect may take up to six weeks. Side effects include drowsiness, a dry mouth, constipation, trembling, blurred vision and weight gain. Tricyclics can also cause abnormalities in the heart's rhythm or an abnormally fast heart rate.

Because the mechanics of depression are not fully understood, the way in which antidepressants work can only be suggested. However, it is known that the tricyclic antidepressants reinforce the action of the neurotransmitters noradrenaline and serotonin.

MONOAMINE OXIDASE INHIBITORS (MAOIs)

Monoamine oxidase is an enzyme (a substance that speeds a chemical reaction within the body) whose function is to break down certain neurotransmitters (noradrenaline, dopamine, and 5-hydroxytryptamine). By inhibiting its action, MAOIs allow the neurotransmitters a longer life span so that they can be more active.

The MAOIs are very effective in the treatment of depression but have a major drawback, in that the patient has to restrict her diet in order to avoid two chemically active substances—dopamine (which is found in broad beans) and tyramine (which is found in cheese, pickled herrings, yeast or meat extracts, some beers and red wines, and any food such as game that has undergone partial decomposition). Both tyramine and dopamine are normally broken down in the wall of the intestine by monoamine oxidases. If, under the influence of MAOIs, they are not broken down but are absorbed unchanged into the bloodstream, they can cause the blood pressure to rise suddenly and dramatically, causing at best a severe headache and at worst a stroke. Some over-the-counter cough and cold medicines also contain substances that may do this and so must be avoided by the patient on MAOIs.

This class of antidepressants has the advantage of starting to work within 24–48 hours and, if the restricted diet is followed, has few side effects.

OTHER DRUGS

In recent years a number of new drugs have emerged that are unrelated to either tricyclics or MAOIs. One of these is flupenthixol, a medication used in the treatment of schizophrenia but that is very effective in considerably lower doses in the treatment of depression when it is associated with anxiety.

L-tryptophan is an amino acid and therefore a natural constituent of the diet. Given in tablet form, it has been found to enhance the action of antidepressants. The main side effects are nausea and drowsiness.

Lithium carbonate is a drug that has been in use for many years in the treatment of manic depression, where long-term medication seems to prevent the patient from relapsing. It is also useful in the prevention of recurrent unipolar depression. Patients who have failed to respond to tricyclics sometimes improve dramatically within two weeks when lithium is given in addition. However, because it can be toxic in overdose, blood tests must be taken every few months to ensure that just the right amount is being absorbed. Side effects include thirst, trembling, weight gain, diarrhea, nausea, swelling of the face, hands, and feet, and hypothyroidism; overdosage causes confusion and staggering. For manic depressive patients who do not respond to lithium, carbamazepine (a drug used in the treatment of epilepsy) has recently been found helpful in preventing severe mood swings.

The newest drug on the market is fluoxetine (Prozac). It is an antidepressant for oral administration and is chemically unrelated to tricyclic, tetracyclic, or other available antidepressants. Fluoxetine works by selectively blocking one neurotransmitter, serotonin, and thus it produces fewer side effects. Many are claiming this to be a "miracle" drug in treating major depression and manic depression. However, side effects have been reported, with some being very severe. They include nausea, nervousness, insomnia, body rash, chills, anxiety, tremor, and sexual problems.

Physical Treatment

ECT is the treatment of first choice for any patient in whom an immediate improvement of mood is essential—for example, one who is seriously contemplating suicide or one who is refusing to eat or drink. It is also used for patients who have failed to respond to drug therapy and can be extremely effective when depression is associated with severe anxiety. It works rapidly and has remarkably few side effects, although some patients complain of problems with memory for a short period after the treatment. The patient is anesthetized and is given a muscle relaxant, then an electric current of about 80 volts is passed, for a fraction of a second, between two electrodes placed on either side of the head. How ECT works is unclear, but results are sometimes quite dramatic.

Psychosurgery is rarely used, and then only for patients whose illness is severely disabling and who have failed to respond to all other forms of treatment. A minute portion of the brain is destroyed, resulting in a marked improvement in mental condition in over 50 percent of cases. This technique has now become highly skilled so that those patients who do not benefit from it rarely end up any worse.

POSTPARTUM DEPRESSION

Like depression that occurs at other times, depression occurring after childbirth can be mild or severe, neurotic or psychotic. Sixty percent or more of women become weepy and irritable two or three days after the birth of a child, but this usually resolves in a matter of days; 10–20 percent develop a mild depression during the first year of their baby's life, usually recovering after a few months. This is often associated with additional stresses such as financial problems, poor family relationships, or being a single-parent family. Support and help from the doctor and other professionals is usually all that is needed and medication is best avoided.

Five percent of mothers develop severe depression during the first three months after the birth. Symptoms usually begin in the first two weeks and gradually get worse. The patient often feels guilty and worthless and worries about her fitness as a mother and about the health and safety of her baby. She may think that her child is ill or deformed in some way or may believe that it is evil, leading her to try to kill it. There is also a danger that she may try to commit suicide. Often a mother says that she is unable to feel love for her baby, although she handles the baby in an obviously loving and caring way. If untreated, some two thirds of patients get better in about six months, but the rest may continue to have symptoms for a further six months or more.

Many psychiatric units now have facilities for mothers and babies to be admitted together and often this is the best course. The most severe cases may need to be treated with ECT, to which the response is generally very good. Less seriously ill patients can be given tricyclic antidepressants, on which they usually start to recover within two weeks, feeling fully well again after about six weeks. However, treatment must be continued for at least six months to avoid a relapse.

Postpartum psychosis occurs in one of every 500 or so births. The patient usually becomes ill during the first two weeks after the birth. The initial symptoms are confusion, fear, distress, restlessness, and insomnia, followed by hallucinations and delusions. Then the condition will resolve into a severe depression, mania, or a schizophrenia-like illness. Fears about the baby are very common—that it has died or is about to, or that another baby has been substituted. One third of these patients have relatives who have suffered from manic depression or schizophrenia.

Treatment of postpartum psychosis involves admission to the hospital where the patient is given a phenothiazine drug (such as is used to treat schizophrenia) to reduce her fear, delusions, and any hallucinations that may occur. ECT is usually the treatment of choice, since it works so quickly, although antidepressant drugs may be used. Unfortunately, the use of drugs usually means that the mother cannot breast-feed.

Most women recover rapidly (mania normally resolving within two weeks, depression within six weeks, and schizophrenia-like conditions within eight weeks). However, because there is the risk of relapse, patients need to continue to take a reduced dose of a phenothiazine drug until the baby is about three months old. Lithium is useful for patients who suffer from mania, but may have to be taken for a year or more.

One third of patients who have a previous history of a major psychiatric illness and one fifth of those whose only mental problems have occurred as the result of a previous pregnancy will have another attack after the birth of their next child. This second attack is usually of the same type as the first and is likely to last as long and respond to treatment in the same way. Sometimes lithium started immediately after the birth may prevent a recurrence of postpartum psychosis in a susceptible patient.

Why some women and not others should suffer from postpartum depression is unknown. It used to be thought that it had to do with the hormonal changes that occur at the time of delivery, but affected women have hormone levels that are no different from those in patients who are unaffected. It seems probable that some people are just more susceptible to depression than others, and that an attack may be triggered by any major life event, of which childbirth is one.

COMPLEMENTARY TREATMENT

Acupuncture
The mind and spirit are, in traditional Chinese theory, aspects of the energy of the heart. Treatment of mental problems involves the use of points that will restore the normal flow of energy to the heart and will calm and strengthen the mind and the spirit.

Aromatherapy
Basil, clary sage, jasmine, rose, and chamomile are among the essences that may be beneficial.

Bach Flower Remedies

Cherry plum may help patients who feel desperate and are afraid of going mad, as well as those who are suicidal. Sweet chestnut may be useful for those who suffer from despair and are extremely negative in their feelings.

Mustard is helpful in the treatment of depression that has developed for no apparent reason.

Olive may be beneficial in postpartum depression since it is for those suffering from mental and physical exhaustion.

Herbalism

Certain herbs are known as nervous restoratives that slowly and steadily improve nervous and mental conditions. They include wild oat, St. John's wort, vervain, scullcap, and lady's slipper. As in the case of traditional treatment, it may be weeks or months before the patient recovers fully.

Homeopathy

Any number of remedies may be appropriate, depending on the individual patient. Aurum may help someone who is suicidal.

Hypnotherapy

In most cases, hypnotherapy is *not* effective in the treatment of depression. In addition, there is a risk that it may lower the patient's mood still further by removing any associated anxiety, which acts as a positive, active factor against the negative, passive depression. Patients who wish to try complementary treatment for depression, therefore, should choose one of the other therapies.

Nutrition

Dr. Carl Pfeiffer of the Brain Bio Center in Princeton, New Jersey, classifies most psychoses into histadelia and histapenia, where the function of the nervous system is impaired, respectively, by excessive or inadequate amounts of histamine. Suicidal depression, blank mind, obsessions, and phobias seem to be associated with histadelia. Such patients also tend to have low pain thresholds, few fillings in their teeth (thanks to a good flow of saliva), frequent headaches, and allergies. Supplements of calcium, zinc, manganese, and the amino acid methionine help to bring down the histamine levels and thus relieve the patient's symptoms.

Postpartum depression may be associated with the rise in copper levels that occurs during pregnancy, because the raised levels of estrogen increase its rate of absorption from the intestines. Copper levels can be lowered by taking supplements of vitamins C, E, and A, and zinc, and by eating apples, which contain pectin. Patients who have postpartum depression should not have copper IUDs (intrauterine devices) fitted, as this may delay recovery. Vitamin B_6 may be helpful but should always be taken together with zinc.

Various amino acids may be beneficial in the treatment of depression. They include phenylalanine, tryptophan (which should be taken with vitamin B_3), and tyrosine. However, neither phenylalanine nor tryptophan should be taken by patients who are taking MAOIs, tryptophan should not be taken before or during pregnancy, and tyrosine should be avoided by anyone who has suffered from a melanoma (a type of skin cancer).

ORGANIZATIONS

Depressives Anonymous: Recovery from Depression
329 East 62nd Street
New York, NY 10021
212/689-2600
(Publishes a newsletter and educational material.)

National Depressive and Manic Depressive Association
Merchandise Mart
Box 3395
Chicago, IL 60654
312/993-0066
(Publishes a bimonthly newsletter and educational material.)

DIABETES

DEFINITION AND INCIDENCE

Diabetes is a condition in which the body's use of carbohydrates is disturbed. Carbohydrates—made up of starches and sugars—are a vital energy source and without them the body cannot function. But in order for dietary carbohydrates to be used by the body tissues, they have to be broken down in the small intestine into glucose, which is then absorbed into the bloodstream. From the blood, under the influence of insulin, the glucose enters all the cells of the body, where it is broken down still further to provide energy. Normally, insulin is secreted by one section of the pancreas—the beta cells—whenever carbohydrates are eaten. Diabetes can be due to a failure of the pancreas to produce this hormone or a failure of the body cells to respond to it in the normal way.

Diabetes is therefore divided into two classes known either as type I and type II, or as insulin-dependent diabetes mellitus (IDDM) and non-insulin-dependent diabetes mellitus (NIDDM), or as juvenile onset and maturity onset. The last of these descriptions has rather dropped out of favor since, although most cases of type I or IDDM occur in young patients and type II or NIDDM in older patients, IDDM can occur at any age and NIDDM can occur in young people.

In IDDM, the patient's pancreas does not function normally and he has to have regular injections of insulin. In NIDDM, the patient continues to produce some insulin and the condition can be controlled by dietary measures or by tablets.

It is estimated that there are some 200 million diabetics in the world of whom three quarters have NIDDM and are middle-age or elderly. In the United States, diabetes affects about 2.4 percent of the population, well over half of whom are overweight, but another 3 percent may be borderline and not know it. Obesity is considered to be a very important risk factor in the development of NIDDM, and during both

137

World Wars, when there was food rationing, the incidence of this type of diabetes fell.

Diabetes seems to run in families and, although it is not inherited as such, it is suggested that patients inherit a susceptibility to it, the disease itself being triggered by other factors such as obesity, pregnancy, surgery, or infection. If one identical twin develops NIDDM when over the age of forty-five, then the other one is likely to as well. In young patients, it is thought that IDDM may be an autoimmune disease in which the immune system attacks the body as it would an invasion by bacteria or viruses. Possibly, an inherited susceptibility allows a viral infection somehow to trigger the body's destruction of the pancreatic beta cells.

Although IDDM tends to develop at an earlier age than NIDDM, it is quite uncommon in the very young, affecting only one child per thousand in the under-sixteen age group. Most cases of NIDDM begin when the patient is in his sixties or older but, in Asians, in whom the disease is four times more common than in Caucasians, the onset is more often between the ages of thirty and sixty.

INSULIN-DEPENDENT DIABETES MELLITUS

The onset of symptoms is often quite sudden, with the patient complaining of excessive thirst and weight loss and passing large amounts of urine. In some cases, however, he may just feel increasingly weak and tired and the weight loss and thirst may be only slight. Occasionally, in children, the illness may start with a chest infection that seems to go on for a very long time, or the first symptom may be constipation due to increasing loss of water from the body through an excessive output of urine. If glucose builds up in the bloodstream, the body will begin to burn fat. Ketones, acidic chemical compounds smelling of acetone, are formed from fat breakdown. The effect of ketones on the body is dramatic and, if the condition is untreated, the patient can start to vomit, develop severe abdominal pain, and kidney failure and, ultimately, will lapse into coma and die. Occasionally, vomiting and abdominal pain may be the first signs of diabetes in a child who previously appeared healthy.

Sometimes the symptoms may come and go for a period of days or weeks before they become constant and, in up to a third of young diabetics, may disappear completely, usually within three months of the first signs of the disease. Unfortunately, this remission is short-lived, sometimes lasting only days but occasionally up to a year. During this period, the patient needs no insulin and may appear to be perfectly healthy.

NON-INSULIN-DEPENDENT DIABETES MELLITUS

Patients who develop this type of diabetes are usually middle-age or older and overweight. The condition may be asymptomatic at first and may only be diagnosed through a routine urine or blood test. Such patients often go on to develop symptoms unless their diet is controlled. First symptoms in NIDDM may include weakness, especially in the elderly, unexplained weight loss, skin problems such as ulcers on the feet or boils, itching of the vulva, visual problems such as the development of cataracts, or numbness, tingling, or pain in the feet and hands.

Although, by definition, NIDDM patients can have their disease controlled by tablets or diet, occasionally an infection or other illness (such as a heart attack) can make their diabetes harder to control and necessitate their having insulin injections. Sometimes this is only a temporary condition, the patient being able to revert to oral medication in due course.

COMPLICATIONS OF DIABETES

Until the discovery of insulin in the 1920s, type I diabetes was a rapidly fatal disease. Nowadays, patients can live long and active lives. However, as they live longer, it has become apparent that, even though their blood sugar levels are controlled by injections of insulin, complications can occur. These are probably more common in those patients (known as "brittle diabetics") who have difficulty in keeping their blood sugar to normal levels, so doctors put great emphasis on maintaining as good a control as possible. There are seven important conditions that the diabetic patient risks developing. These are excess sugar in the blood (hyperglycemia), excess insulin or inadequate sugar in the blood (hypoglycemia), and problems affecting the heart and circulatory system, the nervous system (neuropathy), the feet, the eyes (retinopathy), and the kidneys (nephropathy). The complications that affect individual parts of the body will be dealt with first.

Conditions Affecting the Circulatory System

Atherosclerotic occlusion of the coronary arteries that supply the heart causes angina and heart attacks and is twice as common in diabetics as in nondiabetics. It affects both men and women equally. The arteries supplying the legs may also become involved, causing poor circulation and resulting in intermittent claudication (inability to walk very far because of pain in the legs due to lack of blood), chronic ulcers and, occasionally, gangrene.

Neuropathy

Around 40–60 percent of diabetics have a mild neuropathy, while 5–10 percent have severe symptoms. For 50 percent of patients with NIDDM, the first symptoms they experience are those of neuropathy, pain in the feet being particularly common. Other symptoms may include numbness, tingling, weakness, paralysis, and shaking muscles. The nerves that supply the digestive system may be involved, so that the stomach takes longer than normal to empty, the gallbladder stops functioning normally, or the patient suffers from diarrhea, particularly at night, this often alternating with periods of constipation. Involvement of other body systems may result in impotence or problems with ejaculation, low blood pressure upon lying down (causing dizziness), damaged and swollen but painless joints, and inability to empty the bladder. The commonest form of neuropathy consists of a slight numbness and tingling in the toes and feet and, less often, the fingers, affecting both sides equally and sometimes associated with aching or shooting pains in the feet and legs, especially at night.

One form of neuropathy, in which the patient develops pain and weakness in the legs but no loss of sensation, may progress for weeks or even months before recovering, sometimes completely.

Conditions Affecting the Feet

Normally an injury to the foot is painful, but in patients suffering from diabetic neuropathy sensation is dulled and minor injuries may go unnoticed. Areas with poor circulation heal poorly and, if left unattended, such injuries may develop into ulcers or become gangrenous. However, an ulcer affecting a patient who has circulatory problems but no neuropathy may be very painful.

It is the older male diabetic who is particularly at risk of developing foot ulcers. Ultimately, a gangrenous ulcer may mean amputation, but some specialists believe that 50 percent or more of amputations in diabetics could be avoided if patients followed simple guidelines on foot care (see preventive measures) and visited a podiatrist regularly.

Retinopathy

Of those patients who have been diabetic for thirty years, 10 percent will have lost their sight as a result of retinopathy. This condition affects most patients to a greater or lesser extent in the long term, but fortunately only in a small proportion does it cause total blindness.

The initial abnormality is in the tiny blood vessels that supply the light-sensitive retina at the back of the eye. These become swollen and ultimately leak, producing hemorrhages within the retina itself. As well as blood, fluid that is rich in fats and protein leaks out, forming little patches known as exudates. These may impair vision by preventing light from reaching the retina. In addition, new blood vessels tend to form across the retina. These are often fragile and bleed easily, resulting in the formation of fibrous tissue around them. This, too, obscures the vision and may ultimately pull the retina away from its moorings (retinal detachment) so that the sight is suddenly lost in one eye. Sometimes the earliest symptom of retinopathy is abnormality of color vision. When total blindness occurs it is usually due to retinal detachment, often as the result of a sudden massive hemorrhage into the eye. However, loss of vision rarely happens rapidly and in most cases is a slowly progressive process. Diabetic patients also have a higher than average risk of developing cataracts (opacities in the lens at the front of the eye).

Nephropathy

The function of the kidneys is to extract waste products and excess water from the bloodstream so that they can be expelled from the body as urine. This is carried out by a tiny system of tubes and blood vessels known as a nephron, of which there are about a million in each kidney. One of the most important structures in the nephron is a group of blood vessels known as the glomerular tuft. For some reason, in diabetes a structureless material is laid down at the edge of the glomerular tuft, interfering with its function. When enough of the tufts have been affected, kidney failure results. Some 40 percent of IDDM patients have some degree of kidney failure and, of these, about half are severe enough to need to go on a kidney machine or to have a transplant in order to survive.

The interference with kidney function can also cause high blood pressure (see separate section) and puffy swelling of the body tissues (especially the legs). The urine of most affected patients contains protein. However, not all diabetics with protein in their urine go on to develop renal failure, which is commoner in IDDM than in NIDDM.

Patients who develop nephropathy are usually middle-age or older and have had diabetes for at least ten years. Frequently, other complications have already occurred, notably retinopathy and problems with the circulatory system. Women are more often affected than men.

Hyperglycemia

If a patient with IDDM fails to take insulin regularly, he will become hyperglycemic, develop ketoacidosis (ketones in the blood), as described above, and lapse into coma. Such a coma (termed ketoacidotic, hyperglycemic, or diabetic) may take hours or days to develop and during this time the patient will be thirsty and pass a lot of urine; he may vomit and have abdominal pain and his breathing will become heavy and labored, his breath smelling strongly of acetone. Untreated, he will die. However, some patients whose diabetes is hard to control may have a mild degree of hyperglycemia from time to time without becoming ketoacidotic. This may make them more susceptible to infections and to ulceration of the feet.

Patients with NIDDM rarely develop ketoacidosis since they are usually able to produce some insulin of their own.

Hyperglycemia sometimes occurs when patients develop an infection (which may increase the need for insulin) and think that because they are eating very little they have to omit their injections.

Hypoglycemia

Too much insulin and too little glucose in the blood can also cause coma, which may come on very much more rapidly than a ketoacidotic coma. Usually when patients are newly diagnosed as having IDDM, they are allowed to go slightly "hypo" in order to know how it feels. They are then instructed that if ever they are aware of such symptoms arising—weakness, hunger, nausea, sweating, and trembling—they must take steps to treat them immediately by eating some rapidly absorbable carbohydrate, for example, a piece of hard candy or a piece of chocolate.

Hypoglycemia may occur if the patient accidentally gives himself too much insulin or injects it into a vein instead of muscle, or if he misses a meal or does a lot of exercise to which he is unaccustomed.

Other symptoms of hypoglycemia include mental confusion and abnormal behavior, such as aggressiveness or emotional instability. Because the speech is often slurred, such patients may appear to be drunk. The wearing of a Medic Alert bracelet proclaiming him to be diabetic will avoid the potential tragedy of a hypoglycemic patient being arrested for drunkenness and, later, being found in a coma in a police cell.

During a hypoglycemic coma a patient may have convulsions, so there is a risk that even if he recovers following treatment brain damage may have occurred.

TESTS

Diabetes is usually easily diagnosed by a glucose tolerance test. In this, the fasting patient has blood taken, then has a drink containing a measured amount of glucose. Further samples of blood are taken at half-hour intervals until two hours have elapsed. The results will enable the patient with diabetes to be distinguished from someone who has a low renal threshold—a condition in which the kidneys allow some sugar to pass into the urine, although the patient is perfectly healthy.

All patients who develop diabetic symptoms will have their eyes examined, since many middle-age diabetics have already developed a degree of retinopathy by the time symptoms appear.

Because the onset of diabetes may be precipitated by an infection, it is usual to do a chest X-ray and to send a urine specimen for culture when the condition is first diagnosed.

When complications occur, special investigations may be necessary to determine the extent of the problem. For example, ultrasound may be used to investigate the kidneys in nephropathy, and blood tests and twenty-four-hour urine collections may be taken to assess how well the kidneys are functioning. For patients with retinopathy, a fluorescein angiogram may be necessary—a fluorescent dye is injected into a vein in the arm and is photographed as it travels through the blood vessels in the back of the eye. The investigations described in the section on ischemic heart disease may be appropriate for diabetic patients whose heart and blood vessels are affected.

TRADITIONAL TREATMENT

Insulin-Dependent Diabetes Mellitus (IDDM)

Patients with IDDM will need regular injections of insulin for the rest of their lives. These are given at least twice a day. Either a base level of insulin is provided by a very slow-acting preparation while a more rapidly acting type (known as regular insulin) is used to coincide with the patient's main meals, or a mixture of a moderately slow-acting preparation and regular insulin is given twenty minutes before breakfast and again before the evening meal.

It is very important that the patient should regulate his diet, avoiding sugars, which are rapidly absorbed into the bloodstream. Although about half his calorie intake should be taken as carbohydrates, these should be in the form of starchy foods, preferably unrefined, such as whole-grain breads, high-fiber cereals, and fruit and root vegetables, because these are slowly digested and absorbed. A high level of fiber in the diet may make the diabetes easier to control. Regular meals are very important. Overweight patients should not drink alcohol, which is very fattening, but others can usually have an occasional drink, although they should avoid sweet sherries, liqueurs, and mixers that have sugar in them. Obese patients should also reduce their calorie intake, since diabetes is much easier to control in those who are not overweight.

Any patient who has ketoacidosis requires urgent hospital admission. Treatment consists of fluid given through an intravenous drip to replace that which has been lost, insulin injections, and treatment of any infection that may have precipitated the onset of the condition.

Occasionally, patients who are on insulin react to it, developing painful, red, itching bumps at the injection site that last about thirty-six hours before disappearing. Usually this can be cured by changing to a different brand or type of insulin, but rarely desensitization may be necessary.

Insulin can also cause fat to break down in the area into which it is injected and may therefore produce unsightly hollows in the skin. Most cases occur in women and children, men rarely being affected. However, patients can be taught to inject into their lower abdomen or buttocks where the fat loss will not be seen, or where it may even be welcome.

Non-Insulin-Dependent Diabetes Mellitus (NIDDM)

Many patients with NIDDM can control their diabetes simply by following a suitable diet, similar to that outlined above for IDDM Those who are overweight will also need to go on a reducing diet, since obesity makes diabetes harder to control.

Various types of oral medications are available for those patients who, despite dietary control, continue to have glucose in their urine. The drugs mainly used are the sulphonylureas. They include tolbutamide, glipizide, glyburide, acethohexamide, chlorpropamide, and tolazamide, which are the most frequently used. They act by stimulating the secretion of insulin by the underfunctioning pancreatic cells. Chlorpropamide and glibenclamide may cause hypoglycemia in thin patients, who should always have some food available with which to relieve the symptoms and who should report any such occurrences to their GPs. In a few patients, the sulphonylureas may cause weight gain. In those cases where diabetes is due to a reduced output of insulin by the pancreas, a sulphonylurea is likely to be most helpful.

Treatment of Complications

Renal failure that results from diabetic nephropathy may need treatment on a kidney machine or a transplant.

Infection or ulcers on the feet need urgent and vigorous treatment to try to prevent them from progressing to gangrene. This includes the use of antibiotics and frequent cleansing of the affected area, with removal of any dead tissue.

Gangrene in the foot may require amputation. The level of the amputation will depend on the severity of the arterial disease. The surgeon will wish to remove all the tissue that has an inadequate circulation and in which there is the possibility of gangrene recurring. This may mean, for example, that the amputation is performed at knee level, even though the gangrenous area appears to be confined to the foot.

In recent years, the laser has proved useful in the treatment of progressive diabetic retinopathy. By sealing off the leaking retinal vessels (a technique known as photocoagulation) it can reduce the risk of visual loss by about 50 percent. If cataracts develop in the lens, these can be removed surgically and the sight can be corrected with glasses.

It is sometimes difficult to distinguish between a hypoglycemic and a ketoacidotic (hyperglycemic) coma, but the differentiation is vital since hypoglycemic patients must be given glucose while those who are ketoacidotic must be given insulin. However, as a first-aid measure, it is safe to administer a small amount of sugar. This is unlikely to do much harm to a ketoacidotic patient and may be life-saving for someone who is hypoglycemic. Insulin, on the other hand, must never be given until it is certain that the coma is ketoacidotic, since it could greatly reduce the hypoglycemic patient's chances of recovery. Normally the ketoacidotic patient is dehydrated (dry), flushed, and breathing heavily, and the breath smells strongly of acetone, whereas the hypoglycemic is usually pale, sweating, and restless with dilated pupils and a fast heart rate. Once the patient has reached the hospital, a blood sugar estimation will confirm the diagnosis. A ketoacidotic coma is treated with insulin, usually given both intravenously and intramuscularly to begin with, plus intravenous fluids, while a hypoglycemic patient is given glucose solution by means of an intravenous drip.

DIABETES IN PREGNANCY

Occasionally, a previously healthy woman may become diabetic during pregnancy. Normally, in such cases, the diabetes disappears once the baby has been born although it may recur many years later. Rarely, it persists once the pregnancy has ended.

For those women who are already diabetic, pregnancy can have an adverse effect, causing a worsening of retinopathy, nephropathy, and neuropathy. Conversely, diabetes may affect the pregnancy, increasing the risks for both the mother and her baby. It is therefore essential that all diabetic women, whether longstanding diabetics or "pregnancy diabetics," ensure that they have adequate prenatal care and that their diabetes remains well controlled throughout the pregnancy in order to minimize the risks and complications.

Maternal problems include an increased risk of premature labor and preeclamptic toxemia (rapidly rising blood pressure toward the end of pregnancy) and an increased likelihood of developing cystitis, thrush, or other infections. For the baby, the risks of congenital malformations, breathing problems, and jaundice are higher.

Babies born to diabetic mothers are often much larger than the average and may therefore cause difficult deliveries. A vivid description of the newborn babies of diabetic mothers was given in "The Child of the Diabetic Woman" by J. W. Farquhar (*Archives of Disease in Childhood*, 1959).

> They resemble one another so closely that they might well be related. They are plump, sleek, full faced. . . . During their first twenty-four or more extra-uterine hours they lie on their backs bloated and flushed . . . their lightly closed hands on each side of the head, the abdomen prominent and their respiration sighing. They convey a distinct impression of having had such a surfeit of both food and fluid pressed upon them by an insistent hostess that they desire only peace so that they may recover from their excesses.

Because of the size of the babies, and because there is a slightly increased risk of stillbirth in the last few weeks of pregnancy, diabetic mothers often have labor induced slightly before they reach full term.

However, although the babies tend to be large at birth, they are also likely to grow very slowly during their first three months in the womb. Recent research in Denmark has shown that those children of diabetic mothers who did, indeed, grow slowly at first had impaired abilities in social skills and the use of language by the time they were four years old, compared with other children who grew normally, whether their mothers were diabetic or not. This is another reason, therefore, why strict control of diabetes is so important during pregnancy.

PREVENTIVE MEASURES

All diabetics must monitor their glucose levels by testing their blood regularly. About three times a year, the NIDDM patient will need to have his blood tested by his doctor. However, the IDDM patient will be taught to test his own blood, since this more accurate assessment of glucose levels is needed in order to calculate the dose of insulin required. Meters are now available that will measure the amount of glucose in a drop of blood placed on a paper test strip. The most recent, at the time of writing, is very small and takes only thirty seconds to give a reading.

As well as checking his blood regularly, it is very important that the diabetic checks his feet frequently so that minor injuries or infections do not go unnoticed. This is especially important for older diabetics, among whom the risks of gangrene are greater. The patient should wash his feet with warm (not hot) water every evening and apply an emollient to soften the skin if it becomes dry. He should put a pad of lamb's wool between toes that overlap in order to stop them from rubbing on each other and should never go barefoot. Patients whose eyesight is poor should never cut their own toenails and all should see a podiatrist if they develop corns or areas of hard skin.

Plastic shoes, which do not allow sweat to evaporate, should be avoided, particularly as, early on in the disease, patients' feet tend to sweat excessively. Absorbent socks or stockings made of wool or cotton should be worn in preference to nylon.

According to doctors at the foot clinic of King's College Hospital, Great Britain, patients are at greatest risk of developing foot problems when they are on vacation, but this risk can be avoided by taking simple precautions. On long journeys, whether by plane, train, or car, the patient should walk around for a few minutes every half hour. This will prevent or minimize swelling in the feet and ankles. New shoes, which may rub the feet, should not be worn on vacation when the patient may be walking more than usual. When sitting in the sun, a good-quality sunscreen should be applied to the feet and legs or they should be kept covered. If the feet become dry, an emollient should be used, especially on the heels; if they become moist, they should be dabbed with rubbing alcohol. The normal routine of not going barefoot and of inspecting the feet every day for swelling, sores, or changes in color should be adhered to and any problems should be reported immediately to a podiatrist or medical doctor.

RECENT ADVANCES

It is possible that within the next few years injections of insulin may be used less and less, as new ways of administering it are developed. The insulin pump, which is about the size of a cigarette pack, delivers a constant amount of insulin into the tissues just below the skin, where it is absorbed into the bloodstream. This is equivalent to the long-acting insulin that has to be injected each morning. And instead of an injection before mealtimes, the patient presses a button on the pump, which then gives him the required dose. However, frequent blood tests are necessary in order to monitor the dosages—at least four a day on at least two days a week. But now specialists are working on a new model that will incorporate a glucose monitor, so that the pump itself will adjust the dose of insulin according to the patient's blood sugar levels.

The reason why insulin has to be injected is because it is digested in the stomach and therefore is destroyed if taken by mouth. However, doctors at the Medical College of Ohio have developed a plastic-coated capsule that will pass intact through the stomach and the small intestine. Upon reaching the large intestine, where there is no longer any risk of digestion, the capsule is broken down by the bacteria that reside there and the insulin is absorbed. At present this method seems to be less efficient than injections, but it is still only on its early stages of development.

However, insulin in the form of a nasal spray, which has been tested in Australia and the United States, may be available soon. It has been found to be very much more convenient than injected insulin since it is absorbed within ten minutes and has disappeared from the bloodstream within an hour, which means that mealtimes don't have to be carefully planned in advance. However, nasal insulin would only replace the mealtime doses and not the morning injection, which gives a long-acting base level. Long-term trials of this method of treatment were to begin in 1987, but the major drawback seems to be its expense. Because only 10 percent of each puff is absorbed, ten times the normal dose has to be given.

The development of another nasal spray was reported in the summer of 1988. This contains glucagon, a hormone that stimulates the breakdown of glycogen (which is stored in liver and muscle) to glucose, which is released into the bloodstream. The glucagon nasal spray was found to revive hypoglycemic patients within about seven minutes and could prove to be a piece of lifesaving first-aid equipment. Unfortunately, at present, it is very expensive to produce and lasts only a short time before deteriorating. However, scientists are looking for ways of making it more stable and more absorbable.

The prevention of diabetes and its complications is occupying many researchers around the world. The pharmaceutical company ICI has developed a drug called ponalrestat that may be able to prevent diabetic neuropathy, retinopathy, and nephropathy by stopping the deposition of certain abnormal substances in the nerves, eyes, and kidneys. At the time of writing, a license has not yet been granted to allow marketing of this drug.

Several specialists have been trying out immunosuppressant drugs on newly diagnosed type I (IDDM) patients, based on the widely held theory that type I (IDDM) is an autoimmune disease in which the patient's immune system attacks his own body—in this case, the pancreas. In Canada and Europe, trials showed that patients who were given cyclosporin lost most of their symptoms, although not reverting completely to normal. However, once the drug was stopped, they all eventually relapsed. Some doctors believe that antibodies to the pancreas can be detected up to thirteen years before the patient actually develops diabetes so that, in the future, it might be possible to screen people and then give immunosuppressive therapy to those who seem to be developing diabetes.

Meanwhile, for those patients who suffer from IDDM, surgical treatment is also beginning to offer a complete recovery. Pancreatic transplants seem to be successful, particularly when given to patients before they develop complications of their disease. At the time of writing over a thousand have been done worldwide. And at the Hospital of the University of Pennsylvania, transplants of just the insulin-secreting beta cells have been performed. This treatment is in its early stages, but it seems that the transplanted cells begin to function in the recipient within forty-eight hours of the operation.

COMPLEMENTARY TREATMENT

Treatment by an herbalist, homeopath, or acupuncturist may reduce the diabetic patient's need for medication, either insulin or tablets, and, for the brittle diabetic, may make the disease easier to control.

Nutrition therapy may also be of value. Insulin is more potent when adequate amounts of the hormonelike glucose tolerance factor (GTF) are produced. Some diabetics who secrete normal amounts of insulin seem to lack GTF, which contains chromium, vitamin B_3 (niacin), and two amino acids. Supplements of chromium and B_3 may be beneficial, together with manganese, which is essential for the correct functioning of the beta cells in the pancreas.

ORGANIZATIONS

American Diabetes Association
National Service Center
P.O. Box 25757
1660 Duke Street
Alexandria, VA 22313
703/549-1500
(Publishes books, journals, and newsletters.)

FURTHER READING

Contact the American Diabetes Association (see above) for recommended reading as well as for their own excellent publications.

Two dietary books that are highly recommended are:

The New Pritikin Program, by Robert Pritikin, published by Simon & Schuster, 1990.

Family Cookbook, Vol. IV: The American Tradition, by The American Diabetes Association and the American Dietetic Association, published by Prentice Hall Press, 1991.

DIVERTICULAR DISEASE

INCIDENCE

Diverticular disease is an extremely common condition of the colon (large bowel) that causes no symptoms at all in 80–90 percent of cases. It occurs in people over the age of forty, men and women being affected equally. At post mortem, it is found in over 50 percent of those over the age of sixty and two thirds of those over seventy. In about 95 percent of cases, it is the lowest part of the colon (the sigmoid) that is affected. (See diagram of the colon on page 263.)

DIVERTICULOSIS

Diverticula, or pouches, in the colon arise at points where the bowel wall is weak and result from increased pressure in the bowel itself, due to overdevelopment of the muscles within its walls. It is thought that a major factor leading to the development of diverticulosis is inadequate roughage in the diet and this seems to be borne out by the fact that it is rare in those parts of the world where people eat a large amount of raw food and that it has been produced experimentally in animals by feeding them a diet low in fiber.

However, when symptoms do occur, they may be very similar to those of irritable bowel syndrome, the commonest being left-sided cramplike abdominal pain associated with diarrhea or constipation. One possible cause is that the diverticula tend to get filled up with fecal material and the pain is due to muscle spasm within the bowel wall as an attempt is made to empty them. Patients who tend to be constipated are more likely to develop symptoms than those who have regular bowel movements.

ACUTE DIVERTICULITIS

If fecal material remains for any time within a diverticulum, infection may occur. This is known as diverticulitis. Symptoms develop suddenly and consist of severe central abdominal pain that moves over to the left, associated with diarrhea, vomiting, and fever. It may be possible to feel a vague mass in the left-hand side of the abdomen, which is due to thickening of the colonic wall. Occasionally, the bowel hemorrhages and the patient passes large amounts of blood. Some patients have only a single attack of acute diverticulitis. Others may have repeated attacks at intervals of months or years, or may develop chronic diverticulitis.

CHRONIC DIVERTICULITIS

Symptoms of chronic diverticulitis may include diarrhea alternating with constipation, gas, indigestion, the passage of bright red blood, mucus or melena (stools that are black and sticky because they contain digested blood), and left-sided abdominal pain that is worse upon movement but is relieved by passing gas. Continual loss of small amounts of blood may lead to anemia. A thickened mass is often felt in the left side of the abdomen.

COMPLICATIONS OF DIVERTICULITIS

The outer surface of the inflamed diverticulum becomes sticky and may adhere to the small bowel, causing an obstruction, past which the bowel contents cannot flow. Obstruction of the large bowel may also occur. In either case, the patient develops severe abdominal pain, constipation, swelling of the abdomen, and vomiting. Partial obstruction may occur in which the symptoms are less severe, with some fecal material getting through.

An inflamed diverticulum may rupture, causing peritonitis or producing a localized abscess. It may also perforate into an adjoining structure producing a fistula, or hole, between the two. The commonest is a vesicocolic fistula (between the bladder and colon). The patient may have symptoms of bladder irritation, such as frequency, and then begin to pass fecal material and gas in the urine. The main danger is that the kidneys will become infected.

Diverticulitis is also the commonest cause of massive bleeding through the rectum.

TESTS

In older patients, it is very important to exclude the presence of cancer, which may occasionally produce the same symptoms as diverticular disease. Therefore, full investigations of the bowel will be performed. The first is a barium enema in which a barium-containing substance (that appears white on an X-ray) is gently pumped up the rectum and a series of X-rays is taken enabling the doctor to see the outline of the large bowel. Sigmoidoscopy is also necessary, in which the colon is inspected through a flexible telescope. Sometimes a tiny piece of tissue is removed through the sigmoidoscope to be examined under a microscope.

Occasionally it is necessary to perform an endoscopy in which a flexible telescope is passed into the stomach and duodenum in order to ensure that hemorrhage is not due to a peptic ulcer.

TRADITIONAL TREATMENT

If the symptoms of diverticular disease are mild, they can be relieved by a high-fiber diet, which keeps things moving within the bowel and thus lowers the pressure and spasm. The amount of fiber is slowly increased over a period of about six weeks. A "bulking agent" which absorbs water in the bowel, swells up, and thus helps the patient to pass large soft stools, may also be helpful. Antispasmodic drugs may be necessary in the short term. These include atropine, belladonna, dicyclomine hydrochloride, hyoscine, and propantheline bromide.

In acute diverticulitis, treatment consists of bed rest, painkillers, antibiotics, and plenty of fluids. Solid food is withheld until the patient feels better. In severe cases, the patient may need admission to the hospital and intravenous fluids. Admission is also necessary if complications supervene. An abscess is treated with antibiotics and in most cases will respond. However, sometimes it is necessary to drain the abscess surgically. Small bowel obstruction due to inflammation may settle on a regime of intravenous fluids and suction through a tube inserted into the stomach through the nose, which keeps the digestive system empty. Large bowel obstruction, however, warrants an emergency operation to relieve the blockage.

Peritonitis is also a surgical emergency and, like obstruction, requires removal of the affected part of the bowel (usually the sigmoid colon) and a colostomy, in which the end of the bowel is brought out through an incision in the abdominal wall. Patients with peritonitis are also given antibiotics. After the inflammation has died down, usually within two months, another operation is performed in which the end of the colon is brought down and attached to the remaining section of the rectum, and the abdominal opening is closed.

A fistula is treated in a similar way, with removal of the affected section of the colon, closure of the fistula, and a temporary colostomy. Surgery is also necessary for partial obstruction, persistent or recurrent bleeding, and, sometimes, for recurrent disabling attacks of diverticulitis. However, none of these cases needs treatment as an emergency.

Hemorrhage, when it occurs, is treated with a blood transfusion and most patients stop bleeding spontaneously. Very occasionally it may be necessary to operate to remove the bleeding section of colon.

COMPLEMENTARY TREATMENT

Herbalism
Slippery elm may be used to reduce inflammation, peppermint to reduce pain, diarrhea, and flatulence, and comfrey to heal any damage in the intestinal wall. Chamomile also has antiinflammatory and antispasmodic properties.

SELF-HELP

Patients with diverticular disease may feel better if they eat a diet that is high in fiber, low in fat, and low in sugar. The fiber prevents constipation and stagnation. Fat slows down the passage of food through the intestine and sugar may result in the production of excessive amounts of gas, so reduction in both of these will relieve some of the symptoms of diverticular disease. It may also be necessary to avoid red meat (which also tends to slow down the passage of food), and alcohol, coffee, and strong tea, which may irritate the lining of the digestive tract.

EAR INFECTIONS

MECHANICS OF THE EAR

The ear is a complex piece of machinery made up of three separate compartments known as the outer, middle, and inner ears. The large flaps of skin and cartilage (gristle) that we refer to as our ears are, in fact, the least important part, since we can no longer move them around, as animals can, to pick up the direction of a sound. The flap, which is called the pinna, and the external auditory canal, which leads from it into the ear proper, make up the external ear. The canal ends at the eardrum, or tympanic membrane, which stretches across, dividing it from the middle ear. Sound causes the membrane to vibrate and these vibrations are transferred to a tiny piece of bone, called the malleus, which is attached to it inside the middle ear. The malleus is the first in a chain of three bones, or ossicles, the others being the incus and the stapes. The vibrations travel down this chain and are transferred by the stapes to the fluid-filled inner ear, which contains a complex mechanism controlling balance (the labyrinth) as well as the nerve endings concerned with hearing. Here the vibrations are picked up by the nerves, which translate them into electrical impulses and relay them to the brain, where they are interpreted into recognizable sounds.

The middle ear also communicates with the mastoid process, a bony section of the skull situated just behind the lower part of the pinna, and, via the eustachian tube, with the throat. The purpose of the eustachian tube is to allow the air pressure on both sides of the eardrum to remain equal. That is why, when the air pressure changes, for example, in a descending plane, one's ears feel uncomfortable, but if one swallows, thus opening the tube and allowing air to pass through, the discomfort is relieved.

Ear infections, known as otitis (from the Greek *otos,* meaning "ear") affect either the outer or middle ears. An infection of the inner ear—known as labyrinthitis—is usually due to a virus and often occurs in

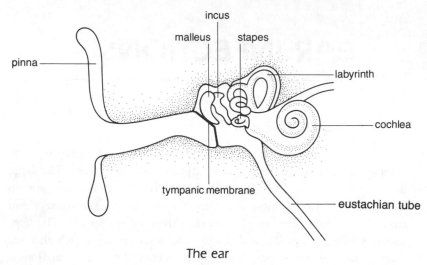

The ear

epidemics. It causes dizziness and vomiting, but normally clears up by itself after about ten days. Bacterial labyrinthitis is rare and is a complication of a middle-ear infection.

OTITIS EXTERNA

This outer-ear infection may be diffuse, involving one or both ears, or may be localized, in the form of a boil in the external canal. A boil in this position causes severe earache that is made worse if the pinna is moved or even touched. The area around the boil becomes red and swollen and this may even extend to the skin behind the ear.

Diffuse otitis externa may be caused by bacteria, fungi, chemical irritants, swimming ("swimmer's ear"), or a generalized skin disorder such as eczema. Sometimes it can be provoked by cleaning out ear wax with an inappropriate instrument (such as a hair pin) that scratches the canal and allows bacteria to enter the skin. The area becomes red, swollen, and very itchy. Pus forms and discharges from the ear and because it blocks the canal the patient often becomes temporarily deaf in that ear.

Tests

Recurrent boils in the ears may be the result of infection from bacteria harbored in the patient's nose. A nose swab will detect any bacteria that may be causing the boils and an antiseptic cream can be used to eliminate them. A blood test may also be taken to test for sugar, since recurrent boils are sometimes the first sign of diabetes.

Traditional Treatment

Patients suffering from boils in the ear are usually given aspirin or acetaminophen to control the pain and an antibiotic (which may be given intramuscularly as an injection) to kill the infection. A small piece of gauze soaked in glycerine and magnesium sulphate paste is put into the ear to draw out the infection. This is changed every day.

The first step in the treatment of diffuse otitis externa is to clean out the external canal. This is done daily until the infection has cleared up. In addition, a piece of gauze soaked in mercurochrome, glycerol, and ichthammol or aluminum acetate may be put in the ear, these preparations all acting to reduce inflammation. Antibiotic steroid drops or creams are normally used; however, these may cause an allergic reaction. Painkillers may be taken if required.

ACUTE OTITIS MEDIA

This is a common complaint in young children, especially during the winter months and among those living in industrial areas. It usually occurs as a result of an infection in the nose or throat. Bacteria may be forced up the eustachian tube if the nose is blown vigorously, infected mucus from the sinuses may flow into the nose and up the eustachian tube, or bacteria may travel up the tube from infected adenoids. Sometimes otitis media follows an attack of measles, scarlet fever, or other infection.

The cells lining the middle ear and the eardrum become inflamed. Pus forms, causing the drum to bulge and then sometimes rupture, which releases the pus into the external canal. With treatment, the drum heals, the inflammation subsides, the eustachian tube opens up again, and the middle ear returns to normal.

The first symptom is usually pain. The child may wake in the middle of the night, screaming. A young baby may just seem unwell without giving any indication of the site of the problem, but may bang his head against the side of the crib or pull at his ear. Usually the patient is feverish and may vomit and have diarrhea. When the drum bursts, there is immediate relief from pain. Sometimes the discharge this causes is the first symptom.

The doctor will look through an instrument (an otoscope) at the patient's eardrum to confirm the diagnosis and, if the drum has burst, may take a swab of the pus.

Traditional Treatment

The external canal is cleaned out daily until there is no longer any discharge. The patient is given aspirin or acetaminophen and antibiotics, which should be taken until the eardrum looks normal again and there is no longer any evidence of deafness in that ear.

Occasionally the infection fails to resolve and it may be necessary to try a different antibiotic or a longer course of treatment.

Sometimes the condition may recur soon after treatment has been stopped or deafness due to mucus or pus in the middle ear may persist. In such cases, a myringotomy may be performed, in which a small incision is made in the eardrum and the fluid is sucked out.

Rapid recurrence may be due to infected adenoids or sinusitis. In such a case, the adenoids may have to be removed or the sinuses washed out.

Complications

Permanent deafness may occasionally follow repeated attacks of otitis media or a single very severe infection. This results from damage to the ossicles, which are no longer able to transmit vibrations to the inner ear. Affected patients will need hearing aids.

Very occasionally, the infection may spread to the mastoid and the area behind the ear becomes inflamed, swollen, and painful. This has to be treated surgically, the bone being opened and the accumulated pus cleaned out.

The facial nerve runs through the middle ear protected by a bony wall in 90 percent of people. However, if someone whose facial nerve is unprotected develops otitis media, there is the chance that the nerve may become temporarily paralyzed. This results in weakness of the muscles on the same side of the face as the infection, but they gradually recover as the otitis media resolves.

Rarely, infection may spread to the inner ear, causing labyrinthitis, with symptoms of dizziness and vomiting.

SECRETORY OTITIS MEDIA (GLUE EAR)

This is a very common cause of deafness in children and one pediatrician has suggested that it may affect up to a third of all children. What causes it is not known, but it may result from a combination of factors such as enlarged adenoids, recurrent respiratory infections, repeated attacks of acute otitis media, or allergies. The mechanism seems to be that the eustachian tubes become blocked so that the air pressure on the two sides of the eardrum can no longer be balanced. Some of the air in the middle ear is absorbed into the surrounding tissues and this creates a vacuum that is resolved by fluid being secreted into the cavity and the eardrum being sucked inward.

Glue ear commonly affects children between the ages of five and eight and usually there are no symptoms other than hearing loss.

Tests

A hearing test is done to assess the loss of hearing and a tuning-fork is used to diagnose the type of deafness from which the child is suffering—this is known as a Rinne test. The tuning fork is placed first in front of the ear and then touching the mastoid behind the ear. If deafness has been caused by the inability of the ossicles or the eardrum to transmit vibrations (as occurs in secretory otitis media) the fork will sound louder when it is on the mastoid than when it is in front of the ear. More formal audiometry (hearing testing) with instruments is commonly done.

The doctor will probably also wish to examine the patient's nose and throat to try to determine whether there is any underlying cause for the condition.

Traditional Treatment

If the patient has enlarged adenoids or sinusitis these will be treated by adenoidectomy or sinus washout. A myringotomy is performed in which the drum is incised and the fluid is sucked out. If the condition recurs, a tiny plastic tube (a grommet) is inserted into a hole in the eardrum for about six months in order to keep the air pressure in the middle ear normal while the eustachian tube recovers its function.

SIMPLE CHRONIC OTITIS MEDIA

If patients have repeated attacks of otitis media, the ossicles and part of the eardrum may eventually be destroyed, resulting in hearing loss. Each time reinfection occurs there will be a discharge, but pain is uncommon unless water gets into the ear.

Tests

When the doctor looks into the ear through an otoscope, he will see a perforation of the eardrum. A hearing test will show the degree of deafness. A normal X-ray of the mastoid looks dark, since the bone is full of little pockets of air, but in a patient suffering from chronic otitis media, the X-ray may appear denser (whiter) than normal as a result of the inflammation.

Traditional Treatment

While the ear is discharging, it needs to be cleaned out daily and a piece of gauze soaked in a mild antiseptic solution should be inserted in the ear. Drops containing a combination of antibiotic and steroid may be prescribed for a period of four weeks or so.

Surgery may be necessary. If hearing loss is slight, the perforation may be repaired. However, if the damage is greater and the hearing loss is more severe, it may be necessary to reconstruct the eardrum and the ossicles. But before an operation can be performed, the patient must have been free of infection for at least three months.

CHRONIC SUPPURATIVE OTITIS MEDIA

If the eustachian tube fails to open properly as it develops during childhood, the air pressure in the middle ear will be constantly lower than that in the external canal. As a result, the softest part of the eardrum can become distorted and form a pouch. Superficial skin cells are constantly dying and being replaced and this same process occurs in the eardrum. However, if there is a pouch in the drum, these dead cells accumulate there, forming a mass known as a cholesteatoma. As this enlarges it presses outward through the bone above the eardrum. Infection then occurs. The cholesteatoma gets larger and destroys the ossicles. It may also erode the bone around the middle ear so that the infection spreads further. As a reaction to the chronic inflammation, a polyp may grow.

The patient has a persistent foul discharge from the ear and if there is a polyp it may bleed. Earache or dizziness may occur, especially if complications set in.

Tests

A hearing test demonstrates that the patient has a hearing loss. An X-ray shows abnormal density in the mastoid bone and sometimes a cavity in the bone surrounding the cholesteatoma, where it has been worn away.

Traditional Treatment

The patient is given a general anesthetic and the cholesteatoma is removed. A mastoid operation is also performed. In a radical mastoid operation (performed if the hearing loss is profound) the damaged remnants of the ossicles are removed together with the eardrum and all the infected tissue within the mastoid. In a modified radical operation (for patients who have been less severely affected) the mastoid is cleaned out, but the ossicles are left intact. After a radical operation, the patient no longer has an outer ear and a middle ear but just one large cavity. He must be seen every week by the ear specialist until the cavity has healed and then every six months to have wax removed from the ear, since a buildup of wax will result in pressure on, and irritation of, the labyrinth, causing dizziness.

Complications

The infection may spread, producing an abscess in the brain or in the layers of membranes that surround it. The patient develops severe headaches and, in the case of a brain abscess, vomiting and drowsiness. The abscess is drained as an emergency operation and the patient is given large doses of antibiotics. When the abscess has resolved, a radical mastoid operation is performed.

Meningitis may also occur. The patient suddenly becomes very ill with a severe headache, vomiting, and fever, and soon lapses into a coma. A lumbar puncture (in which a needle is slipped between two of the bones of the spine and a small amount of fluid is withdrawn from the spinal canal) confirms the diagnosis. Large doses of antibiotics are given as well as intravenous fluids, and a radical mastoid operation is done once the patient is better.

Labyrinthitis is the commonest complication of chronic suppurative otitis media and is due to a spread of the infection into the inner ear. The patient becomes feverish, vomits, and develops severe dizziness or vertigo that is made worse if he moves his head. This, too, warrants emergency hospital admission and treatment with large doses of antibiotics. A radical mastoid operation and removal of the cholesteatoma is performed as soon as possible.

A cholesteatoma may also damage the facial nerve, causing weakness or paralysis of the muscles that it supplies. In such a case, an immediate radical mastoid operation is necessary.

COMPLEMENTARY TREATMENT

Aromatherapy
Lavender essence may help to relieve pain and reduce inflammation in ear infections. Cajuput, chamomile, and other oils may also be used.

Herbalism
Several herbs that are antiinflammatory or antiseptic may be used to treat ear infections. These include chamomile, echinacea, garlic oil, and marigold. Marigold also promotes healing, as does comfrey. Mullein oil can soothe pain in the ear.

Homeopathy
Glue ear may respond very well to treatment with pulsatilla. Hepar sulph. may be prescribed if the pain is sharp and associated with yellow

pus and if the patient wants to be well wrapped up and away from drafts. Aconite is helpful for earache that starts suddenly and is worse at night. Patients who have a throbbing pain in the ear, headache, and pain in the throat and whose skin is hot and dry may find belladonna beneficial. Chamomilla may be prescribed if the pain is stabbing and severe and worse for heat and if the patient is irritable and restless. Sulphur is useful in the treatment of chronic or recurrent infections and merc. sol. is used for patients who have throbbing pain that extends into the teeth, and enlarged glands in the neck. Many other remedies are also available for treating patients with earache.

ECZEMA

DEFINITION

The word *eczema* is derived from the Greek *ekzein,* which means to break out or boil over, and is used to describe a number of conditions in which the skin becomes red, swollen, thickened, or scaly, and may weep, split, or develop blisters. In people with dark skins, the most obvious sign of eczema may be a lightening or darkening of the skin in the affected areas. Eczema is often very itchy and excessive scratching may cause thickening of the skin associated with more pronounced surface markings—a condition known as lichenification. Continual scratching may also cause bleeding into the skin, especially of the legs, although this is uncommon.

Eczema is usually divided into various types, all with similar symptoms but with different causes. These types are exogenous (where the condition is caused by an external agent such as a chemical), endogenous or atopic (the type commonly seen in children), varicose (occurring on the legs, usually in elderly patients whose circulation is poor), seborrheic (a greasy-looking condition that affects the scalp and other hairy areas), nummular (producing small patches, usually in adults), pompholyx (affecting the hands and feet), and diaper dermatitis.

EXOGENOUS ECZEMA

Here the position of the rash will always be related to the causative agent. For example, it may occur under a watch strap (reaction to leather), under jewelry (reaction to metal), or may cover the whole of the hands or the feet if the reaction is to rubber gloves or to shoes. Before the days of tights, "suspender dermatitis" (*suspender* being the British word for "garter") was quite common and was caused by a reaction to nickel, of which most garter belt clips were made. It took the form of small red patches on the thighs where the clips made contact with the skin. Affected women were also likely to have patches of eczema under the metal clips on their bras and were unable to wear nickel jewelry without developing a rash.

Exogenous eczema takes two forms. One is a true allergic reaction whereas the other is purely an irritant reaction in which the chemical in question damages the skin directly (contact dermatitis).

Allergic Contact Eczema

Before an allergic reaction can occur, the causative factor has to be absorbed through the skin, so areas where absorption is easier are more likely to be affected. Such areas include places where the skin is comparatively thin, such as the back of the hands, and where the moisture from sweat increases absorption of foreign substances, such as in the armpits and groins. If contact with the causative agent continues, the rash may later spread to other areas that are not in touch with it—for example, patients with a reaction to nickel often develop eczema around their eyes and in the bend of the elbows. Such a spread may occur days, months, or years after the appearance of the original rash.

The commonest causes of allergic contact eczema are rubber, elastic, metals, dyes, cosmetics, leather, adhesives, and a variety of ointments including those containing anesthetics, antihistamines, antibiotics, antiseptics, or lanolin.

Irritant Contact Dermatitis

Strong irritants may produce a reaction after one or two exposures, but weak irritants require prolonged or repeated exposure. The former include some industrial chemicals and among the latter are household detergents and disinfectants. The resulting rash most commonly appears on the hands; in mild cases it may take the form of redness, dry skin, and scaling; more severely affected patients may have thickening of the skin with painful splits. The palms tend to be affected as well as the backs of the hands.

Diagnosis

Often the diagnosis is obvious from the distribution of the rash and the history given by the patient of contact with an irritant substance.

However, if confirmation of an allergic reaction is necessary or if the diagnosis is uncertain, patch tests can be done. The suspected substances are diluted to a concentration at which they will not act as irritants and are then applied to the skin of the back under specially designed aluminum cups that are taped down with hypoallergenic tape. The cups are left in place for two days, after which time they are removed and the results are inspected. A rash appearing within these two days or up to two days after the cups have been removed suggests that the patient has an allergy to the substance that was applied at that site.

Traditional Treatment

The most important treatment is, wherever possible, to ensure that the patient no longer comes into contact with the substance that has caused the rash. If this is impractical—for example, where the substance forms an integral part of his work—methods must be devised to prevent it from touching the skin. This usually means that the patient must wear some form of protective clothing. For those who have developed a rash on the hands from repeated contact with detergents, the answer is usually to wear rubber gloves, with a pair of cotton gloves inside them or cotton-lined rubber gloves to prevent the skin from reacting to the rubber.

The use of soap on the skin should be avoided and an emollient soap substitute should be used instead. If the hands or feet are affected with a rash that is weeping or blistered, it is helpful to soak them three or four times a day for about ten minutes in a dilute solution of potassium permanganate. When parts of the body are affected that cannot be soaked, compresses of salt solution may be used instead.

The GP or family doctor may prescribe steroid preparations—a lotion when the rash is still moist, followed by a cream, used three or four times a day, once it has started to dry up. If there is any evidence that the rash has become infected, an antibiotic may be necessary. Antihistamines may be prescribed to control severe itching.

ATOPIC ECZEMA

Atopic eczema is a fairly common condition that affects 3 percent or more of children under five. Although it rarely appears before the age of three months, 80 percent of patients develop symptoms before their first birthday; 90 percent of cases occur before the child reaches the age of five. The condition tends to run in families, together with hay fever and asthma; in cases where one parent has suffered from eczema a child has a 30 percent chance of developing it, but if both parents have been affected the figure rises to 50 percent. Around 30 percent of children with eczema will go on to develop hay fever or asthma.

The rash usually appears first on the face or scalp and spreads to other parts of the body. The commonest sites are the bends of the elbows, behind the knees, the wrists, and the area behind the ears. The skin becomes red and rough, and may blister and weep. It is usually very itchy and this may prevent the child from sleeping at night and distract him from his daytime activities. This can be a particular problem for children of school age, whose work may suffer. Scratching the rash can make it very sore and may introduce infection to the already damaged skin whose susceptibility to both bacterial and viral infections is increased. The herpes virus can produce a particularly severe infection known as Kaposi's varicelliform eruption and it is therefore advisable to keep children with active eczema away from people suffering from cold sores.

The rash may be made worse by excessive bathing, rubbing by clothes (especially wool), a warm dry atmosphere, or stress.

In most cases atopic eczema comes and goes; some patients are affected for only a few years and probably half have outgrown it by the time they reach puberty. The vast majority are free from eczema by the time they reach adulthood but some 2–3 percent continue to suffer from the condition for the rest of their lives.

Traditional Treatment

Emollient preparations may be prescribed that soften the skin and alleviate the dryness associated with eczema.

Acute cases may need steroid creams, but these are not used long term because there are considerable risks of side effects (such as stunting of growth) as a result of the steroid being absorbed into the bloodstream. Very rarely, if the condition becomes extremely widespread and severe, steroids may be given by mouth for a period of not more than two weeks. However, although they may be very effective in treating the acute case, they are not curative but suppressive.

Patches of skin that have become lichenified (thickened) may be treated by wrapping them in bandages impregnated with steroids or with tar and zinc ointment. This is particularly useful for treating the legs.

Antihistamines may be needed to relieve itching, but unfortunately they do not work in all cases. Weeping areas can be treated with potassium permanganate or salt solution soaks, as in the case of exogenous eczema. Wet dressings of lead and zinc lotion may also be helpful.

Recent Advances

A concentrate of evening primrose oil, Efamol, is now available for the treatment of eczema. In one study, over 70 percent of patients were able to reduce their dose of oral steroids, nearly 60 percent reduced their use of topical steroids, and over 70 percent were able to stop taking antihistamines when given Efamol. It was found that patients needed to take it for eight to twelve weeks before an improvement was seen and, after that, had to continue taking it in order to prevent a relapse.

Self-Help

Extremes of temperatures and wool worn next to the skin may make itching worse and should be avoided.

Bathing should be regular, but the patient should not remain in the water for too long, and a soap substitute should be used. After bathing, an emollient should be applied to the skin.

Many young children with eczema seem to be allergic to components of their diet, such as eggs or milk. Excluding eggs from the diet or changing from cow's milk to goat's milk may make a considerable difference. Sometimes a particular type of fruit (such as pineapple) may be responsible.

VARICOSE ECZEMA

Also known as stasis dermatitis, this condition affects the lower part of the leg and tends to occur when the blood from that region is not returned efficiently to the heart. Blood travels to the body tissues through the arteries, which have elastic walls to help potentiate the pumping action of the heart. (This can be felt, in arteries that run close to the body surface, as a pulse.) However, once the blood has been through the tissues, it is collected into veins that are not elastic and whose job it is to carry it back to the heart and then the lungs. (See the diagram of the heart and major blood vessels on page 268.) Not only does the venous blood have to return to the heart unaided by any pumping action but the blood returning from the lower part of the body has to flow against gravity. To prevent it from flowing backward, there is a series of valves within the veins and, in the legs, the flow is aided by the pressure exerted by the leg muscles. If these muscles are not used very much—if the patient is inactive or stands still for long periods—it is more difficult for the blood to return along the veins. The long-term effect of this is that the fluid part of the blood leaks out into the tissues, which becomes swollen and susceptible to damage.

The commonest site for varicose eczema is the inside of the leg just above the ankle, but it may spread to affect the foot and the whole of the leg. The skin is scaly and in chronic cases may become darkened and look greasy. Sometimes the skin breaks down and ulcers form. These are dealt with more fully in the section on varicose veins.

Traditional Treatment

Support stockings should be worn to assist the flow of blood upward through the veins.

Ulcers and eczema may be treated by covering them with a bandage impregnated with tar or zinc paste and then applying a firm elastic bandage on top and leaving it in place for one to two weeks. The bandaging is a specialist technique and needs to be done by a nurse.

For acute varicose eczema, bed rest may be necessary, in order to help to reduce some of the pooling in the leg. Compresses of potassium permanganate solution may be helpful, followed by a steroid cream and firm bandaging once the condition has started to subside. Steroids are not used for treating ulcers as they can delay healing.

Antibiotics may be necessary if the eczema becomes infected.

Self-Help

Avoiding long periods of standing, wearing support stockings, lying down with the feet raised for at least half an hour a day, and raising the foot of the bed by about nine inches will all help to get the blood flowing back from the legs.

SEBORRHEIC ECZEMA

This type of eczema often begins on the scalp with itching and scaling, and spreads to the eyebrows, face, ears, and the upper part of the chest. It takes the form of dull red, greasy-looking, scaly plaques and tends to spread to the skin folds, especially in obese patients, where it may become infected with bacteria or Monilia (the thrush organism Candida or yeast infection). The condition is commoner in men and tends to run in families.

On the scalp, seborrheic eczema may remain mild, causing scaling (dandruff) or may become severe with redness, weeping, and crusting. If it is very itchy, continual scratching may cause hair loss, but the hair will grow again once the condition has been treated.

In some patients, seborrheic eczema comes and goes and attacks may be brought on by stress.

Traditional Treatment

When the scalp is affected, medications can be applied in the form of shampoo. Tar shampoos used every two to three days may be helpful, but more severe cases may need the application of a steroid lotion.

Keratolytics such as salicylic acid remove thick scales and smooth the skin. They are usually applied in the form of a cream two or three times a week at night and are shampooed out the next morning.

Steroids, used twice a day, may help to resolve the rash on the face and body but must not be used long term.

Where the skin folds are affected, it is important to keep them as dry as possible in order to avoid infection. Steroid preparations can only be used for a short time as they are more likely to be absorbed into the body through damp skin. Obese patients may be advised to lose weight in order to reduce the area of overlapping skin involved in their skin folds. Antibiotics and antifungal creams may be necessary.

NUMMULAR ECZEMA

Nummular means coinlike and describes a rash that consists of round patches, usually about 2–4 cm in diameter, although sometimes larger than this where several small patches have merged together. Also known as discoid eczema, it is rare under the age of twenty and occurs most commonly in young and middle-age adults, especially those who have had atopic eczema in the past. It usually affects the back of the arms, the front of the legs, the shoulders, and the back. It can be flat or raised and scaly and may blister, weep, or become infected. The rash may persist for several months but tends to clear up of its own accord. However, it may recur from time to time, often in the same place as before.

Traditional Treatment

Small uninfected patches may safely be left without treatment. If there is blistering and weeping, potassium permanganate or salt solution soaks may help to dry the skin and a steroid cream can then be used to reduce the inflammation. Infections will need to be treated with an antibiotic, either in a cream, or taken by mouth if the infection is widespread.

Self-Help

An emollient (bath oil) may help to soften the rough patches of skin. Antiseptics and bath salts should be avoided as these may irritate the rash.

POMPHOLYX ECZEMA

The word *pompholyx,* which is derived from the Greek word for "bubble," has been given to this type of eczema because it is characterized by many blisters on either the hands or feet or both. The hands are more frequently affected—usually the palms and the sides and backs of the fingers. On the feet, the soles and the sides of the toes are most likely to be involved. However, the rash, which seems to be made worse by excessive sweating, may spread across the hands or feet and up the arms or legs.

Usually the blisters are quite small (only a few millimeters in diameter), appearing like little white spots because of the thickness of the skin on the palms and soles. There may be just a few or quite a large number. Eventually they may burst or the fluid may be reabsorbed and the blister will subside. In chronic forms, there may be no blisters but just scaling and splitting of the palms and soles, which may be hard to heal.

Pompholyx eczema can occur at any age, although it is rare in young children. Usually it is self-limiting, resolving within about four weeks of its first appearance, but occasionally it becomes chronic, with new blisters arising as the old ones vanish. Attacks may be recurrent, but the intervals between them may vary from a few months to a few years. Often they seem to be brought on by warm weather or by stress.

Traditional Treatment

Pompholyx eczema is usually very itchy in the early stages and antihistamine tablets may be needed to control the irritation. Potassium permanganate soaks will help to dry the rash if the blisters burst. Steroid creams may be useful in chronic cases. If the skin becomes infected, antibiotics will be necessary, either in the form of a cream or taken by mouth.

Self-Help

When the feet are affected, cotton socks will help to prevent the excessive sweating that can make the rash worse.

DIAPER DERMATITIS (DIAPER RASH)

There are two types of diaper rash that come under this heading. One, which is probably a reaction to the ammonia produced in a soiled diaper, is a typical irritant contact dermatitis. This takes the form of redness and scaling and may affect all the skin covered by the diaper or just the buttocks, where the contact is greatest. The other type looks similar to seborrheic dermatitis, with a dull red rash on which there may be large silvery scales. Both types tend to spread, the contact dermatitic type often affecting the trunk, body folds, and scalp. The seborrheic type responds quickly to treatment and doesn't tend to recur.

Traditional Treatment

If the skin can be kept as dry as possible, by using diaper liners and changing the diaper frequently, all that may be needed is an emollient cleanser to use instead of soap and an emollient to apply to the skin to keep it soft. In severe cases a steroid cream may be prescribed. Infections will need to be treated with antibiotics or antifungal preparations.

Self-Help

The baby should be left out of diapers for as much of the day as is practicable, in order to keep the skin dry. Diapers should be changed at least once during the night. Rubber or plastic pants should be avoided as these make the area even more moist. Disposable paper diapers or coarse towelling ones may irritate the skin and should not be used. Talcum powder should not be used as this, too, may cause irritation. Sometimes diaper rash will respond well if beaten egg white is spread over it and left to dry.

When contact dermatitis occurs as a response to the alkaline ammonia in a soiled diaper, it may help if the diapers are made slightly acidic. After they have been washed, they should be soaked for several hours in a bucket of water containing two or three tablespoons of vinegar. They should then be wrung out and dried without rinsing.

COMPLEMENTARY TREATMENT

Aromatherapy
For dry eczema, geranium or lavender may be recommended, and for a weeping rash, juniper or bergamot. Other oils that are used in the treatment of eczema include chamomile, hyssop, and sage.

Herbalism

Large numbers of herbs are used in the treatment of eczema. Among these are chamomile (which helps to heal the skin and relieve any stress that may be exacerbating the condition), burdock (which is particularly effective in the treatment of dry scaly rashes), chickweed (which is used as a lotion or ointment to soothe, heal, and relieve itching), heartsease (which is used for weeping eczema), red clover (which clears toxins from the skin and helps to restore normal function), and nettle (which is particularly useful for atopic and allergic types of eczema).

Homeopathy

The choice of remedy will depend on the patient's symptoms and the distribution of the rash. Commonly used remedies include graphites (for chronic itchy, moist rashes, especially when in the skin folds or on the head, face, and behind the ears), rhus tox. (for a dry red rash, particularly on the hands, wrists, and in the bends of joints, that is better for warmth, worse for cold and damp, and very itchy especially at night), and sulphur (for a very itchy rash that is rough, worse for heat and for contact with water, and often infected).

Hypnotherapy

This can be very helpful in the treatment of atopic eczema. However, it is not suitable for children under the age of five, because patients need to be able to concentrate on what the therapist is saying and to cooperate in the treatment. Atopic eczema often seems to be made worse by stress so that the irritation of the rash, which itself causes stress, creates a vicious circle. Hypnotherapy can break the vicious circle by teaching the child to relax and giving him suggestions that he will be less aware of the soreness and itching in his skin. Visualizations such as that mentioned in the section on psoriasis may be given and the child is made to feel that he has some control over his eczema. By helping the patient to relax, hypnosis may also be helpful in the treatment of other forms of eczema where attacks seem to be brought on by stress.

Naturopathy

A naturopath is likely to concentrate on finding out whether there is anything in the patient's diet that is making the eczema worse and will then advise on how any aggravating substances may be avoided.

Nutrition
Patients with eczema may have a calcium deficiency and an additional intake may be advised. Healthy skin is dependent on an adequate intake of vitamins A, E, and C, and of zinc, so supplements of these (plus vitamin B_6, which is needed to help the zinc to work) may be recommended.

ORGANIZATIONS

Skin Diseases Branch
National Institutes of Health
5333 Westbard Avenue
Bethesda, MD 20892
301/496-7326

EPILEPSY

DEFINITION AND CAUSES

The nervous system is made up of millions of tiny nerve cells, each of which has long arms or tendrils that allow it to communicate with the cells all around it. Electrical impulses travel from cell to cell, carrying messages that regulate all the body functions. The impulses that occur in the brain produce certain recognized patterns on an electroencephalogram (EEG, or brain wave trace). Their absence is one criterion that may be used by doctors to assess that a patient is dead.

Normally messages are carried correctly around the nervous system, enabling us to breathe, move, see, hear, digest, and so on. But some people may have occasional discharges of abnormal electrical impulses in the brain that send incorrect messages over a limited period of time—this is the condition of epilepsy.

Sometimes epilepsy or seizure disorder may develop as the result of a head injury, but it may also be caused by a number of other conditions including a congenital abnormality in the brain, infection (such as meningitis), a brain tumor (benign or malignant), or addiction to alcohol or drugs. However, in the majority of cases there seems to be no obvious cause and the condition is said to be idiopathic. There are various types of epilepsy, each with different symptoms.

TYPES OF EPILEPSY

Petit Mal

This occurs mainly in children, being slightly more common in girls than in boys. There is no convulsion, but the patient's consciousness becomes impaired for a matter of seconds during which she stares straight ahead and fails to respond to stimuli. In many cases, this is accompanied by twitching of the eyelids and arms or by chewing and swallowing movements or fumbling with the fingers. Usually the pa-

178

tient stays upright and may even continue to walk or to ride a bicycle during the attack, which comes on suddenly and disappears with equal suddenness. When the attack ends, some children are unaware that anything abnormal has happened and just continue to do whatever they were doing previously.

Petit mal rarely occurs before the age of four, with most cases starting between the ages of eight and twelve. The vast majority of patients have stopped having attacks by the time they are seventeen, although in a very few the condition may continue into adult life. Some go on to develop grand mal epilepsy.

The attacks may occur only occasionally or may be very frequent, with a patient having several hundred in a single day. In severe cases, the condition may seriously interfere with the child's schooling and special arrangements may have to be made. Usually an individual attack lasts between two and forty-five seconds, but on rare occasions a patient may go into "petit mal status" in which the attack is greatly prolonged.

Grand Mal

When epilepsy is mentioned, most people think automatically of grand mal convulsions, in which the patient falls to the floor and may thrash around. Grand mal epilepsy is a surprisingly common condition, affecting between four and eight people in every thousand. And it is estimated that as many as three people in every hundred have had a seizure at some time in their lives. However, because in many cases the condition is well controlled by medication and because sufferers don't necessarily like to talk about their illness, most people are not aware of the extent of epilepsy in the population.

Idiopathic grand mal (where there is no apparent cause) usually starts in childhood, often between the ages of eight and twelve. However, about 75 percent of those affected will have stopped having attacks by the time they are twenty. Cases that start when the patient is over the age of twenty usually have an underlying cause.

The seizures often occur early in the morning or even when the patient is still asleep. Indeed, some people only ever have seizures during the night. As in the case of petit mal, attacks may occur rarely or frequently; they may be brought on by late nights or the consumption of alcohol and may be more common in women around the time of menstruation.

For several hours before a seizure, a patient may feel irritable or depressed or, conversely, unusually elated. The seizure itself may begin with an aura in which the patient is aware of certain recognizable sensations, such as discomfort in the upper abdomen, twitches, numbness or tingling, flashing lights in front of the eyes, or a bad taste or smell. The aura only lasts a few moments before the convulsion begins, but may be long enough to enable the patient to get himself into a safe and comfortable position so that he will not hurt himself by falling to the floor.

Whether or not the patient has an aura, the first major sign that the seizure is beginning is a sudden loss of consciousness. All the muscles go into a violent spasm. This is known as the tonic phase. The sudden contraction of the muscles of the chest forces air through the larynx (voice box) and may produce a characteristic cry. It is as he falls that the patient may bite his tongue, and blood and saliva may ooze from his mouth. His face becomes dusky, because the muscle spasm makes it impossible for him to breathe. After a few seconds, the spasm relaxes and is replaced by a series of violent jerking movements, which is known as the clonic phase. It is at this point that the patient may froth at the mouth as air enters the lungs in a series of gasps through the accumulated saliva. Some patients may wet themselves during this stage. After three or four minutes, the movements slow down and eventually stop. The patient is now completely relaxed, breathing deeply but still unconscious. After a few minutes he gradually regains consciousness but may remain confused and drowsy and may have a headache for several hours afterward. Some patients go into an "epileptic fugue" in which they wander off and do things of which they later have no recollection. Most patients sleep after an attack—for anything up to eighteen hours.

Individual patients and individual attacks vary, of course. Sometimes a clonic phase may last for half an hour. Some children may find they are paralyzed after an attack—this usually affects only one side of the body and lasts between twelve and twenty-four hours before disappearing. Some 5–8 percent of patients suffer at one time or another from status epilepticus, a condition in which one seizure is followed by others, without regaining consciousness in between. This may be a life-threatening condition and needs urgent medical treatment.

Psychomotor Seizures

This type of attack usually begins with a sudden alteration in mood and behavior. An aura is common, in which the patient may experience upper abdominal discomfort, nausea, dizziness, hallucinations of various types (hearing, smelling, tasting, or seeing things that aren't there), or the déjà vu phenomenon. The latter is something that many healthy people are aware of from time to time—the feeling that you have been in a particular place or situation before, but at the same time knowing that you haven't. The patient may feel that the world around him has become unreal and he may be aware of a feeling of fear, although he is unable to say what it is that frightens him.

The symptoms may vary according to where in the brain the abnormal discharges start. The patient usually becomes confused and may run around in circles, making chewing movements, smack or lick his lips, and fiddle aimlessly with objects. Sometimes the limbs go into spasm or the head and eyes are turned sharply to one side. The patient may try to remove his clothes and may become violent if restrained. He may shuffle his feet, rub his hands, or wet himself. The attack may end after a few minutes and be followed by confusion, or may progress into a grand mal convulsion. After the attack, the patient may be unable to remember anything about it.

Jacksonian Epilepsy

A Jacksonian attack is one that begins locally and then may become generalized. The first sign may be a change in the patient's behavior, but usually the attack itself begins with twitching of one hand, one foot, or one side of the face. The movements are rhythmic and may occur in bursts. Gradually they spread to other muscles on the same side of the body. They can stop at any point or they may progress to involve the whole body in a generalized fit. Two thirds of all patients who suffer from Jacksonian epilepsy have generalized seizures at some time during their lives. After the attack the muscles that were first involved may be weak or paralyzed for several hours.

Some patients who suffer from Jacksonian epilepsy find that if they very firmly squeeze or press the muscles above those that are twitching, they can stop the attack from progressing.

Febrile Convulsions

Some five children in every hundred will have a seizure during infancy or early childhood as the result of a high fever. A small proportion of these will turn out to be epileptic, the fever just precipitating the first attack, but in the majority of cases the seizure is a result of the fever alone.

A child who has had one febrile seizure is at risk of having another whenever his temperature starts to rise rapidly, but most children grow out of their susceptibility by the age of three. Very rarely, a child may continue to have the occasional febrile seizure until the age of seven or eight. The condition occurs more often in boys than in girls and the commonest cause is tonsillitis. Usually the seizure, which takes the form of a generalized convulsion, is short, although two or three may follow each other in quick succession. After the seizure there is a short period in which the child cannot be roused.

TESTS

If epilepsy is suspected, an EEG, or electroencephalogram, is usually necessary. A number of wires are taped to the patient's head and these then record the brain's activity on a machine. Only the activity closest to the surface is picked up, so if the abnormal focus from which the seizures are starting is deep in the brain, the EEG may appear normal. The test is best done soon after a seizure.

Sometimes, when a generalized convulsion occurs in a previously healthy person, meningitis may be suspected. In such a case, a lumbar puncture will be done to confirm or exclude this diagnosis. Under local anesthetic, a small needle is inserted between two of the vertebrae in the lower part of the back and a small quantity of the fluid that surrounds the spinal cord (the nervous tissue contained inside the backbone) is extracted. If the patient is suffering from meningitis, the fluid may appear cloudy instead of clear and, when tested in the laboratory, will show evidence of infection.

In older patients, when it seems possible that the seizures may be due to a physical abnormality in the brain, such as a cyst, a tumor, or a blockage of a blood vessel, there are a number of tests that may be used. These include CT (computerized tomography) scans, MRI (magnetic resonance imaging), and arteriography. For the latter, a radio-opaque substance is injected into the bloodstream and allowed time to circulate; then X-rays of the head are taken on which the blood vessels of the brain can be seen clearly.

TRADITIONAL TREATMENT

Petit Mal

In most cases, the attacks will be partly or wholly controlled by sodium valproate or ethosuximide, although in some patients the latter may cause drowsiness, dizziness, sensitivity to light, and digestive problems.

An intravenous injection of diazepam may be needed to bring petit mal status to an end.

Medication has to be taken regularly until the patient has had four years without an attack or until he has reached his teens and a considerable amount of time has elapsed since the last attack.

Grand Mal

A number of drugs are available to treat grand mal and in some cases two or more may have to be used together in order to control the condition. All are capable of producing side effects, although some patients react more violently to one drug than another. This, as well as the effectiveness of individual drugs, is an important factor in the choice of long-term medication.

Phenytoin is safe and effective. Side effects are rare; they include skin problems, overgrowth of the gums, hairiness in women, and anemia. Used over a prolonged period, it may cause osteomalacia (softening of the bones). It is probably best avoided during pregnancy as there may be a risk to the unborn child.

Sodium valproate, too, should be avoided during pregnancy, since there is a possibility that it may cause fetal deformities. Its side effects include digestive problems, weight gain, hair loss, rashes, and shaking.

Carbamazepine may cause skin problems, dizziness, fluid retention, and, rarely, anemia. But it has the advantage of being safe in pregnancy. Primidone, too, may cause dizziness and also drowsiness.

Phenobarbital may cause drowsiness and loss of balance but usually only if too much is taken. Rashes may also occur. On the whole this is a very safe drug and is probably the safest to use during pregnancy.

Some female patients find that they have more attacks during pregnancy. So their medication may need to be changed not only to ensure that the baby is not at risk from the drugs but also to control the increased attacks. The contraceptive Pill, too, may increase the incidence of attacks and women suffering from epilepsy should use other methods of birth control.

All epileptic patients need regular follow-up by a specialist for as long as the attacks continue. Once they have been free of attacks for some time, they are usually discharged back to the care of their GP.

Jacksonian Epilepsy

This is the hardest type of epilepsy to control completely and patients may need large doses of the drugs used to treat grand mal in order to prevent generalized seizures.

Febrile Convulsions

Normally all that is required is prompt treatment by the parents if the child's temperature starts to rise rapidly. As soon as they become aware that the child is feverish, they should put him in a bath of tepid water and sponge him continuously until he appears to have cooled down. Older children may be given the sponge and allowed to play with it, which usually has the same effect.

If it seems likely that the fever is the result of a bacterial infection— for example, tonsillitis or an ear infection—the child should be seen as soon as possible by the GP so that a course of antibiotics may be started.

In some cases, where a child has had a prolonged seizure, the GP may think it advisable to prescribe phenobarbital, to be taken on a regular basis until the child reaches the age of three.

COMPLEMENTARY TREATMENT

Acupuncture
The points used in treatment will depend on the individual symptoms. Febrile convulsions, for example, are seen as being due to an invasion of the body by wind that stirs up inner heat. The therapist will use specific points to expel wind, eliminate heat, relieve spasm, and clear mental clouding.

Bach Flower Remedies
It has been observed by a doctor that giving a patient who is having an epileptic seizure the compound Rescue Remedy will bring him around quite quickly. Indeed, this doctor has even found it possible to cut short status epilepticus by putting a few drops of this remedy into the patient's mouth. As a first-aid measure it is certainly worth trying, since it can have no harmful effects whatsoever.

Herbalism
Treatment may be given to reduce the severity and frequency of attacks. Scullcap is commonly used for this.

Homeopathy
A wide range of remedies may be appropriate, but belladonna may be particularly useful in the treatment of febrile convulsions, and cuprum may be given to a patient whose attack begins with twitching in the fingers and toes.

Hynotherapy
Hypnosis may help to reduce the frequency of epileptic attacks. Occasionally, when a patient has warning that an attack is coming on, the

use of self-hypnosis or of techniques learned while under hypnosis may help to abort the full attack.

Nutrition

Epileptic patients are often found to have a deficiency of manganese and a supplement of this mineral may be beneficial. The amino acid taurine may help to control attacks in some patients. It is taken initially in doses of 1 g daily, but because it accumulates rapidly in the body, this can soon be reduced to a maintenance dose of around 50 mg a day.

SELF-HELP

Attacks may be brought on by overbreathing or by watching flashing lights, so patients should avoid both of these.

As a first-aid measure for a patient in petit mal status, a paper bag placed over the mouth and nose may be helpful. This makes the child rebreathe the carbon dioxide that has been exhaled and this may help to bring the attack to an end.

It is a common belief that during an attack of grand mal epilepsy a patient is at risk of swallowing his tongue and that something should be pushed into his mouth to hold the tongue in place. However, there is, in fact, very little risk of the tongue being swallowed and if it is bitten this occurs right at the start of the attack and cannot be prevented. On the other hand, forcing something into a patient's mouth during a seizure could seriously damage his teeth or his jaw and therefore should be avoided.

Anyone who has epilepsy is banned from driving a car, but may reapply for a driver's license once six months to a year have elapsed since the last seizure. But no one who has ever had a seizure is allowed to drive a truck or bus.

ORGANIZATIONS

Epilepsy Foundation of America
4351 Garden City Drive
Landover, MD 20785
301/459-3700
(Publishes a newspaper, newsletter, and educational materials.)

Epilepsy Concern Service Group
1282 Wynnewood Drive
West Palm Beach, FL 33409
305/586-4804
(Publishes a newsletter.)

FIBROIDS

INCIDENCE AND DESCRIPTION

Fibroids are benign growths of muscle and fibrous tissue that occur in the uterus (womb). They affect about 20 percent of women over the age of thirty, although in many cases they produce no symptoms. When symptoms do arise, they are likely to do so between the ages of thirty-five and forty-five. Fibroids are commoner in black women than in white, but although they may cause infertility in between 25 and 35 percent of white women, they do not have this effect in black women. Why this should be is not known. Nor is the cause of fibroids known. However, they are to some extent dependent on the woman's hormonal status, since they tend to enlarge during pregnancy and shrivel up after the menopause.

Fibroids may be single or multiple and vary enormously in size, although they grow only slowly. Usually they occur within the muscle of the uterus itself (interstitial or intramural fibroids). But they may arise on the outside of the uterus (subserous fibroids) or on the inside (submucous fibroids) and in these positions they may become pedunculated (grow out on stalks). Rarely, they grow within the cervix (neck of the womb). Also rare is the so-called wandering fibroid. This is a large subserous fibroid that becomes attached to a band of tissue lying in the abdomen called the omentum. The omentum carries in it a number of blood vessels and eventually the fibroid may develop a blood supply from it. When this occurs, it may break off from its stalk so that it is now separated completely from the uterus.

SYMPTOMS

To a certain extent, the symptoms depend on where in the uterus the fibroids are situated. Submucous fibroids have abnormally large blood vessels stretched over their surface and they increase the surface area of the inside of the uterus, so they often cause heavy periods (menorrhagia), although the periods themselves are not prolonged. Anemia is a common result of this. These fibroids may also become infected, producing a discharge. Irregular vaginal bleeding may occur if they become ulcerated. A large pedunculated fibroid may descend through the cervix (neck of the uterus) and in this position may cause quite heavy bleeding. Pedunculated fibroids may cause colicky pain, as the uterine muscle tries to push them out. This may be particularly severe during a period (dysmenorrhea). Large polyps may cause urinary symptoms of discomfort in the rectum because of the pressure they exert on the surrounding organs. Patients may also suffer from infertility or recurrent miscarriage.

Intramural fibroids may first be noticed as a mass in the abdomen. Like submucous fibroids they may cause menorrhagia, pressure symptoms, and infertility.

Women who have subserous fibroids frequently have no symptoms, although they may become aware of a mass in the abdomen. Occasionally they may develop severe abdominal pain due either to bleeding or to twisting of the stalk. Hemorrhage may occur either inside the fibroid itself or into the abdominal cavity. If the stalk of the fibroid twists (torsion), the blood supply to the fibroid is cut off and the pain persists until the fibroid dies.

Fibroids within the cervix are rare. They may be associated with urinary symptoms (pain upon passing water, frequency, or stress incontinence), bleeding, infection, pain during intercourse, and infertility.

COMPLICATIONS

As well as torsion of a pedunculated fibroid, there are several other complications that may occur. All of them are uncommon.

Pregnant women who have fibroids may develop severe pain in the second trimester of pregnancy (the middle three months) due to red degeneration caused by the fibroid losing its blood supply so that it shrinks. However, this only occurs with large fibroids.

Pressure on the bladder or ureters may cause acute retention of urine, repeated urinary tract infections, or partial obstruction of urinary flow from the kidneys to the bladder.

Malignant change occurs in about one in two hundred patients with large fibroids, which is why doctors always recommend that large fibroids be removed. Symptoms of malignant change include sudden rapid growth of the fibroid, pain, and fever.

Fibroids may also interfere with pregnancy, producing recurrent miscarriage, premature labor, and postpartum hemorrhage or infection. They may also prevent normal vaginal delivery and necessitate a cesarean section.

TESTS

Fibroids are first diagnosed by a vaginal examination. Their presence can then be confirmed by ultrasound investigation. Sometimes fibroids become calcified, especially in older patients, and in this case they will show up on X-ray. If the patient has been having irregular vaginal bleeding, a scrape of the uterus (D & C) is necessary to rule out a diagnosis of cancer.

TRADITIONAL TREATMENT

Surgery is usually unnecessary if the patient has few or no symptoms and if the fibroids are small and either intramural or subserous. It is also avoided during pregnancy.

If the patient has been bleeding heavily, iron supplements may be necessary and, rarely, a blood transfusion. Infection is treated with antibiotics. It may be possible to control excessive bleeding in younger patients by prescribing progesterone or other drugs used for the treatment of menorrhagia.

When an operation is necessary, the simplest is a hysterectomy. However, for those women who dislike this idea or who wish to become pregnant in the future, it is possible to remove the individual fibroids (myomectomy), leaving the womb intact. Unfortunately, myomectomy carries the risk of post-operative bleeding and infection, and fibroids recur in between 5 and 20 percent of cases.

RECENT ADVANCES

Researchers have recently been trying to shrink fibroids with hormone manipulation, specifically using analogs of gonadotropin releasing hormone (Gn-RH). Significant improvement occurs, but once the drug is stopped the fibroids regrow. Since estrogen levels drop with this treatment, menopausal symptoms can develop. More research is needed, but currently this treatment is being used in women who can't have or don't want surgery, or it is used to shrink fibroids preoperatively and to help prevent surgical complications and excess blood loss.

COMPLEMENTARY TREATMENT

Herbalism
Some herbs may help to prevent fibroids from becoming any larger and may relieve the patient's symptoms. Helonias root improves the function of the ovaries and helps to maintain menstrual regularity. Agnus castus also has a hormonelike effect, acting on the pituitary gland in the brain, whose hormones control other glands in the body, including the ovaries. Life root relieves spasm in the uterus as do blue cohosh, motherwort, and black cohosh.

Homeopathy
The remedy chosen for an individual patient will depend on her symptoms and may include any of those mentioned in the section on menstrual problems.

ORGANIZATIONS

Hysterectomy Educational Resources and Services Foundation
422 Bryn Mawr Avenue
Bala Cynwyd, PA 19004
215/667-7757

GALLBLADDER DISEASE

THE FUNCTION OF THE GALLBLADDER

Because fat cannot be dissolved in water, a special system has evolved for its digestion and its absorption through the intestinal wall. Bile is an essential factor in this, since it contains substances that allow fats to be emulsified. It also stimulates the secretion of an enzyme concerned with the breakdown of fats. Bile is secreted by the liver and stored in the gallbladder until needed. When fat is eaten, this stimulates the gallbladder to contract and bile flows down the cystic duct, into the common bile duct and through the ampulla of Vater into the intestine.

As well as acting as a storage vessel, the gallbladder concentrates the bile within it by removing water through its wall. Thus, if the gallbladder is removed, although bile still flows into the intestine from the liver, fat digestion may be less efficient because the bile is not concentrated.

GALLSTONES (CHOLELITHIASIS)

The commonest disorder of the biliary tract (gallbladder and bile ducts) is gallstones. This occurs very frequently in developed countries and may be associated with eating a diet that is high in fat and refined carbohydrates and low in fiber. Probably 10–20 percent of the population over the age of forty have gallstones, but only in a minority do symptoms occur. If gallstones are found by chance on an X-ray taken for some other reason it is standard practice to leave them alone if they are causing no symptoms, since the risk of developing problems is slightly less than the risk from a major operation. However, if a patient with symptomless gallstones is having an abdominal operation for another reason, the gallbladder may be removed at the same time.

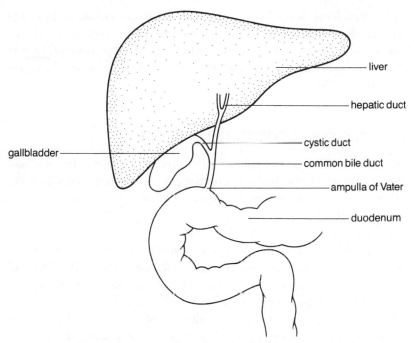

liver

hepatic duct

cystic duct

gallbladder

common bile duct

ampulla of Vater

duodenum

The relationship between the liver, gallbladder, and duodenum

Medical students learn that the typical patient with gallstones is "fair, fat, female, fertile, and forty." However, this is rather a simplification. Certainly obese patients have a greater risk of developing gallstones, as do women, especially those who have had a number of children. Taking the contraceptive Pill also increases the risk. But the condition becomes commoner with increasing age and, although it is rare in Asians and Africans, it is especially common among the Mediterranean races.

Gallstones are made up of the substances contained in the bile and may be described as cholesterol stones, pigment stones, or mixed. About 20 percent contain pure cholesterol and may occur as single large stones. The majority of stones (about 75 percent) are mixed (usually containing a large amount of cholesterol) and multiple. About 10 percent contain enough calcium to be visible on X-ray. Why and how gallstones form is not fully understood, but it is thought that in some cases an abnormality in function causes the gallbladder to remove an excessive amount of water from the bile so that some of its constituents can no longer remain in solution.

The problems that gallstones can give rise to are various and include cholecystitis (inflammation of the gallbladder), choledocholithiasis (stones in the common bile duct), cholangitis (inflammation of the bile ducts and gallbladder), and gallstone ileus (obstruction of the intestines by a gallstone).

CHRONIC CHOLECYSTITIS (BILIARY COLIC)

Both these names are somewhat of a misnomer, since this is not a chronic inflammatory condition and the pain it produces is not colicky. (True colic comes and goes in waves, but the pain of biliary colic is constant during the attack.)

Of those patients who have symptoms from their gallstones, the majority will suffer from chronic cholecystitis. The attacks are caused by a stone becoming stuck either in the junction of the gallbladder and the bile duct or in the duct itself. The muscle in the wall of both gallbladder and duct contracts in an effort to move the stone and this produces intense pain usually felt under the ribs on the right-hand side of the abdomen. However, the pain may also be felt under the V of the ribs or may extend right across the abdomen and spread around to the back, below the right shoulder blade. The patient may vomit and is usually restless. After several hours, the stone either falls back into the gallbladder or, by virtue of the muscle contractions, is passed down the bile duct and into the intestine.

Some patients suffer from a constant dull ache in the upper abdomen and many complain of discomfort and flatulence after eating a fatty meal.

Traditional Treatment

Patients who are otherwise healthy should have a cholecystectomy (removal of the gallbladder) to prevent further recurrences. If an operation is inadvisable because the patient is frail, elderly, or has severe heart or lung disease, it may be possible to control the symptoms with painkillers and antiemetics (drugs to stop vomiting), but ultimately surgery may still be necessary if the pain becomes intolerable or if complications, such as jaundice, occur. A low-fat diet and weight reduction will also help these patients and those who are waiting for surgery.

In some patients who are not fit for surgery, it may be possible to dissolve the stones by giving them chenodeoxycholic acid or ursodeoxycholic acid. These preparations are taken by mouth and are excreted in the bile. However, they will only work if the gallbladder is seen by testing to be functioning (see below) and if the gallstones are very small and contain very little calcium (making them invisible—or radiolucent—on a plain X-ray of the abdomen). This treatment is not suitable for women of childbearing age or for those with any form of liver disease. It has the disadvantage that, although 80 percent of stones may be dissolved after six months' or a year's treatment, they frequently re-form after the medication has stopped.

ACUTE CHOLECYSTITIS

Twenty percent of those who develop gallbladder symptoms suffer from this condition, which most frequently affects women between the ages of twenty and forty. Like chronic cholecystitis it is caused by a stone becoming jammed either in the junction of the gallbladder and duct or in the duct itself, and many patients have previously suffered from biliary colic, indigestion, or flatulence. The pain of acute cholecystitis stems from inflammation that is probably caused at first by the chemicals in the bile. However, a bacterial infection then supervenes in 50 percent or more of cases.

The pain comes on suddenly and is severe and constant. It is felt across the right and central parts of the upper abdomen and under the right shoulder blade. The patient usually vomits and is quite ill and feverish. If the common bile duct becomes swollen, slight jaundice may occur as bile from the liver is prevented from passing into the intestine and enters the bloodstream instead.

Traditional Treatment

At least 90 percent of cases settle on a regime of bed rest, painkillers, and antibiotics. Rarely, complications may occur that include abscess formation, peritonitis, and septicemia.

The patient is admitted to the hospital and is given fluids intravenously. If she is vomiting, a tube is passed through the nose into the stomach in order to keep it empty.

If complications occur, emergency surgery is necessary. In most cases, however, the symptoms are allowed to settle down and an operation is performed to remove the gallbladder at a later date. Nowadays many surgeons like to do this two or three days after the patient's admission to the hospital. Some, however, prefer the traditional gap of two or three months between the acute attack and surgery. Waiting for a few months has the advantage that obese patients have the chance to lose some weight, reducing the risks of surgery, and that the surgeon can be certain that all the inflammation has settled. However, 10 percent of patients get another attack while waiting for their operation.

CHOLEDOCHOLITHIASIS (STONES IN THE COMMON BILE DUCT)

Some 10 percent of patients who have gallbladder symptoms have stones in the common bile duct. Some of these stones actually form in the duct itself whereas others originate in the gallbladder and then pass into the duct where they gradually enlarge. This condition occurs more frequently in older patients.

Various complications may arise as the result of stones becoming lodged in the common bile duct. They may prevent bile from getting through, causing jaundice as the bile escapes into the bloodstream. They may result in an infection in the gallbladder (suppurative cholangitis) in which the patient has a high fever and becomes extremely ill. Occasionally, acute pancreatitis (inflammation of the pancreas) may occur. Rarely, the back pressure that builds up in the duct may affect the liver and cause liver failure (biliary cirrhosis).

Because some of these complications may be life-threatening, it is usual to remove ductal stones when they are diagnosed, even if they are not producing any symptoms. When symptoms occur, they are usually recurrent, lasting for a few hours or days at a time, and consisting of pain, jaundice, and fever. The pain, which is felt in the right upper abdomen and under the V of the ribs, is usually severe and the patient may vomit. While the patient is jaundiced, the stools are pale and the urine is dark because the pigments from the bile that normally color the stools can no longer get through to the bowel and are being excreted in the urine.

Traditional Treatment

Usually the acute episode is allowed to settle before surgery is performed, although a very ill patient with jaundice may need an emergency operation. Painkillers are prescribed and, if necessary, antibiotics. Once the symptoms have subsided, the patient is taken to the operating room, the common bile duct is opened, and all the stones are removed. Because it is easy to miss stones, a cholangiogram (see below) is performed during the operation to see whether the duct has indeed been cleared. During the operation a T tube is inserted into the duct. This is a piece of plastic tubing in the shape of a T. The crossbar is inserted into the duct and stitched in snugly using catgut, which will then slowly dissolve. The long vertical part of the T is brought out to the surface and is anchored to the skin with a stitch. Bile drains from the tube and is collected in a plastic bag. About nine or ten days after the operation, a substance that will show up on X-ray is injected down the tube and into the bile ducts and an X-ray is taken. If there is no evidence of any stones or blockage in the duct, the skin stitch is removed and the T tube comes out easily. Within about a day the tiny hole left in the bile duct has closed up and bile is flowing normally again. If, however, the X-ray shows that there are still stones in the duct, it is usually possible to remove them through the T tube, either physically or by injecting the solvent, mono-octanoin. Another operation is only rarely necessary.

Elderly or frail patients who are at increased risk from a major operation may be treated by endoscopic sphincterotomy rather than by surgery. This technique, which has a 90 percent success rate, consists of inserting a flexible telescope through the mouth down into the small intestine. The muscular band at the mouth of the common bile duct is cut into and large stones can be removed.

CHOLANGITIS

This bacterial infection involving the gallbladder and bile ducts may be mild or severe. It often occurs as a result of an obstruction in the ducts—from a gallstone, congenital narrowing, scarring from a previous operation, or malignant growth. The patient has severe pain in the gallbladder area, fever, shivering fits and, often, jaundice. The right upper section of the abdomen is very tender.

Complications include the development of a liver abscess and liver failure. If the symptoms continue despite treatment, septicemia may occur. This condition is known as acute suppurative cholangitis.

Traditional Treatment

Acute suppurative cholangitis needs emergency treatment. The patient is admitted to the hospital and is given intravenous fluids and large doses of antibiotics. As soon as she is in a fit condition, an operation is performed at which the obstruction to bile flow is relieved and bile is drained out. The simplest and quickest procedure possible is used, in order to minimize the risk to the patient. (Various methods are available to the surgeon.) Once the patient has fully recovered, another operation may be necessary to ensure that further episodes do not occur.

The treatment of milder forms of cholangitis consists of antibiotics and, if necessary, intravenous fluids; the operation to relieve the obstruction can be delayed until the patient has recovered from the acute attack.

Patients who have recurrent attacks of mild cholangitis but who are not suitable for surgery may be helped by long-term courses of antibiotics.

Because cholangitis may be precipitated by operative procedures, any patient who is to have surgery on the biliary tract or tests such as ERCP or PTC (see below) will be given a course of antibiotics as a preventive measure.

GALLSTONE ILEUS

This uncommon condition usually occurs in older women. The gallstone responsible is an inch or more across. Having taken some years to achieve this size, it ulcerates through the wall of the gallbladder into the duodenum. It passes down the small intestine and then becomes lodged lower down where the intestine becomes narrow. The patient develops a colicky pain, as the muscles of the intestinal wall contract in an attempt to dislodge the stone, and vomits profusely. Often the symptoms settle and then recur, because the obstruction of the intestine is not complete. The vomit contains food at first, then bile, and finally material from the lower part of the bowel consisting of the waste left over after food has been digested.

An operation to remove the stone is essential.

CANCER OF THE BILIARY TRACT

Cancer of the gallbladder is rare. Cancer of the bile ducts is rarer. Gallbladder cancer usually occurs in elderly women and the first symptom is jaundice or pain in the gallbladder area. The outlook is not good since the tumor has usually spread by the time symptoms develop.

Cancer of the bile ducts usually occurs in men over fifty and more frequently in people who suffer from ulcerative colitis, although the reason for this is not known. Symptoms include jaundice, pain in the gallbladder region, and weight loss. As with cancer of the gallbladder, the outlook is poor, but radiotherapy is sometimes helpful and, if the tumor is entirely confined within the liver, a liver transplant may be possible.

TESTS FOR DISEASE OF THE BILIARY TRACT

There are a number of tests that are in use to diagnose gallbladder and bile duct disease and to differentiate the various conditions from each other.

Three types of blood test are used. The first is a complete blood count. A raised number of white cells in this suggests that the patient has an infection (although not necessarily in the biliary tract). Thus, the count will be raised in acute cholecystitis and cholangitis but will be normal in chronic cholecystitis or if there is a stone in the bile duct.

Blood may also be taken for liver function tests. These measure certain enzymes and other substances produced by the liver. Various abnormalities suggest different biliary tract problems.

If a patient is thought to be suffering from acute cholecystitis or cholangitis, blood may be cultured in order to detect whether there are any bacteria in it.

There are also three types of X-ray in use. The first is the plain abdominal X-ray, which will demonstrate the 10 percent of gallstones that are radio-opaque because they have a large amount of calcium in them. A cholecystogram is a test that has been in use for many years. The patient is given a radio-opaque dye that she takes by mouth the night before the X-ray. This is absorbed from the intestine and excreted by the liver into the bile. An X-ray will show the gallbladder full of the dye and if there are stones present these will appear as dark holes. However, if the gallbladder is not functioning, the dye will not be concentrated by it and nothing more will be seen than was apparent on a plain X-ray. Other reasons for the gallbladder not being shown are the loss of the dye from vomiting or diarrhea before it can be absorbed from the intestine.

The third type of X-ray is intravenous cholangiography. In this, the radio-opaque dye is injected into a vein. It is excreted in a concentrated form by the liver and often it is possible to see the bile ducts as well as the gallbladder. It is particularly useful when the biliary ducts need testing after the patient has had the gallbladder removed.

More recent techniques include ultrasonography, biliary scintigraphy, endoscopic retrograde cholangiopancreatography, and percutaneous transhepatic cholangiography. The first of these consists of using a small instrument that sends an ultrasound beam through the body tissues and analyzes the beam that they reflect back. It is an extremely safe and easy procedure and, since it is as accurate as a cholecystogram and can provide more information, it is tending to replace the older investigation in many hospitals. In acute cholecystitis it often demonstrates gallstones and an inflamed, distended gallbladder. It also shows up the bile ducts and the liver. It is particularly useful in patients in whom cholecystography is useless (those with a nonfunctioning gallbladder and those who are jaundiced) and in patients in whom it is inadvisable (such as pregnant women who should avoid all unnecessary X-rays).

Biliary scintigraphy involves the use of a radioactive chemical that is injected into the bloodstream and is then excreted into the bile. A scan shows the bile ducts and gallbladder.

Endoscopic retrograde cholangiopancreatography (ERCP) is used to examine the bile ducts and the pancreatic ducts and is especially useful in patients who are jaundiced. A flexible telescope (endoscope) is passed through the patient's mouth into the small intestine and a radio-opaque dye is injected through the ampulla of Vater. This travels up and flows into the biliary and pancreatic ducts. X-rays are then taken that allow diagnosis of abnormalities within the ducts.

Percutaneous transhepatic cholangiography (PTC) consists of an injection given under local anesthetic through the skin into the liver, using a very fine flexible needle. A radio-opaque dye is injected and this outlines the bile ducts within the liver and the larger ducts that arise from them. This investigation can be especially helpful in locating the position and determining the cause of an obstruction in the biliary tract and it is used particularly for jaundiced patients who have been shown on ultrasound to have abnormally dilated bile ducts within the liver.

RECENT ADVANCES

A technique known as extracorporeal shock-wave lithotripsy (ESWL) that has for some time been used in the treatment of kidney stones has recently been used for gallstones. A shock wave is transmitted through water to the gallstone region and this causes the stones to shatter. The gravel that remains passes easily down the bile duct into the intestine. A German trial in which 200 patients were treated found that over 90 percent remained free of stones a year later. Since then, a new machine had been developed. When this is used together with ultrasound to locate the stones, the treatment takes less than an hour, an anesthetic is usually unnecessary, and the patient need only stay in the hospital for two days. It is thought likely that this form of treatment will be suitable for about 25 percent of all patients.

Attempts to dissolve stones using chenodeoxycholic acid and ursodeoxycholic acid, mentioned above, have not been very successful due to the high rate of recurrence after treatment is stopped. However, at the Mayo Clinic in Rochester, Minnesota, another substance, methyl tert-butylether (MTBE), was injected into the gallbladder. After several treatments, the stones were found to dissolve rapidly. This technique was used in a modified form by doctors in Glasgow, Scotland, who inserted a long fine tube into the ampulla of Vater, using an endoscope with its upper end protruding from the patient's nose. MTBE was then injected down the tube. The subjects were ten elderly patients whose stones were too large to be removed endoscopically. In eight, the bile duct was found to be completely free of stones after an average of eight hours of treatment. The other two patients were operated on and were found to have stones low in cholesterol which, it seems, are less likely to respond well to MTBE.

COMPLEMENTARY TREATMENT

Acupuncture
Jaundice is said to be due in some circumstances to damp heat in the Gallbladder channel and specific points will be used to eliminate this and to remove the obstruction to the flow of Chi.

Aromatherapy
Several oils may be recommended for patients with gallstones, such as bergamot, eucalyptus, chamomile, and hyssop.

Herbalism
Certain herbs known as cholagogues stimulate the flow of bile, helping to prevent stagnation within the gallbladder. Dandelion leaves, for example, stimulate the liver and help to reduce cholesterol levels. Echinacea may be prescribed for an infection in the biliary tract.

Homeopathy
A large number of remedies may be suitable for the treatment of biliary colic, including berberis, dioscorea, and chelidonium, and may help to prevent further attacks.

Nutrition
Lecithin, which is a natural emulsifier, can be taken as a supplement to help keep cholesterol in solution in the bile and prevent the formation of stones. Globe artichokes stimulate the flow of bile and may prevent stagnation in the gallbladder.

HAIR LOSS

THE MECHANISM OF HAIR GROWTH

The average person has about 100,000 scalp hairs and loses between 20 and 100 of these each day. Hair growth is not continuous—a hair will only grow to a certain length before dropping out and being replaced by another. The length of hair varies according to its site and according to the individual. Thus, the eyebrows and body hair are shorter than the scalp hair and, whereas some people can grow their hair until they can sit on it, with others it will never grow much beyond shoulder-length.

Each hair follicle, from which the hair itself grows, goes through a cycle that starts with great cellular activity (the catagen phase). This is followed by the anagen or growing phase in which the hair develops and lengthens, and, finally, the telogen phase during which the hair is shed and the follicle rests before once again entering the catagen phase. In a normal person about 85 percent of the scalp hairs are in anagen at any one time.

Hair loss can be divided into two main groups—diffuse and patchy. Patchy hair loss can then be broken down into primary hair loss, in which the problem lies in the hair or its production, and secondary hair loss, in which hair cannot be produced because the follicles have been damaged.

PRIMARY DIFFUSE HAIR LOSS

MALE PATTERN BALDNESS

Cause and Symptoms

This is the commonest form of primary diffuse hair loss, affecting many men in middle age, although it may begin as early as the teens. It is

203

an inherited condition, but only occurs in the presence of male hormones, so that a eunuch would not go bald. (Perhaps this underlies the popular idea that bald men are sexy!)

Once the hair loss has begun, it is usually progressive, but the length of time over which it occurs is very variable. Some men become quite bald over a period of two or three years, whereas others gradually lose some hair but never become completely bald. Hair is lost at the front of the scalp and on the temples and also on the crown. However, even in the most severe cases, a ring of hair always remains at the base of the skull and the sides.

Traditional Treatment

Until recently, traditional medicine had little to offer the balding man, although hair transplants have proved effective for some. Hair plugs are taken from the area at the base of the skull which, it seems, are unaffected by the male hormones, and are inserted into the bald areas, where they continue to grow.

However, a new drug has been produced that can induce regrowth of hair in bald areas. Known as Rogaine, its active ingredient is minoxidil, which is used, in tablet form, to treat high blood pressure. One side effect of these tablets is increased hairiness in some patients and it was this observation that led to the research resulting in the production of Rogaine. Unfortunately the preparation does not work for everyone. It is most likely to be effective in men who have recently started to go bald and it is unlikely to help those who have been balding for more than ten years or whose bald patch is more than 10 cm (4 inches) across. It comes as a fluid that must be applied twice a day to the bald patch for at least four to six months. If it has not worked within this time, it is unlikely to do so. Once it has started to work, it must continue to be used, as stopping treatment will allow the baldness to take over again. Several trials of minoxidil have shown that over 50 percent of patients have significant regrowth of hair within a year of starting treatment, and many of the other patients notice a slowing down or stopping of the balding process. Side effects include irritation and redness of the bald area and, because some of the drug gets absorbed through the scalp into the bloodstream, increased hair growth in other areas such as the beard or the ear. Minoxidil is available only by prescription and is quite expensive.

FEMALE BALDNESS

Some middle-age and elderly women tend to lose their hair, but the loss is usually just from the crown and rarely proceeds to total baldness of the area. It may occur in young women, in which case it is often associated with an excess of male hormones and can be treated with hormone therapy.

Sometimes baldness can result from underlying diseases, the commonest being thyroid disorders and iron-deficiency anemia. Tension on the hair caused by styles involving tight braiding or by wearing rollers for prolonged periods may produce bald patches, and both perming and bleaching may damage the hair.

TELOGEN EFFLUVIUM

Sometimes a large number of hair follicles suddenly go into the resting phase (or telogen) so that the hair is shed. The reason for this is unknown, but the condition is most commonly precipitated by a severe illness or by childbirth. Hair loss usually begins three or four months after the event and may be quite severe. Nail growth may also be affected. However, the hair cycle returns to normal within a few months and the hair starts to grow again. Other conditions that may be associated with telogen effluvium are thyroid disease, iron deficiency, and rapid weight loss from dieting.

Drug-Induced Alopecia
Some drugs may cause hair loss. Commonest among these are the cytotoxic drugs used in the treatment of cancer. Others include anti-coagulants, thyroid drugs, allopurinol (used in the treatment of gout), the contraceptive Pill, and the retinoids used in the treatment of skin conditions such as acne and psoriasis. Hair growth usually begins again when the patient stops taking these drugs.

ALOPECIA AREATA

This is a fairly common condition, affecting both sexes and producing small or large patches of hair loss. It usually affects children and young adults, only 25 percent of patients being over the age of forty. One quarter of those affected have a close relative who has also suffered from the condition. Many patients have had atopic conditions (eczema, asthma, or hay fever), or these diseases may run in the family. Alopecia is sometimes seen in patients suffering from autoimmune diseases (in which the body is attacked by its own immune system), such as thyrotoxicosis, Addison's disease, and pernicious anemia, and this has led to the theory that a disorder of the immune system may be involved in this type of hair loss.

Women are affected as often as men. Usually there is a fairly sudden onset, with the discovery of a round or oval bald patch, frequently on the head but occasionally in the beard area or elsewhere on the body. The hair loss may be complete or there may be so-called "exclamation mark" hairs visible. These short hairs, usually seen at the edges of the patch, derive their name from their appearance, since they taper toward their base. If they are pulled with tweezers, they come out easily. In children, it is more common to see black dots on the bald surface, indicating the position of the abnormal hair follicles. The skin itself is normal, although sometimes it may be a little pinker than usual. Sometimes the nails become pitted and deformed and, in the most severe cases, may be lost completely.

Rarely, all the scalp hair is lost—this is known as alopecia totalis and is commonest in children who have had atopic conditions. Even more rarely, loss of all the body hair may occur as well—alopecia universalis. In one study of alopecia areata, it was found that 54 percent of children and 24 percent of adults who had the disease progressed to alopecia totalis and, of these, 21 percent of children and 30 percent of adults did not get their hair back again.

In most cases, however, the hair begins to regrow—often within two to three months and usually within a year. At first the new hair is fine and downy and often white, but it becomes stronger and pigmented with time. In some cases, as the hair regrows other bald patches appear.

The more extensive the hair loss, the less likely is a complete recovery. However, sometimes hair may start to grow again after many years of baldness.

Traditional Treatment

Steroids given by mouth will induce regrowth of hair in many cases, but patients often relapse once the treatment is stopped. In addition, it is inadvisable to give children steroids unless it is unavoidable. Injection of steroids into the scalp (by a special technique that uses pressure to force the fluids in and is therefore painless) is often helpful. Some cases respond to PUVA (see section on psoriasis) and others to minoxidil (see above).

TRICHOTILLOMANIA

Some patients (usually children) develop bald patches because they get into the habit of rubbing a particular area of the scalp or pulling a section of hair. The hairs can be seen to be broken off close to the surface. Most children grow out of the habit, but if it is associated with other anxieties or problems, patients may need psychiatric help.

SECONDARY HAIR LOSS

DESTRUCTIVE OR SCARRING ALOPECIA

This may result from burns, severe infections of the scalp, or X-ray therapy to the scalp. Some skin disorders such as lichen planus, scleroderma, and discoid lupus erythematosus may also cause localized baldness. Scarring may be seen but is not always apparent. When a bald patch is small and due to a nonrecurring cause, such as a burn, plastic surgery may be possible.

COMPLEMENTARY TREATMENT

Aromatherapy
Oils of lavender, sage, or thyme may be recommended.

Herbalism

Because alopecia areata often seems to be brought on by stress, herbs with relaxant properties, such as chamomile, balm, and vervain, may be helpful.

Homeopathy

Phos. ac. or staphysagria may be helpful if hair loss follows emotional problems, and cinchona if it appears after an illness.

Hypnotherapy

Because alopecia areata may sometimes be precipitated by an emotional upset, hypnosis may speed recovery by relieving anxiety and teaching the patient how to cope with stress.

HEMORRHOIDS
(Piles)

DEFINITION AND SYMPTOMS

Hemorrhoids are varicose veins that occur in the anal canal (the lowest part of the rectum). Here there is a network of veins that forms a soft pad inside the canal. Pressure inside the abdomen, such as may be caused by pregnancy, a tumor, or chronic constipation, may impair the blood flow out of these veins so that they swell up, forming hemorrhoids. However, in many cases no specific underlying cause can be found.

Hemorrhoids are usually classified as first, second, or third degree. First-degree hemorrhoids are usually painless but cause bleeding. This is slight at first, and may remain so for months or years, just a small amount of bright red blood being seen when the patient passes a stool. Later on, the condition may progress to second degree, in which defecation (passing a stool) brings the hemorrhoids down through the anus so that the patient is aware of soft swellings protruding out of his anus. These prolapsed hemorrhoids usually slip back by themselves, or the patient may have to give them a gentle push. Eventually, they begin to prolapse at other times, such as upon exertion or when the patient is tired and, finally, they become third-degree hemorrhoids, which are permanently prolapsed. These may cause great discomfort together with a feeling of heaviness in the rectum and may be associated with a discharge and itching around the anus.

Chronic excessive bleeding from hemorrhoids may result in anemia. The other major complication is thrombosis, in which the blood inside a prolapsed hemorrhoid clots. The hemorrhoid becomes swollen, purple, and very painful. Without treatment it may become infected or may ulcerate, but usually starts to shrivel up after two or three weeks.

TESTS

Because bleeding from the rectum can sometimes be a sign that there is a serious disorder in the bowels, a doctor should always be consulted when this occurs. He will examine the patient's abdomen to see whether he can feel any abnormal masses and will also examine the rectum. A small instrument called a proctoscope can be inserted into the rectum to enable the hemorrhoids to be inspected. Usually there are three prominent ones, situated at three, seven, and eleven o'clock when the patient is lying on his back. In order to rule out any other problems, the doctor may use a flexible telescope (sigmoidoscope) to see higher up the bowel or may send the patient to have a barium enema (described in the section on irritable bowel syndrome).

TRADITIONAL TREATMENT

Because hemorrhoids may be associated with constipation and the resultant straining that is necessary to pass a stool, a high-fiber diet and avoidance of straining are effective preventive measures that will also help to stop first-degree hemorrhoids from getting any worse.

The treatment of choice for troublesome first-degree hemorrhoids is injection. This is done in an outpatient setting, since it is painless and fairly quick. Phenol in oil is injected into the area above each hemorrhoid, and this shuts down the blood vessel, cutting the vein off and allowing it to shrivel up. This treatment controls bleeding in about 90 percent of patients, but up to a third of these may find that their symptoms return after a while. Sometimes several injections are needed, at monthly intervals. Injections may also be used for more advanced hemorrhoids if the patient is frail, elderly, or otherwise unfit for an operation.

If the patient is young and fit, stretching (dilatation) of the muscle band inside the anus (the anal sphincter) under general anesthetic is a quick, simple procedure that has very good results. It can be used in the treatment of all degrees of hemorrhoids, although prolapsed hemorrhoids may not respond well. Afterward, some patients find that they are unable to control their bowels completely, but this is a short-term side effect that corrects itself fairly soon.

Other treatments include drying up the hemorrhoids with heat (infrared photocoagulation) or with cold (cryosurgery). The former, used for first-degree hemorrhoids, is effective and painless, but about 18 percent of patients need further treatment. The latter is less often used since, although it is useful in the treatment of prolapsed hemorrhoids, it may cause discomfort and a discharge for up to two weeks afterward.

The treatment of choice for second-degree hemorrhoids is to tie them off (ligation). Sometimes the hemorrhoids are injected at the same time. The results are good and up to two thirds of patients with third-degree hemorrhoids may also be helped by this procedure. Four percent of those treated develop pain as a result and 1 percent may have bleeding that occasionally is bad enough to warrant readmission to the hospital.

For third-degree hemorrhoids, the usual course of action is hemorrhoidectomy in which they are actually removed. The results are excellent, with symptoms recurring in only 5 percent of patients over a period of five years. Occasionally patients may have problems such as pain, bleeding, or acute retention of urine after the operation. Urinary retention is treated with catheterization (insertion of a tube into the bladder to drain it until it regains its function). If the bleeding is severe, it may be necessary to take the patient back to the operating room and pack the bowel with gauze around a large rubber tube. This is then removed after forty-eight hours.

Specialists differ on the correct way to treat thrombosed prolapsed hemorrhoids. Some put the patient to bed with the foot of the bed raised, give painkillers, and put ice packs on the hemorrhoid and allow the condition to settle by itself. Others prefer to do an immediate hemorrhoidectomy or anal dilatation.

PERIANAL HEMATOMA (THROMBOSED EXTERNAL HEMORRHOID)

Strictly speaking, this is not a true hemorrhoid but a ruptured vein at the edge of the anus. It develops suddenly, often after the patient has been straining to pass a stool. There is pain and a lump that, if untreated, either subsides over the course of a few days or else bursts and releases a small amount of clotted blood.

Treatment consists of opening the hematoma under a local anesthetic and removing the clotted blood inside. If, however, it has already started to resolve, frequent hot baths are all that is necessary.

COMPLEMENTARY TREATMENT

Aromatherapy
Myrrh and cypress are among the oils that may be recommended.

Herbalism
Witch-hazel ointment or lotion will relieve itching and soothe inflammation around the anus. The appropriately named pilewort in ointment form will relieve pain and reduce inflammation. Chamomile suppositories, which are inserted into the rectum, may be soothing. A number of other herbs are also used.

Homeopathy
Nux vomica may be prescribed for patients who have large hemorrhoids that prolapse during defecation and who suffer from constipation and from burning pains that are worse at night. Burning and itching at night, relieved by lying down and associated with hard stools and sometimes diarrhea in the early morning, may respond well to sulphur. Patients with very large prolapsed hemorrhoids that bleed and burn and feel better when bathed with cold water may benefit from aloes. Hamamelis is helpful if there is profuse bleeding. Various other remedies may also be appropriate.

HERPES SIMPLEX

THERE ARE TWO TYPES of herpes simplex virus, known as HSV 1 and HSV 2. Both are very common. HSV 1 is mainly responsible for causing cold sores and HSV 2 produces genital herpes. However, approximately 5 percent of cases of genital herpes are due to the HSV 1 virus, the infection probably having been transmitted during oral sex.

COLD SORES

A large percent of the population have antibodies to HSV 1, which means that at some time they must have been infected with the virus. However, only a minority—about 20–40 percent of the U.S. population—have recurrent symptoms.

The first attack, or primary infection, usually occurs in childhood. Mothers who have HSV 1 antibodies pass them through the placenta to their infants, who are thus protected for the first year or so of their lives. But after this, the immunity dwindles and primary infection is commonest between the ages of one and five.

In a large number of cases, no symptoms at all occur at the time of the primary infection. However, some children react quite severely to the virus. The mouth and throat become painful and the child is feverish, unwell, and unwilling to eat. The gums swell and may bleed. Shallow white ulcers develop on the tongue, gums, and the lining of the mouth and throat, and saliva may dribble from the mouth if the child finds it painful to swallow. The lymph glands in the neck may become swollen and tender. In mild cases, the worst is over within three to five days, but in more severe cases the infection may take up to two weeks to subside. If the child is unable to drink because of the pain from the ulcers, hospital admission may be necessary so that fluid can be given by an intravenous drip.

213

Occasionally one of the fingers may be the site of primary infection in the form of a herpetic whitlow. The area becomes swollen and painful and then blistered over a period of seven to ten days, finally subsiding over the next month.

Once the herpes virus has gotten inside the body it can lie dormant in the tissues, ready to cause trouble if the patient's resistance drops, through stress, injury, or illness. Fortunately, the recurrences are never as severe as the primary infection can be. Attacks may also be brought on by cold, exposure to strong sunlight, or menstruation. A group of small blisters appears, usually on the lips or around the mouth; after a few days, they burst and then scab over. Healing normally takes ten to fourteen days.

GENITAL HERPES

This is a very common infection that is usually sexually transmitted. In 1979 the incidence was about 30 per 100,000 people in the United States. As in the case of cold sores, the primary infection is usually the most severe, although in women there may be no symptoms if all the blisters develop high up in the vagina.

In genital herpes, either in the primary infection or the recurrence, blisters may occur in the vagina, on the cervix, and on the vulva in women, on the shaft of the penis in men, around the anus or even on the buttocks and thighs. In male homosexuals they commonly involve the anus and rectum. The patient may be aware of a burning, tingling, or itching sensation in the affected skin for a few hours before the blisters appear. These then break down to form shallow, very painful ulcers. Female patients may have a watery vaginal discharge. The lymph glands in the groins may become enlarged and tender, and, if there is an ulcer close to the urethral opening, passing water may be very painful. Indeed, this may be so severe as to cause complete urinary retention, which needs urgent medical treatment.

An individual attack lasts between three and five days, and patients may have many attacks during the course of a year, although the average is three to four. The infection may continue to recur over a number of years before eventually dying out.

COMPLICATIONS OF HERPES INFECTIONS

The commonest complication, especially of cold sores, is bacterial infection. If this occurs repeatedly, there is a risk that the affected skin will become scarred.

Patients who suffer from eczema (even if it is quiescent at the time) may react very severely to a herpes infection, developing eczema herpeticum or Kaposi's varicelliform eruption, in which there is a widespread rash and fever. In severe cases, the blisters cover a large amount of the body surface and if untreated almost 10 percent of patients will die. This type of infection may also occur in people who are suffering from burns. It is therefore vital that anyone with an active cold sore should avoid all contact with patients who have eczema or burns.

One of the most worrying complications of cold sores is the development of ulcers on the surface of the eye, since not only are these painful but they can cause scarring that may lead to blindness.

If a patient's resistance to infection is very low, he may develop a generalized herpes infection that in severe cases can cause death from hepatitis or encephalitis. This is most likely to occur in patients whose immunity has been lowered by intensive cancer therapy or by AIDS, or in newborn babies whose mothers are suffering from a genital herpes infection at the time of delivery. In the case of a baby, the first symptoms of fever, vomiting, diarrhea, breathing problems, jaundice, and convulsions usually appear on the fifth day of life. Often the infection is fatal. It is standard procedure, therefore, to do a cesarean section for any mother who is suffering from herpes when her pregnancy comes to term, rather than allow a vaginal delivery.

TESTS

These are usually unnecessary since the diagnosis is obvious in most cases. However, a swab taken from a blister can be cultured to show the virus.

TRADITIONAL TREATMENT

Drying agents such as rubbing alcohol encourage the ulcers to crust over and help to diminish the pain. Povidone-iodine also works in this way as well as having a mild antiviral action and its use may help to prevent bacterial infection from occurring.

In recent years, specific antiviral agents have been developed, including vidarabine and acyclovir (ACV). Both of these, in ointment form, have been used in the treatment of herpes eye infections, while ACV, given as tablets or intravenously, has been found to reduce considerably the mortality from generalized herpes. Intravenous ACV may also be necessary for patients whose genital herpes has caused retention of urine. Applied locally, ACV can be useful in the treatment of both cold sores and genital herpes but needs to be used as soon as symptoms begin and before the blisters appear. Patients who suffer from frequent severe recurrences of genital herpes can be treated with ACV taken orally over a period of several months.

RECENT ADVANCES

Doctors at the University of Birmingham Medical School, England, and others in the United States, notably in Atlanta, Georgia, have been working on the possibility of producing a vaccine against herpes. In Britain, the sexual partners of some patients with herpes have been successfully treated with such a vaccine as a preventive measure. The vaccine has also been shown to be of use for patients if given after the first attack of herpes. And in the United States, recent research suggests that it may be possible to develop a vaccine which will modify recurrences of herpes in infected patients.

COMPLEMENTARY TREATMENT

Aromatherapy
Lavender, lemon, and geranium are among the oils that may help to dry up a cold sore.

Herbalism
Echinacea may be used to promote the body's defenses against viral infection. Golden seal, St. John's wort, myrrh, or calendula tinctures may be applied topically to act as an antiseptic and to promote healing. St. John's wort is also a painkiller.

Homeopathy

Any number of remedies may help to prevent recurrences of cold sores or genital herpes, but the prescription depends very much on the individual patient.

Nutrition

The herpes virus needs the amino acid arginine in order to thrive; lysine, however, will prevent it from flourishing. A diet that is low in arginine and high in lysine is therefore likely to be recommended during an attack, plus a supplement of lysine. Arginine is found in peanuts, cashew nuts, pecan nuts, almonds, chocolate, edible seeds, peas, nontoasted cereals, gelatin, carob, coconut, whole-wheat and white flour, soya beans, wheat germ, garlic, and ginseng. Fish, chicken, beef, lamb, milk, cheese, beans, brewer's yeast, and mung bean sprouts are high in lysine and low in arginine.

SELF-HELP

Because it seems as though there may be a link between genital herpes infection and cancer of the cervix, all women who have recurrent attacks should have a Pap smear every year.

Female patients with cold sores should take care when applying or removing makeup to avoid spreading the virus. All patients should, when washing, dry their eyes before drying the infected area and should also avoid kissing or sharing cups, cutlery, towels, or washcloths during the course of the infection.

Fresh lemon juice applied to a cold sore as soon as the itching begins may promote rapid healing.

ORGANIZATIONS

Herpes Network
P.O. Box 267
Framingham, MA 01701
617/879-0409
(Publishes *New Day Register.*)

Herpes Resource Center
Box 100
Palo Alto, CA 94302
415/328-7710
(Publishes *The Helper*, quarterly.)

HIGH BLOOD PRESSURE (Hypertension)

DEFINITION

In medical terminology, high blood pressure is known as hypertension, tension in this respect meaning pressure. Blood pressure is measured using an instrument known as a sphygmomanometer ("sphyg" for short) of which there are now various types available. The traditional sphyg has a column of mercury that travels up a graduated glass tube to show the pressure that is being exerted on the patient's arm by an inflatable cuff. Blood pressure is therefore measured in millimeters of mercury (abbreviated to mm Hg). Two readings are taken as the pressure in the cuff is slowly released. The first is where the doctor, listening with a stethoscope over an artery at the patient's elbow, starts to hear the sound of a pulse and the second is where that sound becomes muffled or disappears. The first reading is known as the systolic pressure and corresponds to the pressure in the arteries when the heart contracts, pumping blood through them. The second reading is the diastolic pressure, which corresponds to the pressure in the arteries when the heart relaxes, allowing it to fill up with more blood.

Normal blood pressure is usually said to be 120/80 but, in fact, there is a range of values that could be taken as normal. For example, 110/70 or 125/85 are normal for many people. Because of this range, it is difficult to say exactly where high blood pressure begins. The World Health Organization defines hypertension as a level of 165/95 or more, recorded in a sitting patient. Below 140/90 is defined as normal and the range between 140/90 and 165/95 is regarded as "borderline."

Usually, when trying to diagnose hypertension in a patient, a doctor will take a series of readings, since there are many factors that can affect the level of the blood pressure. For example, anxiety or excitement can

219

cause it to rise, but it will drop when the patient is very relaxed or asleep.

ESSENTIAL AND SECONDARY HYPERTENSION

In the vast majority of cases, no underlying illness can be found to account for the patient's hypertension, which is therefore said to be "essential." It has been suggested that the condition of the blood vessels and their response to a number of hormonal and nervous stimuli may be partly responsible, but it seems likely that in any one case a combination of many factors is involved. In many cases, hypertension and atheroma (hardening of the arteries) seem to go hand in hand. Each seems to make the other worse and it is hard to say whether one condition initially caused the other (a chicken-and-egg situation) or whether a third factor is responsible for causing both.

Essential hypertension usually begins during the thirties or forties and very often there is a family history of the condition. It is particularly common in black people, in whom it may be quite severe. However, in some 5 percent of patients, some definite abnormality can be found that has resulted in "secondary" hypertension. This may occur at any age.

Twenty percent of all cases of secondary hypertension are due to kidney disease. Because it is vital that blood flows steadily through the kidneys to have its waste products and excess water removed, the kidneys have a special mechanism for controlling their own blood flow. If the blood pressure drops, a substance known as renin is released that acts on a protein in the blood (angiotensin I) to produce angiotensin II. This latter substance not only acts directly on the blood vessels, constricting them and thus raising the blood pressure, but also stimulates the secretion of the hormone aldosterone, whose effect is to raise the blood pressure. Thus, the flow of blood through the kidneys returns to normal and, when it has done so, no more renin is secreted. It is thought that kidney disease causes hypertension by interfering with this mechanism and causing a steady excretion of renin.

The commonest form of kidney disease to produce hypertension is chronic pyelonephritis (described in the section on urinary tract infections). When only one kidney is affected, its removal may bring the blood pressure back to normal. Another condition that can be treated surgically is renal artery stenosis. In this, the artery that supplies blood to the kidney is constricted, so that the blood flow is reduced.

A similar condition affecting the aorta (the main artery leading from the heart) is known as coarctation and, like renal artery stenosis, it is commoner in males than in females and can be corrected surgically. Coarctation is rare and only causes hypertension in the upper part of the body, making it relatively easy to diagnose. It is usually apparent before the patient reaches the age of thirty.

Other causes of secondary hypertension (all of which are rare) include conditions in which the adrenal glands produce an excess of hormones that have the effect of raising the blood pressure. In Cushing's syndrome excessive quantities of steroids are secreted. In the very rare Conn's syndrome the hormone produced is aldosterone. And the tumor known as a pheochromocytoma (or "pheo" for short), which may occasionally be found outside the adrenals, produces large amounts of adrenaline and noradrenaline.

In Cushing's syndrome, the patient may become obese, although the legs remain thin, and his face becomes moon-shaped and flushed. Women may notice that they are becoming hairy. Patients suffering from Conn's syndrome may complain of weakness, headache, cramps, and tingling, and may pass large amounts of urine. The symptoms of a patient with a pheochromocytoma are often intermittent, as is the hypertension, and attacks may be precipitated by a number of things, such as emotional upsets or exertion. The symptoms include severe headache, nausea, vomiting, abdominal pain, sweating, and a rapid heart rate. Fortunately, removal of the tumor will cure the condition.

TESTS

Because hypertension can be secondary to other conditions, it may be necessary to do a number of tests before making a definite diagnosis of essential hypertension. This is especially the case if the patient is relatively young.

Examination
The doctor may feel the pulses in the patient's groins—if they are less full than they should be, this may be a sign of coarctation of the aorta. An abdominal examination will enable him to feel whether the pa-

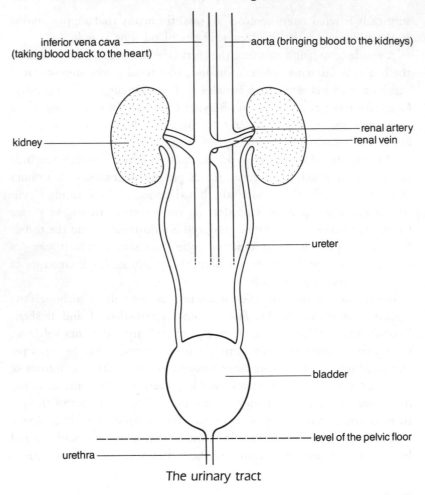

The urinary tract

tient's kidneys are abnormally large. He may also listen to the abdomen with a stethoscope, since a murmur can be heard in 50 percent of the patients who have renal artery stenosis.

Urine
The urine may be examined for protein and blood since these may be found in kidney disease or in advanced cases of hypertension. It may also be tested for sugar, which is sometimes found in the urine of patients who have Cushing's syndrome or a pheochromocytoma. If

protein is detected, a collection of the total urine passed over twenty-four hours may be required for an assessment of kidney function.

Blood

Blood may be taken to test for urea (a waste product whose level rises in kidney failure) and for potassium (which may be low in Conn's syndrome, Cushing's syndrome, and renal artery stenosis). It may also be taken when the patient is fasting to test for cholesterol and fats, since high levels of these may be associated with hypertension and an increased risk of heart attack.

Ophthalmoscopy

The doctor may examine the back of the patient's eyes with an ophthalmoscope, since this is the one place in the body that a clear view can be obtained of the blood vessels. Early signs of hypertension include spasm of the arteries, which appear narrowed. As the condition advances, the vessel walls become thickened and opaque, which gives them, at first, a coppery appearance and, later, a silvery look. Little patches of blood may be seen where the vessels have leaked. In the severe form of high blood pressure known as malignant hypertension (see below), the optic disc that is visible as a light-colored circle at the back of the eye becomes swollen and its edges become blurred. Small hemorrhages and fluffy-looking white patches, or exudates, formed by protein leaking from the vessels may also be visible.

Aortography

This is done only if renal artery stenosis is suspected. A catheter is inserted into the aorta (usually through a needle in the femoral artery in the groin) and a dye is pumped in that will show up on X-ray. The renal artery branches off from the aorta and will be clearly outlined by the dye.

X-rays

A chest X-ray may be done, since it will show up any enlargement of the heart that has resulted from longstanding hypertension. (Such enlargement will also be shown by an electrocardiogram or ECG.) Occasionally an X-ray of the kidneys may be performed.

Tests for Cushing's, Conn's, and Pheochromocytoma
Various specialized tests are available to diagnose these conditions, most of which involve collection of the urine over twenty-four hours, plus blood tests.

SYMPTOMS OF HYPERTENSION

In the early stages, patients may have few symptoms. Indeed, it is not at all uncommon for hypertension to be discovered during the course of a routine medical examination, the patient having been quite unaware that his blood pressure was raised.

Among the symptoms that may occur are headaches that are often at the back of the head and present upon waking and that tend to wear off during the course of the day. Nosebleeds are not uncommon. Patients may also complain of noises in the head, dizziness, irritability, visual problems, or palpitations.

As the hypertension progresses, further symptoms may arise as a result of the damage that it causes to various parts of the body.

DANGERS OF HYPERTENSION

High blood pressure is always treated, even if the patient has no symptoms, because of the damage that it can do. Borderline hypertension is usually treated if the patient has symptoms.

Surveys have shown that patients with hypertension have an increased risk of stroke, heart failure, coronary heart disease, and kidney disease. Treatment has been shown to reduce the mortality from strokes and kidney failure and, although there is less evidence that it protects patients from heart attacks, the newest medications have not been in use for long enough to be assessed in this respect.

Left Ventricular Failure (LVF)
Hypertension puts strain on the left side of the heart, which receives blood from the lungs and pumps it out to the rest of the body. As a result, the left side of the heart enlarges (left ventricular hypertrophy) and ultimately may be unable to cope with the work, in which case its function deteriorates (left ventricular failure). Patients who have LVF may experience shortness of breath due to the pooling of blood in the

lungs. This is commonest when they lie down and they make wake feeling breathless during the night.

Coronary Heart Disease

One of the commonest sites at which atheroma (hardening of the arteries) occurs is within the coronary arteries that supply the muscle of the heart with blood. The rate at which atheroma is formed is speeded up in patients with hypertension and may cause angina or a heart attack.

Cerebrovascular Disease

The arteries supplying the brain may also get occluded (blocked). High blood pressure may result in weaknesses appearing in the walls of these arteries, which can then hemorrhage, causing a stroke or even death.

Kidney Damage

The kidneys may be damaged by high blood pressure, even when kidney disease has had nothing to do with causing the condition. In severe cases, kidney failure may occur.

Malignant Hypertension

In some 2 percent of cases, the blood pressure rises very high and can cause widespread damage, resulting in death within about a year if it is untreated. Fortunately, the introduction of modern drugs now means that the life expectancy for these patients is almost normal once they are on treatment.

Malignant hypertension is commoner in men than in women and usually occurs between the ages of forty and sixty. The small blood vessels in the kidneys, eyes, and brain are severely damaged, resulting in renal failure, deteriorating eyesight, and mental confusion. Left ventricular failure also occurs. If untreated, the patient may have seizures, lapse into a coma, and die from renal failure or from a stroke.

TRADITIONAL TREATMENT

Secondary Hypertension

Treatment will depend on the underlying cause. Often, as in the case of coarctation of the aorta and renal artery stenosis, it is surgical.

Surgery also has a part to play in the treatment of Cushing's and Conn's syndromes and pheochromocytoma, when the tissue responsible for the excessive hormonal secretion may be removed, after which any residual hypertension is treated with drugs. Kidney disease that is causing hypertension may require the kidneys to be removed and either dialysis or a transplant will be necessary.

Essential Hypertension

The GP may suggest some or all of the measures given under "Self-Help" below. They are all worth trying, since it is sometimes possible to reduce the blood pressure to normal levels without the use of drugs.

Thiazide Diuretics
These are often the first drugs to be given to a patient with hypertension. Their main action is to make the kidneys excrete more water, thus reducing the volume of blood circulating around the body, but they probably also cause a relaxation in the blood vessels, both of these actions resulting in a drop in the blood pressure.

Although they may take up to eight weeks before their full benefit is felt, the thiazide diuretics have many advantages. They have minimal side effects, which may be elevated blood sugar and LDL (low-density lipoprotein) cholesterol, and rarely need to be stopped because of these. They can be used in combination with other blood-pressure drugs and will enhance their effect. In addition, they are useful in the treatment of black patients, who often don't respond to some of the other drugs, such as beta blockers.

The main disadvantage of thiazide diuretics is that they cause the body to lose potassium. Although this may not be a problem in the short term, it may ultimately produce symptoms such as weakness and muscle cramps. Patients who are on the heart drug digoxin are particularly likely to develop abnormal heart rhythms if they become short of potassium, and so will always be given a potassium supplement if they are put on thiazide diuretics. Some doctors like to give all patients on thiazides a potassium supplement and combined preparations are available.

Thiazide diuretics may cause a buildup of uric acid in the blood and so are unsuitable for patients who suffer from gout. They may also precipitate gout in those who have not previously suffered from it. Rashes may occur and, occasionally, dizziness and tiredness during the first few weeks of treatment.

The drug most commonly used is hydrochlorothiazide (HCTZ).

Loop Diuretics

These work in a different way from the thiazide diuretics and are not commonly used in the treatment of hypertension. However, they are useful for patients who are suffering from kidney disease. They, too, may cause the potassium level to fall and the uric acid level to rise, and they may cause disturbances in the levels of fats, calcium, and other minerals in the blood. They include furosemide and bumetanide, which are also available combined with a potassium supplement.

Potassium-Sparing Diuretics

These diuretics, which include amiloride and triamterene, have the advantage that they do not cause a drop in potassium levels in the blood. They are also less likely than the other diuretics to cause a rise in uric acid, although this may still occur. They are unsuitable for patients with kidney failure and may cause sexual side effects such as impotence. Weakness, cramps, swelling of the breasts in men, and disturbance of the menstrual cycle in women may also occur.

Beta Blockers

These are probably the commonest drugs to be used in the treatment of hypertension. Although they may sometimes produce unpleasant side effects, they have been available for a considerable time and are therefore tried and tested.

The way in which beta blockers act to reduce blood pressure is not absolutely clear. It is known, however, that they prevent the hormones adrenaline and noradrenaline from acting on so-called beta receptors in the brain, heart, and lungs, and in the muscle layers in the walls of the blood vessels. Stimulation of the beta receptors in the brain causes a rise in blood pressure, of those in the heart (known as beta-1 receptors) an increased rate and force of heartbeat, and of those in the blood vessels and lungs (known as beta-2 receptors) relaxation of the vessels and of the bronchioles of the lungs. Beta blockade produces the opposite effect. The earliest beta blockers prevented all beta stimulation and therefore were unsuitable for use in asthmatic patients, since they could cause constriction of the bronchioles and precipitate an asthmatic attack. These nonselective blockers, which can also cause cold hands, fatigue, and unpleasant dreams, include propranolol and nadolol, which are still used for suitable patients. However, propranolol seems to work less well in smokers.

Selective beta blockers block only the beta-1 receptors and include metoprolol and atenolol. They are more suitable for asthmatics and can be used for insulin-dependent diabetics, whereas the nonselective blockers may mask hypoglycemic attacks and are therefore not suitable.

Side effects of the beta blockers include a slow heart rate, fatigue—especially during exercise—dizziness, sexual problems such as impotence, and a lowering of HDL (high-density lipoprotein) cholesterol.

Vasodilators

Vasodilators—drugs that cause dilation of the blood vessels—are normally used in combination with a diuretic or a beta blocker or both.

HYDRALAZINE

Although vasodilators are useful drugs, they have a considerable range of side effects that may, however, be reduced if they are used in combination with other types of antihypertensive therapy. Hydralazine may cause headache, a rapid heart rate, palpitations, tremor, nausea, dizziness, weakness, tiredness, and flushing of the skin. However, it is safe in pregnancy. A derivative of hydralazine is minoxidil.

PRAZOSIN

This is less likely to cause palpitations than hydralazine, but patients may faint after the first dose due to a sudden drop in the blood pressure. Advice is usually given, therefore, to take the very first dose when going to bed at night. It is customary to start with a small dose and gradually increase it during the following weeks.

ALPHA BLOCKERS

Prazosin is thought to prevent constriction of the blood vessels by blocking stimulation of the so-called alpha receptors in their walls. Another drug, labetalol, is both an alpha and beta blocker. At the time of writing a preparation called doxazosin has been developed but not yet licensed for use. It seems to give effective control of the blood pressure in both black and white patients and has the advantage of lowering the blood cholesterol while raising the levels of HDL, which appears to have a protective effect against atheroma. It seems to be safe for use in patients with diabetes, asthma, or gout, and unlike beta blockers, does not cause impotence. There may be side effects, however, and these include tiredness, dizziness, fluid retention, blurring of vision, headache, and constipation.

Calcium Antagonists

These drugs, which include nifedipine and verapamil, have only recently come into general use, but are becoming increasingly popular. Originally they were thought to act by controlling levels of calcium in the body fluids, but the mechanism has been shown to be a great deal more complicated than this.

They can be used in patients who have diabetes or angina, and indeed they seem to have a preventive effect against the development of atheroma. They also seem to relieve spasm in the coronary arteries that supply the heart muscle and are therefore useful in the treatment of patients with angina. Unfortunately, they produce an effective lowering of blood pressure in only about 50–60 percent of patients, although others may respond if one of the drugs is combined with a beta blocker or an ACE inhibitor (see below). The main side effects include headache, palpitations, nausea, swelling of the ankles, and flushing, but these are less likely to occur with slow-release preparations. A recent discovery is that the calcium antagonists may also cause swelling of the breasts in men, although this will subside once the drug is stopped.

ACE Inhibitors

These, too, are recently developed drugs. ACE stands for angiotensin-converting enzyme, an enzyme that plays a vital role in the conversion in the blood of angiotensin I into angiotensin II. The action of the drugs is to prevent this reaction from taking place. Angiotensin II has a powerful constricting effect on the blood vessels and its production is stimulated by the excretion of renin from the kidneys (see above).

The ACE inhibitors, which include captopril and enalapril, are effective in about 90 percent of patients, but may need to be used together with a loop diuretic or a calcium antagonist.

Older Drugs
Before the beta blockers came on the market, the drugs in use for the treatment of hypertension worked in a fairly crude way on blood-pressure-controlling receptors in the brain. As a result, they had many side effects and, since the development of newer therapies, they have tended to be used less and less. However, two—methyldopa and clonidine—are still used in certain situations and like other older drugs they continue to be used for patients who have been taking them for years and are happy on them.

Methyldopa is the drug of choice in pregnancy, since it is known to be perfectly safe. Indeed, if a woman who is hypertensive is planning to get pregnant, her GP may decide to change her medication so that she is already established on methyldopa by the time she conceives. There will therefore be no risk to the baby. It may be combined with hydralazine, which is also safe in pregnancy.

Methyldopa and clonidine are useful drugs for patients with renal problems because they do not reduce the flow of blood to the kidneys. In the United States, clonidine is now available as a transdermal patch—a sticking patch that contains the drug and slowly releases it into the skin over a period of time.

Side effects of methyldopa and clonidine include drowsiness, dizziness, and a dry mouth. Methyldopa may cause headaches and clonidine may cause constipation. An additional problem with clonidine is that it must not be stopped suddenly after a prolonged period of therapy, since this may result in the blood pressure rising rapidly. It is important, therefore, that patients who take clonidine never run out of their tablets.

COMPLEMENTARY TREATMENT

Acupuncture
Hypertension is said to be due to hyperactivity of the yang (or masculine, positive) aspect of Chi or to an accumulation of phlegm and damp. Treatment consists either of reducing yang and stimulating yin (the balancing, feminine, negative aspect) or of expelling phlegm and damp. There are also some specific points whose use will bring down the blood pressure.

Aromatherapy

Clary sage, lavender, melissa, lemon, and ylang ylang are some of the oils that may be prescribed.

Herbalism

Mistletoe, hawthorn, lime blossom, and garlic are among the remedies used by herbalists in the treatment of hypertension. Mistletoe dilates the blood vessels, slows and steadies the heart rate, and is a diuretic. Hawthorn dilates the coronary blood vessels and slows and stabilizes the contraction of the heart. Lime blossom is particularly useful for patients who are anxious or tense, since it has a relaxant effect as well as dilating the blood vessels and being a diuretic. Garlic dilates the blood vessels and also reduces the amount of cholesterol in the bloodstream.

Homeopathy

The choice of remedy is vast since there is no set pattern of symptoms for patients with hypertension. However, glonoine may be effective for patients who suffer from pounding headaches, palpitations, and a feeling of fullness in the chest, whereas those complaining of weakness, dizziness, and a fear that they will collapse may respond well to gelsemium.

Hypnotherapy

By teaching the patient to relax and to cope with stress, hypnotherapy can be useful in the treatment of hypertension.

Manipulation

This may help insofar as it can relieve physical tension and muscle spasm.

Nutrition

Vitamins C, B complex, and E will help to keep cholesterol levels down and regulate blood clotting; vitamin C also keeps the arteries healthy.

SELF-HELP

There are a number of steps that the hypertensive patient can take that should help to control his blood pressure. Indeed, in some cases of mild hypertension such self-help measures may be all that is necessary and the use of drugs may therefore be avoided.

Blood pressure tends to be higher in overweight, sedentary people and in those who smoke. The patient should therefore try to keep relatively slim, give up smoking, and exercise regularly. Recent studies have shown that reducing alcohol intake is beneficial for hypertensive patients. The role of salt in the development of hypertension is still being debated by specialists. However, studies have shown that in communities where the salt intake is low throughout life, high blood pressure tends not to occur. Some studies have shown benefits in reducing the amount of salt in the diet, but the effects seem to be a highly individual thing—possibly genetically determined. It is worth reducing one's salt intake, therefore, to see whether it is helpful in one's own case. A low-fat diet is also beneficial, but a study done in the United States has shown that a certain amount of olive oil in the diet can help to reduce the blood pressure. Fresh fruit and vegetables contain potassium and this, too, seems to have a lowering effect on the blood pressure.

Naturopaths may recommend excluding sugar, coffee, and red meat from the diet.

Certain drugs may contribute to a rise in blood pressure. It is usually recommended that women whose blood pressure rises while they are on the contraceptive Pill should stop taking it. If necessary, they may take the progestogen-only Pill, since it is the estrogen component that is responsible for the rise. Nonsteroidal antiinflammatory drugs (NSAIDs), which are taken by arthritic patients, may also affect the blood pressure, but substituting a simple painkiller such as acetaminophen may bring it down again.

Anything that will help to reduce stress and promote relaxation, such as yoga or meditation, will also be beneficial.

IMPOTENCE

DEFINITION

Impotence is defined as the inability to achieve or sustain an erection adequate for satisfactory intercourse. It is extremely common, affecting about one man in every ten at some time or another.

CAUSES

Both erection and ejaculation are reflex involuntary actions, governed by nerves running from the spine to the genitalia. However, they are also controlled to some extent by psychological stimuli and are dependent on an adequate output of male hormones (androgens). But because they are reflex actions, they cannot be made to happen voluntarily—a man cannot decide to have an erection in the same way that he can decide to raise his arm or open his mouth.

It is thought that just over half of all cases of impotence are psychogenic—that is, they are due to psychological problems. Temporary impotence is common during any illness or if the patient is anxious, depressed, or under stress. Very often, one episode of impotence occurs when the man is tired or has had too much to drink and as a result he begins to worry about his sexual performance. This makes it more difficult for him to have an erection the next time he tries, and a vicious circle arises in which his impotence causes anxiety and his anxiety causes impotence.

Of those cases that are due to a physical cause, 27 percent are caused by diabetes, and 32 percent by injury. Long-term or permanent impotence may be due to disease of the blood vessels, hormonal abnormalities, diseases involving the nervous system (particularly diabetes), alcohol or drug abuse, certain prescribed medicines, damage to the spine or pelvic area, unavoidable damage during a prostatectomy or operations on the bladder or rectum, or problems affecting the penis itself.

The penis contains two spongy compartments that fill up with blood

233

when a man becomes sexually excited, causing it to become stiff. If the blood vessels that run into the penis are badly affected by atheroma (hardening of the arteries), blood cannot flow as readily and this may be a cause of impotence. When atheroma is widespread, resulting in inadequate amounts of blood being delivered to the legs and causing pain when walking and poor healing, the condition is referred to as peripheral vascular disease. Fifty percent of men who suffer from this will be affected by impotence.

To achieve an erection a properly functioning nervous system is necessary, since this controls the initial dilation of the blood vessels supplying the penis and the relaxation of the muscles in the spongy compartments, which allows blood to flow in. It is probably also responsible for closing down the outflow of blood from the penis, thus helping to keep it erect. Diseases that interfere with this will cause impotence. Diabetes is the commonest of these (see section on diabetic neuropathy). Other causes include multiple sclerosis and damage to the lower end of the spinal cord, from which the nerves run to the penis.

Patients who have low circulating levels of male hormones will suffer from impotence, but because the hormonal lack will also reduce their libido (sex drive), they rarely complain about their impotence. Medication with estrogen, in the treatment of cancer of the prostate, for example, will have the same effect.

Both illegal and prescribed drugs may cause impotence. Those that most commonly do so are cannabis, opiates (such as morphine and heroin), barbiturates, drugs that lower the blood pressure (particularly bethanidine, guanethidine, methyldopa, and beta blockers), diuretics, and the tricyclic antidepressants. Alcohol frequently has the same effect.

Peyronie's disease is a problem affecting the penis in which fibrous plaques develop, so that it is no longer soft and mobile. When an erection occurs, the penis can't stretch correctly and becomes deformed. This may be associated with pain. The cause is unknown, but some cases seem to resolve after a few years.

DIAGNOSIS

It is very important that impotence due to a psychological cause should be differentiated from that due to a physical cause. Sometimes this will be apparent from the history. A patient who still has early-morning erections and who can masturbate satisfactorily has psychogenic impotence. This type usually has a sudden onset whereas physical impotence, in which an erection becomes impossible under any circumstances, is more likely to come on gradually.

Impotence may also be classified as primary or secondary. A man with primary impotence has never been able to have intercourse whereas secondary impotence comes on later in life, after a previously satisfactory sex life. The type of onset, however, gives no clue as to the cause.

TESTS

If it is suspected that a man has physical impotence, there are various tests that may be used to determine the cause. Initially, the doctor will examine the penis and testes, looking for signs of any abnormality, and will take the patient's blood pressure. He will also check the pulses in the legs and feet, since absence of these will suggest that there is a problem with the blood vessels. The urine will be tested for sugar in case impotence is the first sign of diabetes. Checking the reflexes in the legs and testing the genital area for sensation to touch and vibration will indicate whether or not the problem is one involving the nervous system.

If a hormonal problem is suspected, blood will be taken to test for hormone levels. If the patient is referred to a specialist, further tests may be undertaken, including the use of a special stethoscope to measure the blood pressure in the penis. The ability to have an erection while asleep can also be determined. Normally, some degree of erection will occur during periods of rapid eye movement (which correlate with episodes of dreaming). This is known as nocturnal penile tumescence or NPT. Patients with psychogenic impotence will continue to have normal NPT, whereas in those whose impotence is due to a physical cause it will be reduced or absent. NPT is usually measured by a small device called a mercury strain gauge, consisting of a piece of mercury-filled tubing put around the penis and attached to a measuring instrument.

The injection of papaverine into the penis will always cause an erection unless the blood supply is seriously impaired or blood is leaking out of the penis as fast as it is flowing in. Patients who fail to have an erection after such an injection may then be investigated by more sophisticated tests to determine the exact problem that affects their blood vessels. These include the injection into the bloodstream of a substance that shows up on X-ray. Screening then shows whether the failure of the erection is due to blood leaking out of the penis.

TRADITIONAL TREATMENT

If impotence is due to psychological causes these have to be treated. In simple cases, where impotence has occurred as a result of the man's anxieties about his own performance, reassurance may be all that is necessary. In other cases, psychosexual counseling may be very helpful in restoring the patient's sexual function to normal. However, where there is a longstanding problem or the cause is a very deep-rooted one, it may be a considerable time before the patient responds to therapy.

Various substances can be injected into the penis to produce an erection, the most popular of these being papaverine. As mentioned above, this will not help patients whose impotence is due to disease of the blood vessels, but all others will respond, including those with psychogenic impotence. It is sometimes prescribed for patients whose problem is psychological, since it can be remarkably effective in restoring their self-confidence. Usually they only need to use it a few times but have the assurance of knowing that they can resort to it again if it is ever necessary. Patients with physical problems, however, need to continue with the injections long term. Once they have been taught how to inject themselves, most patients find it very simple. It is important that the correct dose is determined from the start, since an overdose can produce a prolonged erection (priapism) that after a number of hours can become very painful. There is then the risk of the blood clotting and gangrene occurring. Fortunately, only 4 percent of those using the injection develop a prolonged erection and this can be treated by an injection of metaraminol and heparin, which will counteract the papaverine and get the blood flowing again.

In young men whose impotence is due to problems with the blood vessels leading to the penis, surgery is now available that attempts to restore the blood flow. This is a very specialized technique and has about a 50 percent success rate. For those patients whose blood flow is poor because of atheroma in the larger blood vessels supplying the lower part of the body, an operation on these vessels may restore potency as well as improving the blood supply to the legs. Surgery may also be able to prevent blood leaking from the penis during an erection.

When a patient is unsuited to any of these forms of treatment, a penile implant may be the answer. These devices are of two basic types—those that are semirigid and those that can be made rigid by pumping fluid into them. One type has a fluid-filled reservoir implanted into the patient's abdomen and a pump into the scrotum. Squeezing the pump causes an erection and at the end of intercourse pressing a valve releases the fluid back to the reservoir. The simplest, semirigid implant makes the penis permanently erect, but can be bent into position. The implant does not interfere with ejaculation or with the patient's fertility.

RECENT ADVANCES

Research in Canada has shown that a new drug, called yohimbine, now available by prescription, may be helpful in the treatment of both psychogenic and physical impotence.

A device known as ErecAid has been produced that may be a practical alternative to a penile implant for some patients. It consists of a type of condom that is placed over the penis and it uses suction to bring on an erection. The erection is then maintained by placing a constriction band around the penis. The device is being used in the United States and a study of its use by ten diabetic patients at Leeds General Infirmary showed that most of them found it easy to use and effective. People in the United States can ask about various devices, including ErecAid, by consulting a urologist.

COMPLEMENTARY TREATMENT

Acupuncture
Impotence is said to be due to a lack of the yang (positive, male) aspect of the Chi of the kidney or to damage to the Chi of the heart, spleen, and kidney, which may result from emotional problems. Points are

chosen that will strengthen the yang of the kidney or the Chi of the heart, spleen, and kidney.

Aromatherapy

Various oils may be recommended, including cinnamon, clove, mint, and pine.

Herbalism

Certain herbs have a hormonelike effect on the male reproductive system and may be used in the treatment of impotence. They include damiana and saw palmetto. Ginseng, too, may help to improve the hormone balance. Other herbs with a relaxant effect may be helpful for patients with psychogenic impotence.

Homeopathy

Impotence in the elderly or impotence that has occurred as the result of an illness may respond well to sabal serrulata. If it follows injury, arnica may be helpful. In the early stages agnus castus may restore the patient's sexual function to normal, but for chronic cases lycopodium may be prescribed. If impotence is associated with anxiety, arg. nit. may be appropriate.

Hypnotherapy

Hypnosis can be very valuable for treating any complaint that is triggered or made worse by anxiety and so may be appropriate for the patient with psychogenic impotence. Not only can techniques be used to teach the patient to relax and to relieve him of his anxiety about his sexual performance but analytical techniques may in certain cases be used to try to find out the underlying reasons for his problems.

Nutrition

Impotence may be associated with low levels of zinc, so supplements of this mineral may be recommended, together with vitamin B_6, which works with it in the body.

ORGANIZATIONS

I-Anon (Impotents Anonymous)
Impotence Institute of America
119 South Ruth Street
Maryville, TN 37801
615/983-6064
(Publishes educational material.)

INCONTINENCE

INCIDENCE

Incontinence of urine is a very common problem, mainly involving women. It is estimated to affect about 5 percent of young women who have never been pregnant, 10 percent of all young to middle-age women, and 20–40 percent of older women. But in a recent survey, over 50 percent of those women suffering from incontinence said they were too embarrassed to discuss the problem with their GPs. Many thought it would clear up by itself and nearly a third waited over five years before seeking help. This is a sad state of affairs, since, if left, the condition will not improve and may get worse, whereas treatment offers an excellent chance of cure.

HOW THE BLADDER WORKS

(See the diagram of the urinary tract on page 222.) The bladder receives urine from the kidneys in frequent small spurts. Two rings of muscle, or sphincters, at the base of the bladder prevent leakage into the urethra, the tube that leads to the outside. One of these rings, the internal sphincter, is under the control of the autonomic nervous system that regulates automatic reactions over which we cannot exert willpower, such as breathing and digestion. The second ring, the external sphincter, is under voluntary control and it is this that we consciously relax when we wish to pass water. During urination, the muscle in the bladder wall (the detrusor muscle) contracts and helps to push the urine out. For this system to function normally, the entire bladder and the upper part of the urethra have to maintain their position above the muscle layer that makes up the "pelvic floor"; if the pressure becomes raised in the abdomen (for example, by coughing, sneezing, laughing, straining, or other exercise), it will affect the urethra as well as the bladder. However, if the bladder drops, any rise in pressure will affect the bladder alone and will force urine through the sphincters and down the urethra. Women are more likely to suffer from incontinence than men because the muscles of the pelvic floor and the urethral sphincters can be damaged during childbirth.

CAUSES OF INCONTINENCE

Stress incontinence is a condition in which any rise in intraabdominal pressure (from coughing, laughing, and so on) causes a slight loss of urine. This happens when the urethral sphincters are not functioning correctly and is usually due to damage to the sphincters themselves or to the ligaments that hold the bladder in position, or both. In mild cases, vigorous activity or a bad fit of coughing may be necessary for incontinence to occur, but in severe cases a slight cough or even a change of posture may result in urinary loss. Patients are usually women over forty who have had one or more children. The condition may, however, appear for the first time during pregnancy, although it usually clears up after the baby is born.

Urge incontinence is the condition in which the patient suddenly feels the need to pass water and may be unable to get to the toilet in time. This is due to abnormal contractions in the detrusor muscle of the bladder, which increase the pressure within the bladder above what can be controlled by the urethral sphincters. It may occur as a result of urinary infection, diabetes, or a disease of the nervous system, but in many cases the cause is unclear. Very occasionally, it may be produced by a slipped disc pressing on the nerves that supply the bladder.

Some patients suffer from a combination of stress incontinence and urge incontinence. In such cases, the urge incontinence usually disappears once the stress incontinence has been treated.

Incontinence may also be due to retention in the bladder of abnormally large amounts of urine. As more urine flows into the bladder from the kidneys, the pressure overcomes the urethral sphincters and overflow occurs in which some urine is passed but the bladder is not completely emptied. Usually this condition results either from an inability of the bladder to contract and expel its contained urine or from an increased resistance that prevents normal emptying. If the pressure within the bladder becomes abnormally high, there may be back-pressure on the kidneys, which can be damaged as a result. Retention with overflow may be due to damage affecting the nerves that supply the bladder, for example, injury to the spinal cord, multiple sclerosis, or extensive surgery in the pelvic area, so that the patient can no longer sense when the bladder is full. Increased resistance, preventing normal emptying, may be due to an enlarged prostate gland in men or a large fibroid or ovarian tumor (benign or malignant) in women.

Rarely, patients may have an abnormal exit (fistula) between the ureter, bladder, or urethra and the skin surface or the vagina, which means that they are permanently wet. This may be due to a congenital abnormality or may result from injury or surgery.

TESTS

An initial assessment can be made by the GP and sometimes this is all that is necessary for a diagnosis to be made. He will test the nervous system by looking in the patient's eyes and checking her reflexes and the strength of her muscles, and will examine the abdomen to see whether the kidneys are unduly large or whether any abnormal mass can be felt. An examination of the rectum will allow the doctor to assess the size of the prostate gland in a male patient and will also tell him whether there is any fecal impaction—a condition of chronic constipation in which rock-hard feces (stools) accumulate in the rectum. This can cause transient incontinence in patients of either sex, particularly in the elderly. In a woman, an internal examination through the vagina will allow the doctor to detect any degree of prolapse, which may be associated with stress incontinence. The patient may be asked to cough and if this causes a leak the doctor may proceed to do Bonney's test in which he places two fingers high up in the vagina, so that they are supporting the bladder neck. The patient is then asked to cough again. If, under these circumstances, there is no leak, it suggests that an operation that lifts the bladder neck back up above the pelvic floor will cure the condition.

For patients in whom the diagnosis is not so clear, further tests may need to be undertaken by a specialist. Uroflowmetry necessitates the patient attending the hospital with a full bladder and then passing water, in privacy, into a special machine that records the rate of flow.

Somewhat less sophisticated is the pad test in which the patient drinks a large amount of fluid and then, wearing a special pad that will absorb the urine, performs various physical exercises over a period of thirty to sixty minutes. This may be useful if the patient is uncertain about the degree of activity that causes her to be incontinent.

If it seems that a neurological disorder may be the cause of the patient's problems, measurements can be taken of the activity of the muscles of the pelvic floor, using a special instrument.

A slightly uncomfortable but very useful test is cystometry, which actually measures the pressure within the bladder and can differentiate between excessive resistance at the bladder neck and an underactive or overactive detrusor muscle. A fine tube (catheter) is passed into the bladder and another into the rectum, through which the intraabdominal pressure is measured. A known amount of fluid is put into the bladder and the level at which the patient feels a desire to pass water is noted. In a normal bladder, the desire is first felt when it contains about 150 ml and becomes strong at around 400 ml. The pressure within the bladder is measured and, when the pressure in the rectum is subtracted, this gives an estimate of the pressure being exerted by the detrusor muscle. Finally, the patient is asked to pass water into a special machine that measures the rate of flow. The whole test takes about thirty minutes. Sometimes the fluid instilled into the bladder can be seen on X-ray and a film can be taken of the whole sequence. This is known as voiding cystourethrography, or VCU.

TRADITIONAL TREATMENT

The treatment of incontinence depends on the cause. If there is any evidence of infection, this will be treated with antibiotics. If the patient has a fistula, this can be treated surgically.

For patients who are suffering from stress incontinence, particularly younger women, exercises that increase the strength of the pelvic floor may be useful. After the menopause, weakness in these muscles may be due to a lack of estrogen, so hormone replacement therapy may be effective.

A comparatively new method of treatment that seems to be proving successful is the use of a series of vaginal cones. These are made from plastic, are 5 cm long, and contain different metal weights. One is inserted into the vagina with its pointed end downward. It tends to fall out, so the patient has to use her muscles to keep it in place. When she becomes skilled at retaining the cone, she replaces it with another that is heavier. By the time she can keep the heaviest cone in place, her pelvic muscles will be working well.

In the postmenopausal patient, incontinence may result from thinning of the tissues of the urethra. The use of an estrogen cream, applied to the vagina, can sometimes be remarkably effective in such cases, as mentioned in the section on the menopause.

For those in whom these methods fail, there are several types of operation available that raise the bladder up into the abdomen, either by passing a sling (about 1 cm wide) under the bladder neck or by attaching the vagina walls to tissues higher up in the pelvis, so that the urethra is lifted. About 80 percent of patients are cured by operation, good results being less likely in those who are obese. However, even after an initial failure, a second operation may be successful. Following an operation, patients must be very careful to avoid heavy lifting or straining as these may undo the good results.

Urge incontinence may be helped by drug treatment in about 60 percent of cases. The drugs used have an effect on the nervous system, reducing the excessive activity of the detrusor muscle. They include propantheline and imipramine (which is also used in the treatment of bed-wetting in children). Unfortunately, many patients complain of side effects including a dry mouth, blurred vision, and constipation. Occasionally, an injection into the bladder wall of local anesthetic or phenol solution may reduce its irritability.

For a patient who has no apparent neurological cause for her urge incontinence, bladder retraining may be helpful. For seven days, she keeps a diary in which she records how much she drinks, how often she passes water, and how much urine she produces. Then she tries to increase the length of time she can go without urinating and over several weeks works at developing better control of her bladder. Another method is biofeedback, in which the patient has up to eight one-hour treatment sessions during which a catheter is inserted into her bladder and, as fluid is instilled into it, she is taught how to use various techniques to reduce her feeling of needing to pass water. Both these methods can be very successful, but may have a high relapse rate if patients do not continue to practice the techniques.

The treatment of retention with overflow is the treatment of the primary cause. When no specific treatment (such as prostatectomy) is appropriate, surgical enlargement of the urethra may be helpful. Various drugs may be used, including prazosin, bethanechol, and antibiotics if necessary. Some patients may have to practice intermittent self-catheterization in which they insert a tube into the bladder in order to empty it completely.

If all else fails, or if the patient is unsuitable for or refuses surgical treatment, there are two alternative methods of treatment. In mild cases, incontinence pads or appliances may be appropriate. The most modern versions are well designed so that discomfort and smell are reduced to a minimum. For more severe cases, the patient may need a permanent catheter linked to a collecting bag taped to the upper leg.

Recently an artificial urinary sphincter has been developed that has proved revolutionary in the treatment of some patients who had seemed condemned to a life of catheters. It consists of an inflatable cuff that goes around the bladder neck and is connected by a fluid-filled tube first to a pump near the skin surface and then to a reservoir of fluid in the pelvis. The patient can activate the pump, which deflates the cuff and the bladder, then empties slowly over a couple of minutes. After this, the cuff automatically reflates. Unfortunately the device is very expensive and the surgeon needs special training in order to be able to insert it, so it is not widely available. Complications include a breakdown of the mechanism, so that the bladder cannot be emptied, and irritation of the surrounding tissues by the cuff. However, in over 80 percent of cases, the device has proved successful.

RECENT ADVANCES

In Norway, doctors have found that electrical stimulation of the pelvic floor by a device inserted into the rectum for several hours a day over a period of nine months produced a significant improvement in over 60 percent of the 121 women taking part. All had been incontinent for a considerable number of years and 40 percent had regained complete continence by the end of the course.

COMPLEMENTARY TREATMENT

Acupuncture
Incontinence is said to be caused by a deficiency of Chi in the kidney and spleen. Treatment consists of using specific points to strengthen Chi in these organs and their related channels.

Aromatherapy
Oils of cypress or pine may be recommended.

Herbalism
Various herbs may be used in the treatment of incontinence, including agrimony, horsetail, marshmallow root, and yarrow.

Homeopathy
Gelsemium may be helpful in the treatment of men whose incontinence is associated with an enlarged prostate. For stress incontinence or a slow stream with dribbling, causticum may be effective. Baryta carb. and cantharis may be appropriate for elderly patients.

SELF-HELP

Because the intraabdominal pressure may be raised by constipation or obesity, these should be avoided. A high-fiber diet containing plenty of fresh fruit and vegetables is helpful. Patients with incontinence tend to reduce the amount they drink, but this may be counterproductive, since it may result in constipation or urinary infection. They should therefore drink plenty, although reduced amounts at night may be sensible. Another reason for drinking plenty is that dilute fresh urine has very little smell. Therefore, patients using pads who change them regularly and who do not allow their urine to become concentrated need have little fear of having a detectable odor.

Advice on laundry services and home-help services for the incontinent is available from local social services departments (addresses in the phone book).

ORGANIZATIONS

Help for Incontinent People
P.O. Box 544
Union, SC 29379
803/585-8789
(Publishes a quarterly newsletter.)

INFERTILITY

INCIDENCE

For many who find that they cannot have a family, the discovery can be very traumatic. Nowadays, infertility is not an uncommon occurrence—it affects some 10–15 percent of all couples. The increased incidence may be due to a number of causes, not least of which is the fact that many women are delaying their first pregnancy until their late twenties or early thirties and many of them have used contraception such as the Pill or the IUD (intrauterine device) for several years beforehand. It is thought that the Pill may interfere with the hormone balance in susceptible women—indeed, in a few, it may cause long-term loss of periods (amenorrhea). The IUD may act as a focus of infection, resulting in pelvic inflammation and blocked tubes. Even if she has not used these methods, an older woman may find it harder to get pregnant, since fertility declines after the age of thirty-five and after forty-five pregnancy is rare.

However, if one looks at 100 women who have just started trying to get pregnant, 25 will be successful during the first month, another 38 in the following five months, a further 12 in the next three months, and by the end of a year between 80 and 90 of the group will have become pregnant. The more frequently a couple has intercourse, the greater the likelihood of pregnancy, with 83 percent of those having intercourse more than three times a week being successful within six months. However, during the same period, only 16 percent of those who have intercourse less than once a week will get pregnant.

CAUSES OF INFERTILITY

In those couples who do not conceive, there may be one or more reasons for their failure. The man may have too low a sperm count; the woman may not be ovulating, or the egg, when produced, may not be able to travel down the Fallopian tube to the womb. The womb itself may be

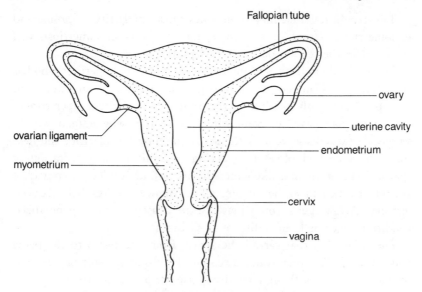

The female reproductive system

abnormal—for example, there may be fibroids present, which can interfere with the implantation of a fertilized egg. Or the sperm may be unable to swim into the womb because of hostile secretions in the vagina. In some 10 percent of cases, the cause of infertility is never established.

Ovulation—the maturation of an egg and its release from the ovary into the Fallopian tube—is dependent on normal hormone levels, each stage of the egg's development being under hormonal control. Because the sex hormones are themselves controlled by other hormones produced by the pituitary gland in the brain, anything that disrupts the working of this gland may interfere with the reproductive cycle. It may also interfere with the activity of the adrenal glands and the thyroid, which, like the ovaries, are under pituitary control.

Some 5 percent of cases of infertility that occur in young women are caused by a condition known as the Stein–Leventhal (or polycystic ovary) syndrome in which large numbers of cysts develop on the ovaries, preventing ovulation. Patients may also have problems with their periods (which can be scanty or infrequent), may become hairy or overweight, and may develop acne.

Blockage of the tubes, so that an egg cannot travel through to the womb, is usually due to a previous infection.

Two conditions that may sometimes cause infertility—fibroids and endometriosis—are dealt with in separate sections (endometriosis will be found in the section on menstrual problems).

In one third of all cases of infertility, it is the male partner who has the problems. Damage to the testes, from mumps or an injury, for example, may result in a low sperm count. Raising the temperature of the testes may have the same effect, which is why a man with a varicocele (a varicose vein in the scrotum) may be infertile, the heat from the increased blood flow acting to inhibit the maturation of sperm. Male hormones, like female hormones, are under the control of the pituitary gland so, here again, an imbalance may result in reduced fertility. A low sperm count may also be caused by more generalized conditions such as kidney disease or diabetes.

The tube (vas) that carries the sperm from the testes to the penis may, like the Fallopian tubes, become blocked as a result of infection or trauma so that, although healthy sperm are produced, they don't get through into the ejaculate.

TESTS

Before any investigations are performed, the doctor will need to take a full history from the couple involved to try to see whether this gives any clues as to what may be causing the problem. Rarely, there may be some obvious abnormality. For example, if the woman has never had a period this suggests that her reproductive system could be underdeveloped or even absent. This may result from a defect in her chromosomes, which can be determined from a blood test.

However, in most cases, the first test to be done is a sperm count. The male partner has to produce a specimen of sperm that must be delivered very rapidly to the local hospital laboratory. Because it is essential that the specimen is kept warm and is looked at within two hours of ejaculation, most hospitals provide facilities for the specimen to be produced on the premises.

If the sperm count is normal, the woman will then be tested. This usually begins with a full examination, a cervical smear, and swabs taken from the vagina and neck of the womb to ensure that there is no infection present. Repeated blood tests may be taken at different stages of the monthly cycle to see whether her hormones are rising and falling

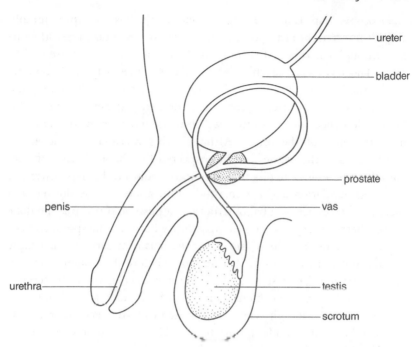

The male reproductive system, prostate, and bladder

correctly, and she may be asked to take her temperature upon waking every morning, since ovulation is often preceded by a rise in temperature.

If it seems that she is not ovulating, other tests may be done to find out why. One reason may be an excessive secretion of the hormone prolactin by the pituitary. This hormone is normally secreted during pregnancy to suppress ovulation and, if excessive amounts are produced when a woman is not pregnant, it will have the same effect and may also interfere with the menstrual cycle. It is a condition that may be brought on by stress and it may also be due to an enlarged pituitary gland, certain drugs, thyroid deficiency, and kidney disease. If a prolactin excess is suspected, blood may be taken for thyroid function tests and the skull may be X-rayed to see whether there is any evidence of enlargement of the pituitary gland.

Ultrasound may be used to check the ovaries, to detect cysts, or to follow the development of an egg before its release. In order to discover whether or not the tubes are blocked, a hysterosalpingograph or a laparoscopy ("lap") and dye may be done. In the hysterosalpingograph, a dye is injected into the womb, and X-rays are then taken to follow its flow through the tubes. If there is an obstruction, the exact site will be seen. The advantage of this test is that no anesthetic is necessary, unlike the lap and dye, in which a dye is injected into the womb and a small telescope is inserted into the abdomen just next to the umbilicus. The gynecologist can then watch to see whether the dye emerges from the ends of the tubes. Although this method has the added advantage that the ovaries can be inspected for abnormalities, it does not allow the exact site of a blockage in the tubes to be demonstrated.

If both ovulation and sperm production appear to be normal and there is no evidence of tubal obstruction, a postcoital test may be done to see whether there is some incompatibility between the sperm and the mucus in the neck of the womb. For this, it is necessary for the couple to have intercourse not more than six hours before the woman comes in for examination. The test is usually done at midcycle, when the cervical mucus should, under hormonal influence, be in such a condition that sperm can pass through easily. A specimen of the cervical mucus is taken and examined under a microscope. The sperm should be seen in considerable numbers, swimming vigorously.

In cases where the man is found to have a low sperm count, the woman will usually be investigated too, to ensure that her reproductive system is functioning normally, but additional tests are carried out on the man. Follicle-stimulating hormone (FSH) is produced by the pituitary gland and its secretion is controlled, via a feedback mechanism, by hormones from the testes. If a man with a low sperm count has high levels of FSH in his blood, it suggests that his testes have been damaged; however, if the levels are normal, this may indicate that there is a blockage in the vas, preventing sperm from being ejaculated. In such a case, a biopsy of the testes may be taken under anesthetic in order to determine whether or not they are functioning normally.

TRADITIONAL TREATMENT

A variety of drugs have been developed to stimulate ovulation in the nonovulating woman. One of these is clomiphene citrate, which is given for five days at the beginning of each cycle. Side effects include hot flashes, palpitations, blurring of vision, abdominal discomfort, and depression, which may be quite severe. There is also a risk that if a woman gets pregnant using clomiphene she will have more than one baby—15–20 percent of cases result in a multiple birth. Another drug, tamoxifen, seems to have fewer side effects, but many gynecologists prefer not to give either of these drugs for longer than a few months.

Gonadotropins—hormones that stimulate the ovaries into action—may be given by injection. They are usually given daily for five days or so to bring about the rise in the level of estrogen necessary for the egg to mature, and then a final injection of a different hormone is given to trigger ovulation. This form of treatment may be continued for up to six months, if necessary, and some 60 percent of patients get pregnant this way. Again, multiple pregnancy occurs in about 20 percent of cases.

If an excessive secretion of prolactin from the pituitary is suppressing ovulation, it can be controlled with bromocriptine. Side effects of this drug include dizziness, depression, nausea, vomiting, and headache, although these tend to diminish as treatment progresses. If a tumor of the pituitary is responsible for the excessive secretion, bromocriptine may be able to shrink it. However, in some cases, surgery may be necessary.

Patients with the Stein–Leventhal syndrome may respond to treatment with clomiphene, but the most successful treatment seems to be to remove a section from each ovary. This restores normal function in up to 80 percent of cases.

Any infection that is discovered in the course of testing will, of course, be treated, but treatment of blocked Fallopian tubes is seldom satisfactory.

If the male partner's fertility has been reduced by the increased heat generated by a varicocele, an operation may be performed to tie off the vein, so that the testes can return to their correct temperature.

IVF (in vitro fertilization) is used for women whose tubes are blocked, who have been unable to conceive over a long period of time for no apparent reason, or whose cervical mucus remains hostile to sperm. It is also used in some cases of male subfertility. The mature egg is removed from the ovary, fertilized, and allowed to grow a little before being replaced into the womb where, with luck, it will implant. The egg can be removed either at laparoscopy, the surgeon using the same telescope as in the lap and dye, or by needle, which he inserts through the vagina, using ultrasound to guide him. Ovulation is usually stimulated by clomiphene and gonadotropins.

Another form of treatment is gamete intrafallopiana transfer (GIFT), in which the egg is mixed with the sperm and immediately transferred back into the Fallopian tube so that fertilization occurs there. This technique may be used in cases of unexplained infertility or sperm problems.

AIH (artificial insemination by husband) is used where the only problem preventing pregnancy is a mechanical one—impotence or an inability to ejaculate on the part of the man. AID (artificial insemination by donor) may be used where the male partner is severely subfertile or where a hereditary disorder makes the likelihood of an affected child very probable. The medical history of a potential sperm donor is investigated thoroughly before he is accepted and no one in poor health, with a family history of inherited disorders or with an increased risk of catching AIDS, is allowed to become a donor. Once accepted, donors have regular HIV antibody (AIDS) tests, their sperm only being used after each test is shown to be negative. The donor's semen is deposited in the neck of the womb around the time of ovulation. Sixty percent of women treated become pregnant within the first three months, but this form of treatment can be very stressful psychologically.

COMPLEMENTARY TREATMENT

Acupuncture
The reproductive system is said to be under the control of the kidney and points may be used to stimulate the kidney and the flow of energy through its meridian.

Aromatherapy
Geranium, melissa, jasmine, and rose may be prescribed.

Herbalism
A mixture of herbs may be indicated to promote normal function in the reproductive organs and to ensure a proper hormone balance. Among those used are helonias (or false unicorn) root, blue cohosh, and agnus castus, which work on the ovaries, pituitary, and womb, and, for men,

damiana and saw palmetto, which stimulate the function of the testes. Other herbs, such as black cohosh and licorice root, are useful for both male and female patients.

Homeopathy
Conium may be given if infertility is associated with scanty periods, sepia when it is accompanied by a loss of sex drive, apathy, and irritability, or aurum when the patient is depressed. Other remedies may also be used depending on the patient's symptoms.

Hypnotherapy
A woman who is unable to conceive easily may become very anxious as a result. Unfortunately, this anxiety may make matters worse by affecting the patient's hormone balance. Hypnotherapy may help to reduce her anxiety levels by teaching her how to relax.

Nutrition
Zinc is vital for fertility in both sexes and, since many people are mildly deficient, a supplement of 15 g a day, or more, may be recommended. In addition, vitamin C supplements may help to increase a low sperm count and to promote fertility. Octacosanol and essential fatty acids, which are found in cold pressed vegetable oils, are also important to the normal functioning of the reproductive system. A tablespoon each day of cold pressed vegetable oil, in the form of a salad dressing, is an adequate supplement.

The amino acid arginine may be helpful in cases where sperm motility is reduced. (Not only do sperm have to be plentiful but they also have to be mobile in order to enter the womb and fertilize an egg.) Up to 8 g a day may be prescribed, but arginine should not be taken by anyone with a history of schizophrenia.

Radionics
Some radionics practitioners have a very good record for treating infertility.

SELF-HELP

Recent studies have shown that men tend to be less fertile if they smoke and that women's fertility can be reduced by a high caffeine intake (from coffee, tea, and carbonated drinks). Stopping smoking and cutting down on caffeine is probably advisable for any couple wishing to start a family.

Women whose periods are irregular may find it very hard to know when they are at their most fertile. They, and other women who are having difficulty conceiving, may find an ovulation prediction test helpful. This simple test can be bought at a pharmacy without a prescription, but unfortunately it is quite expensive. However, it is capable of predicting ovulation thirty-six hours in advance, by measuring a hormone whose level rises just before an egg is released. Brand names include First Response and Clearplan Easy.

ORGANIZATIONS

American Fertility Society
2131 Magnolia Avenue
Suite 201
Birmingham, AL 35256
205/251-9764
(Publishes a journal and newsletter.)

INSOMNIA

INCIDENCE AND DEFINITION

Insomnia is a very common problem, affecting almost all adults at some time in their lives, but women twice as frequently as men. The average adult sleeps between six and eight hours a night, but sleeping patterns change as we get older and most elderly people sleep less than this. It is understandable, therefore, that it is among the elderly that most complaints of insomnia are to be found.

Insomnia can be described as transient (when it is due to some unusual experience that interferes with sleep—for example, sleeping in a strange bed), short term (when it is often due to worry or stress), and long term (when it may be due to a variety of factors such as depression, alcohol abuse, drug dependency, pain, or habit). A recently recognized form of insomnia is known as sleep apnea, in which the patient (frequently an obese man) wakes repeatedly during the night as a result of his airway being temporarily cut off by the fat around his neck.

Insomniacs complain that it takes them a long time to get to sleep, that once they are asleep they wake often, and that they don't feel refreshed in the morning. Patients with sleep apnea also complain of nodding off frequently during the day.

TRADITIONAL TREATMENT

Doctors are far less willing than they used to be to prescribe sleeping pills, or hypnotics. Barbiturates fell out of favor because they were dangerous in overdose and were addictive. The newer drugs, benzodiazepines, have also been shown to cause dependence, although they are somewhat safer in overdose. However, it is estimated that patients can become tolerant to them (need a larger dose for the same effect) after only a few days of continuous use and it is usually recommended that they are taken for no longer than a few weeks. The patient who is

257

stopping benzodiazepines needs to do so slowly, since stopping suddenly may cause insomnia that is worse than it was before treatment. Some specialists recommend that patients who need benzodiazepines for insomnia take them only every other night or every third night. In this way they can be sure that they will get two or three good nights of sleep a week, but will reduce their risk of becoming dependent on the drug. Benzodiazepines may also produce hangover effects, although this is less likely with the newer, short-acting preparations.

The longer-acting benzodiazepines include diazepam, flurazepam, and orazepam. The shorter-acting preparations include alprazolam, temazepam, and triazolam. The latter group may be less suitable for patients who wake early in the morning and are unable to get back to sleep.

Other hypnotics include chloral hydrate (a tried and trusted medication but less pleasant to take than the benzodiazepines) and its derivative dichloralphenazone. Elderly patients are often given short-acting benzodiazepines or antidepressants. Children should not be given hypnotics, but if absolutely necessary an antihistamine with a sedative effect such as promethazine or trimeprazine may be used for a short period.

For patients whose insomnia stems from depression, treatment with an antidepressant drug may bring rapid relief. The tricyclic antidepressants such as imipramine and trimipramine have a particularly sedative effect.

Sleeping pills should not be taken by patients with sleep apnea, since they can make the problem worse. Patients are advised to lose weight, avoid alcohol after 6 P.M., and stop smoking. In severe cases, a special device can be provided by a chest physician, which consists of a mask placed over the patient's nose and a pump that forces air through and keeps the airway open.

COMPLEMENTARY TREATMENT

Acupuncture
Classical Chinese theory says that insomnia may result from a number of different causes. These include a deficiency of energy in the spleen resulting from anxiety, a lack of yin (the negative, feminine aspect of

Chi) in the kidney resulting in fire in the heart, mental depression causing fire in the liver, and retention of phlegm and heat due to indigestion. Other causes are a weakness of the heart and stomach, an imbalance between the liver and gallbladder, and a disturbance of the Chi of the spleen and stomach. Whichever organ is affected, the aim of treatment is to restore a normal flow of Chi through it. Fire and phlegm are eliminated where necessary. Where Chi, or its yin aspect, are lacking, these are stimulated. The spirit is said to reside in the heart and points along the Heart channel are used, in appropriate cases, to calm the spirit.

Aromatherapy
Oils of chamomile, lavender, neroli, rose, basil, and marjoram are among those that have a relaxant effect and that may be helpful in the treatment of insomnia.

Bach Flower Remedies
Patients who are suffering from mental and physical exhaustion may be helped by olive. However, when exhaustion has resulted from overeffort by a highly strung person who finds it hard to relax, vervain may be appropriate. White chestnut may be beneficial if the patient's mind is unable to relax and thoughts continue to go around and around endlessly.

Herbalism
Many herbs have a relaxant or sedative effect. These include chamomile, balm, St. John's wort, lime blossom, passiflora, and hops. Vervain and scullcap are useful when insomnia results from nervous tension. On the whole, herbal remedies are nonaddictive, but valerian, which is a powerful relaxant, may be habit-forming and so is reserved for severe cases and is usually used for only a short period.

Homeopathy
If insomnia is associated with restlessness and anxiety, aconite may be helpful. If it results from overwork and lack of exercise or from indigestion or excessive alcohol, nux vomica may be appropriate. Sulphur may be prescribed for the patient whose insomnia is worse in the early hours and who is awakened by the slightest noise. If insomnia is

associated with nightmares when the patient does fall asleep, belladonna may help. Coffea cruda may be beneficial for the patient who is unable to sleep because her mind is going endlessly. For children, chamomilla is often the remedy of choice. For the patient who is unable to sleep until after midnight and then wakes at about 3 A.M., often getting up to have a snack or a drink, pulsatilla may be helpful. A number of other remedies may also prove useful in the treatment of patients suffering from insomnia.

Hypnotherapy
Hypnosis can be remarkably effective in the treatment of insomnia. There are three ways in which it may be used. First, it can teach the patient to relax so that she is less likely to be kept awake by anxieties or muscular tension. Second, she can be taught how to hypnotize herself and can be given the suggestion that if she does this when she is in bed, she will very quickly fall asleep. In fact, if a patient is left quietly in a hypnotic trance for any length of time, it is quite natural for her to fall asleep, so the suggestion just reinforces this. Third, if there are deep-seated reasons for the patient's insomnia, these can be investigated under hypnosis and she can be helped to resolve them.

Nutrition
Calcium, magnesium, and vitamin B_6 have a tranquilizing effect. Calcium and magnesium are combined in tablet form as dolomite and are also found in seeds, nuts, and vegetables. Vitamin B_6 must always be taken with zinc, since the two work together in the body. The amino acid tryptophan is a very effective treatment for insomnia, is nonaddictive, and has no known side effects in the short term. However, its long-term use is not recommended. It takes about an hour to work and is effective for up to four hours. It must not be taken by pregnant women or by those hoping to become pregnant or by patients who are taking MAOI (monoamine oxidase inhibitor) antidepressants.

SELF-HELP

Insomnia may start as a transient phenomenon and may become long term simply because the patient begins to worry about it. It is important, therefore, to remember that a few nights of sleeplessness do no harm and that most people sleep longer than they think they do.

Patients should go to bed only when they are sleepy—going to bed at a set time will almost inevitably result in lying awake on some nights. The bedroom should be warm and quiet. Alcohol and caffeine should be avoided in the hours before bedtime. Some quiet relaxation in the form of a hot milky drink, some music, or a good book is helpful. Very often when children can't sleep it is because they have gone to bed in an overstimulated state, having been watching an exciting program on television or playing an exciting game right up to bedtime.

People who wake in the night should, once they are sure that they will not drop off again right away, get out of bed and do something— read, listen to the radio, write letters, or make a hot drink—until they feel tired again.

IRRITABLE BOWEL SYNDROME (Spastic Colitis)

DEFINITION AND SYMPTOMS

Irritable bowel syndrome (IBS) is a very common condition that can cause recurrent bowel disturbances and attacks of abdominal pain over a long period of time. The cause is unknown, but some authorities suggest that it may result from an initial attack of food poisoning or dysentery that makes the bowel hypersensitive, whereas others think that some of the cases are due to an allergy to a certain foodstuff or to a deficiency of fiber in the diet. Recently it has been suggested that the disorder may lie in the nerves that supply the bowel. The section of bowel affected is the colon (which is why this condition used to be called spastic colitis or spastic colon). Normally, in order to pass its contents along, the muscles in the wall of the colon gently contract and relax, an action known as peristalsis. However, in patients with IBS the colon contracts more than is usual and is also unduly tender.

Although in about 20 percent of cases painless diarrhea is the only symptom, most patients with IBS complain of abdominal pain. Classically, this is in the lower left side of the abdomen and is usually relieved by passing a stool or gas. However, the pain may appear on the right lower side of the abdomen, mimicking appendicitis, or on the right side under the ribs, mimicking gallbladder disease. It may occasionally take the form of indigestion and may be associated with nausea. It can be dull or colicky (coming in spasms) and can sometimes be quite severe. It may be brought on or be made worse by eating and during an attack fatty or gas-forming foods (such as vegetables) may make it considerably worse. Cow's milk products may produce symptoms in some.

The patient may also have constipation or diarrhea, or both alternately. Sometimes there is mucus in the stools, which may be small, like pellets, or long and thin. After passing a stool, the patient may still feel that he needs to go. Occasionally, there is pain in the anus, although this may occur at any time, not necessarily during defecation. Between attacks, the bowels may be normal.

Almost invariably, attacks can be brought on or made worse by stress or anxiety.

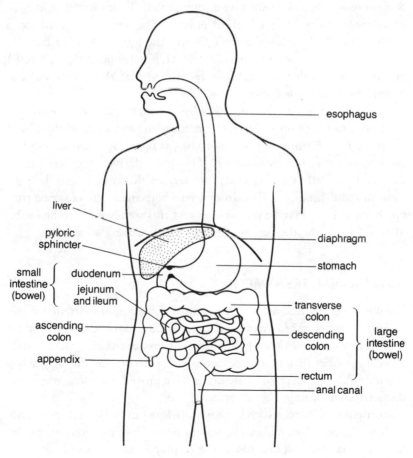

The digestive system

TESTS

IBS is a benign disease that causes no obvious bodily changes. Therefore, the diagnosis is made on the history and by ruling out other possible diagnoses.

Upon examination of the abdomen, it may be possible to feel the outline of the colon, which in some cases is tender. The doctor will usually examine the rectum and ask for a sample of stool, which will be tested to see whether there is blood in it (the presence of blood may indicate that the patient has an inflammatory bowel disease). A blood test may be taken to check for anemia, which can result from the loss of minute amounts of blood over a long period. Following this, it may be necessary to perform a barium enema. The patient is given some medication that he takes the night before the test to clear his bowels. Then a substance containing barium, which is radio-opaque, is pumped gently into the colon through the rectum so that the outlines of the bowel can be seen on X-ray.

Another useful test is sigmoidoscopy in which a flexible telescope is inserted into the colon through the rectum and the walls of the bowel are inspected. A tiny piece of tissue (biopsy) may be taken in order to exclude an inflammatory disorder. This is a relatively painless procedure and, as well as ruling out more serious diseases, it may help to confirm the diagnosis of IBS. In order to help the sigmoidoscope pass up the bowel, air may be pumped in and this sometimes produces the identical pain that the patient with IBS feels during an attack.

TRADITIONAL TREATMENT

Various types of treatment are recommended. It is important for the patient to try to avoid stress and occasionally psychotherapy may be appropriate for a particularly anxious person. Between attacks a balanced high-fiber diet should be eaten and patients should only avoid specific foodstuffs if repeated incidents have proved that they cannot eat them without bringing on an attack.

Antispasmodic drugs such as propantheline can be helpful. A "stool-bulking agent" that makes the stools larger and firmer is useful in reducing diarrhea and also has a role to play in constipation, since by making the stools softer it allows them to be passed more easily. Such agents, which include ispaghula husk, methylcellulose, and psyllium seed, come in the form of granules or drinks.

One study of patients with IBS showed that after a time 30 percent stopped having attacks, 60 percent had recurrent mild symptoms with which they could cope, and in 10 percent the condition continued to cause problems.

RECENT ADVANCES

In 1986 doctors in Italy tried the antiallergic drug cromolyn sodium (which is used in the treatment of asthma) on twenty-eight patients suffering from IBS. These patients seemed to have allergies to certain foods and their symptoms had improved when they cut these foods out of their diets. Twenty of them responded well to treatment with this drug. However, it is unlikely to become a universal treatment for IBS since it is probably only in a small proportion of patients that the symptoms are due to allergy.

In 1988 doctors at the University Hospital in Manchester, United Kingdom, acting on the theory that calcium has a lot to do with the contraction of the muscle in the bowel, gave some patients with IBS an injection of nicardipine. This is a calcium antagonist, used in the treatment of high blood pressure. Another group of patients was given an injection of saline and the contractions in each patient's bowel were measured after he had consumed a 100-calorie liquid meal. In the patients who had been given the saline, there was increased contraction over a period of several hours whereas there was no increase in those who had been given nicardipine. The drug seemed to have little in the way of side effects, but more work needs to be done before it is offered generally to treat IBS.

COMPLEMENTARY TREATMENT

Herbalism
Meadowsweet, marshmallow root, bayberry, slippery elm, and comfrey can all be used to reduce irritability in the wall of the intestine. Linseed may be prescribed for constipation.

Homeopathy

Ignatia may be prescribed for patients who have spasms of abdominal pain and diarrhea after emotional upsets. For those who suffer from pain that is relieved by passing offensive-smelling wind and whose stools are bulky and may contain mucus, graphites may be appropriate. A patient who suffers from sudden cramplike pains that are relieved by bending over but made worse by eating or drinking may respond to colocynthis.

Hypnotherapy

Because attacks of IBS are often brought on by anxiety or stress, hypnosis can be an effective treatment. Patients are taught how to relax and how to cope with stressful situations and suggestions are given while they are under hypnosis that their bowel symptoms will no longer trouble them.

ISCHEMIC HEART DISEASE (Angina and Heart Attacks)

DEFINITION, MECHANISM, AND INCIDENCE

The word ischemic means having an inadequate blood supply and is used to describe heart conditions caused by blockages of the coronary arteries. These arteries carry blood containing oxygen to the muscle of the heart; having released its oxygen, the blood absorbs and removes the waste products that are formed as a result of the heart's work. If the blood supply is inadequate, the muscle receives insufficient oxygen to be able to work efficiently, while waste products accumulate that further interfere with the heart's function and that cause pain by stimulating nerve endings within the muscle.

By far the commonest cause of ischemic heart disease is atheroma (atherosclerosis), or hardening of the arteries. Atherosclerosis (whose name derives from the Greek word for porridge) is caused by a fatty substance laid down in plaques along the inside of arteries. Not only does it narrow the artery but there is the risk that thrombi (clots) may form on it, shutting off the blood flow altogether. No one is quite sure what initiates atherosclerosis, but there are a number of risk factors that make its development more likely. These including smoking, obesity, an unbalanced diet, high blood pressure, a high level of cholesterol in the blood, physical inactivity, and diabetes. There is also some evidence that drinking soft water, more than six cups of coffee a day, or large amounts of milk may increase a person's chances of developing severe atherosclerosis.

Atherosclerosis is found to a certain extent in everybody. Although

267

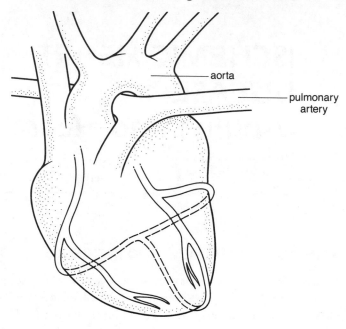

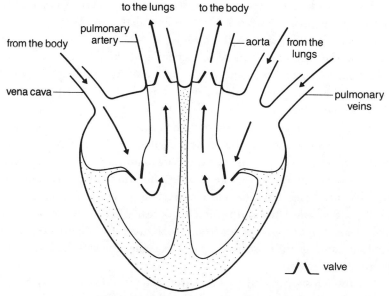

The blood flow through the heart

it is rare in childhood, fatty streaks, which are the beginning of atherosclerosis, are commonly found at postmortem exams in children; postmortem examinations of young men between the ages of twenty and thirty often show evidence of some atherosclerosis. A "high-risk" man (that is, one whose lifestyle and medical condition include several risk factors) has a one in three chance of developing angina or having a heart attack within ten years. Asians living in the United States probably have less ischemic heart disease if they continue their rice-based, low-fat diet. Blacks have a high incidence of this disease. There is also a small group of people who have hyperlipoproteinemia running in the family. This is a condition in which there is an excess (hyper-) of fats (lipoproteins) in the blood (-emia) and these tend to cause the deposition of atherosclerosis at an early age.

Ischemic heart disease has a great deal to do with lifestyle—it is the leading cause of death in all affluent countries and yet was hardly known before the turn of the century. Diseases of the heart and blood vessels account for about half of all deaths in the United States; three fourths of these deaths are due to ischemic heart disease, which kills approximately half a million people each year. Women seem to be protected by their hormones until the menopause and in the forty to fifty age group ischemic heart disease is six times more common in men. After the menopause, however, the proportion of women with the disease steadily increases and eventually catches up.

ANGINA PECTORIS

Symptoms

The literal translation of the Latin term *angina pectoris* is "a strangling sensation of the chest." Patients usually complain of a constricting or crushing pain that may be felt right around the chest but is worst across the front or beneath the breast bone. It may travel up into the shoulders, the neck, and the jaw, and is commonly associated with a heavy sensation, tingling, or pain down one or both arms. If only one arm is affected it is usually the left. Rarely, pain may also be felt in the teeth or in the abdomen. Occasionally there may be pain in the arms and not in the chest.

There are several types of angina of which "classical" or "exertional" angina is by far the commonest. This, as its name implies, is brought on by exertion. It is particularly likely to occur if the patient is walking uphill or against the wind or has just eaten a meal or if the weather is cold. Some patients can walk long distances on flat land and only develop pain if they try to walk up a slope. Anger, excitement, or mental stress can also bring on an attack, which may last up to twenty minutes. However, if the pain has occurred during exercise, it will usually disappear within five minutes if the patient sits down to rest. Some people find that the pain disappears if they continue walking, but this may be dangerous and the onset of an attack should always be a signal to rest.

Other types of angina include angina decubitus (which may be associated with exertional angina), in which pain comes on when the patient lies flat and is eased by sitting up, and the rare Prinzmetal's angina, in which the pain occurs at rest, especially during the night or early morning, being caused by spasm in a coronary artery.

Unstable angina is a term used to describe a condition that is steadily worsening, being provoked more easily and responding less readily to treatment than before. Vigorous treatment is needed for such patients in order to avoid the onset of a heart attack.

Tests

Many conditions can cause chest pain and it is very important that an accurate diagnosis is made. It is not unknown for a patient suffering from angina to think that his pain is due to indigestion. Usually the patient's description of the pain, together with the details of when it occurs and how long it lasts, will indicate to the GP that he is dealing with a case of angina. However, in the majority of cases, there is nothing abnormal to find during examination, although some patients may have a raised blood pressure. Most cases of angina are confirmed by an ECG (electrocardiogram). Wires are attached to the patient's ankles, wrists, and chest, and a record of the electrical impulses received from them, which reflect the impulses occurring in the heart, is traced out on a strip of paper. Very often, the ECG is normal and it is not until the patient is asked to perform some gentle exercise that changes are seen on it that suggest the heart muscle is ischemic. Resting electrocardiography will only be abnormal if the person is having symptoms at rest. Stress tests are usually required to diagnose angina.

In cases where there are few changes even during exercise, but where the history strongly suggests a diagnosis of angina, further tests may be performed. Ultrasound can be used to assess how well the heart muscle contracts. Radionuclide ventriculography consists of injecting a mildly radioactive substance into the bloodstream and scanning it as it travels through the heart, a technique that allows the heart's function to be measured accurately. In nuclear imaging another mildly radioactive substance, thallium 201, is injected and this is absorbed into the healthy heart muscle, leaving a blank "cold spot" on the scan in any area that is ischemic. The thallium is usually given during exercise and a scan is taken soon afterward and then again after another three to four hours, when the disappearance of the cold spot confirms that the ischemia was brought on by exercise and relieved by rest.

If the diagnosis is still uncertain, or if the patient is suffering from severe attacks and surgical treatment is being contemplated, coronary angiography may be performed. In this, a substance that is radioopaque (shows up white on X-rays) is introduced into the coronary arteries and X-rays are taken to try to demonstrate the position of the blockages.

Traditional Treatment

The general condition of a patient with angina is very important. He will therefore be advised to stop smoking and, if he is overweight, to go on a diet. Regular gentle exercise is encouraged since it may help to open up the smaller vessels that bring blood to the heart muscle, but vigorous exercise and overexcitement should be avoided.

An acute attack of angina is normally treated with nitroglycerine. This comes in the form of little tablets that are dissolved under the tongue. Once the pain has been relieved, the tablet is spat out, to try to avoid the main side effect of nitrates—a pounding headache. Unfortunately, once a bottle of tablets has been opened they deteriorate within a few weeks and in recent years sprays have been developed that have the same effect when applied to the tongue, but that can be kept much longer.

Nitrate preparations are also used in the long-term treatment of angina and patients are advised to take them before embarking on something that might provoke an attack, rather than waiting for symptoms to appear. Long-acting preparations include isosorbide dinitrate or isosorbide mononitrate, buccal pellets that are allowed to dissolve between the upper lip and the gum, and ointments or patches applied to the skin and from which nitrate is slowly released. They all have the effect of relaxing the blood vessels and therefore reducing the work that the heart has to do by decreasing the resistance it has to overcome.

In an acute attack of angina, 75 percent of patients get immediate relief from taking a tablet of nitroglycerine, and another 15 percent have a slightly delayed response. Fortunately, nitroglycerine is not addictive and its effect does not diminish even if taken repeatedly over a long period. However, it has recently been ascertained that, for nitrate preparations to work maximally, the patient should have a "nitrate-free" period of about eight hours a day. Thus, patches should be removed at bedtime and the last dose of the isosorbide preparations should be taken in the early evening.

A nitrate preparation is usually the first that a patient with angina receives. For patients whose pain is not controlled adequately by this, beta blockers or calcium antagonists are added. (These drugs are more fully described in the section on high blood pressure.) Some doctors like to prescribe beta blockers routinely with nitrates.

The effect of beta blockers, of which propranolol is probably the most widely used, is to reduce the heart rate, the blood pressure, and the force with which the heart contracts, and, as a result, to reduce the amount of work that the heart has to perform and its need for oxygen. Calcium antagonists, such as nifedipine, verapamil, and diltiazem, also reduce the heart's force of contraction and its need for oxygen, at the same time relaxing the coronary arteries, thus allowing more oxygen to be brought to the heart.

Unfortunately, all these drugs have side effects. The nitrates can cause headaches, facial flushing, dizziness, nausea, and light-headedness. Beta blockers can cause tiredness, muscle weakness, impotence, sleep disturbance, and cold hands and feet. (This last effect is less likely with labetalol, which has some alpha blocking action—see the section on hypertension.) Calcium antagonists may cause headache, dizziness, flushing, and palpitations, all of which may be reduced by using a slow-release preparation. Nifedipine may cause ankle swelling and diarrhea; verapamil may cause constipation.

For patients with high levels of cholesterol in the bloodstream, medication such as clofibrate may be needed in order to lower it. Drugs now more frequently used than clofibrate are corastatin, gemfibrovil, and niacin.

When the attacks of angina continue to be frequent and severe, surgical treatment may be suggested. The simplest form is coronary angioplasty. A very thin catheter (tube) with a balloon on its end is inserted into an artery and fed through into the partially blocked coronary vessel by the doctor, who uses an X-ray screen to guide him. Once in place, the balloon is inflated with a substance that shows up on the X-ray. It is deflated and inflated a number of times and the pressure it exerts on the atheromatous plaques cracks and demolishes them, clearing the obstruction. This treatment is especially useful for patients in whom atherosclerosis is limited to one or two patches. It is successful in 60–80 percent of cases, but patients need to have follow-up arteriography after six to twelve months because in 20–30 percent of those helped the condition will recur. Angioplasty has the great advantage that patients can return to work within a few days, whereas those who have bypass surgery usually have to convalesce for several months.

Two types of bypass surgery are performed. In one, a vein is removed from the leg and sewn into place between the aorta (the large vessel that carries blood from the heart to the arteries) and the section of the coronary artery that lies beyond the obstruction. In the other, the internal mammary artery, which runs down the inside of the chest wall, is loosened and fed into the far end of the blocked artery. There is a slight risk associated with the operation, which has a 1–2 percent mortality rate—this is usually considered to be an acceptable risk. Results are very good, with about 90 percent of patients being free of symptoms in the year following the operation. This falls to 75 percent after five years, since some of the grafts gradually become blocked. However, a bypass operation offers a patient not only an improved quality of life but also an increased life expectancy.

Complementary Treatment

Acupuncture
Chest pain is divided into two types by acupuncturists—the shi type in which there is an excess of energy (Chi) and the xu type in which Chi is deficient. In both types the channels of the heart are obstructed. Treatment consists of using points that will restore the flow of Chi to normal, overcoming the obstruction.

Aromatherapy
Aniseed may be recommended.

Herbalism
There are a number of herbs that have an effect on the heart and blood vessels. Hawthorn dilates the arteries, including those supplying the heart muscle, and slows the heart rate. Yarrow, too, can dilate arteries. Garlic not only dilates arteries but also helps to reduce cholesterol levels in the blood and acts to prevent abnormal blood clotting.

Homeopathy
The remedy prescribed will depend not only on the patient's symptoms but on his general personality. For example, nux vomica may be suitable for someone who is outwardly calm but bottles up anger, whereas arsenicum may be appropriate for an overanxious perfectionist who finds it hard to express emotions or fears. Aconite may be of value during the acute angina attack when there is severe pain that is made worse by activity.

Nutrition
Eicosapentenoic acid (EPA) is an extract obtained from fatty fish that has remarkable effects on the cardiovascular system. The reason why heart attacks are rare among Eskimos seems to be that they eat large amounts of raw fatty fish. EPA prevents abnormal blood clotting, stops arteries from going into spasm, and reduces the triglyceride level and, to a lesser extent, the cholesterol level. EPA is available in capsule form and is nowadays prescribed by doctors as well as by nutrition therapists.

HEART ATTACK (MYOCARDIAL INFARCT OR INFARCTION)

Mechanism and Symptoms

This is the commonest cause of death in the United Kingdom and other developed countries, and is nearly always due to the sudden deposition of blood clots on an atheromatous plaque inside a coronary artery. This is usually an end result of an obstruction that has caused the blood to run more and more sluggishly through the artery until it comes to a standstill. The section of heart muscle that is supplied by the artery dies and, if the patient survives, is replaced by scar tissue. However, if the area of muscle is a very large one, the heart may cease to function and the patient dies suddenly at the time of the infarction.

The symptoms are similar to those of angina but are more severe, continue when the patient is at rest, and may last for a day or more. However, a few patients (usually among the elderly) may have no symptoms at all or may develop breathlessness or an abnormal heart rhythm without any pain occurring. Half the patients who have heart attacks have had increasingly severe angina during the previous weeks, but for the others the attack is the first indication that they are suffering from ischemic heart disease. As well as the pain, the patient may feel sick and faint, and may vomit, sweat, and become short of breath.

Tests

Usually it is fairly clear from the condition of the patient that he has suffered a heart attack and this can normally be confirmed by an ECG. He is likely to be transported to the hospital solely on the basis of his symptoms and all tests will be done once he has arrived there.

When heart muscle dies, it releases chemicals known as cardiac enzymes into the bloodstream. These enzymes, which include lactic dehydrogenase (LDH), aspartate aminotransferase (AST), and creatine phosphokinase (CPK), can be measured by a blood test to confirm the results of the ECG. This test is particularly useful in the 5 percent of cases where the ECG remains normal for a few days after the attack.

A scan may be helpful in distinguishing a heart attack from a bad attack of angina. The thallium nuclear-imaging technique mentioned above will continue to show a "cold spot" after several hours if an infarct has occurred. A pyrophosphate scan uses the chemical pyrophosphate labeled with a mildly radioactive substance that is taken up by recently dead heart muscle. It is injected into a vein between one and five days after the attack and a few hours later a "hot spot" will be seen on the scan at the site of the infarct.

Prognosis

Once over the first two or three hours following the attack, the patient has a very good chance of survival. However, complications may occur, the most important of which are abnormalities of heart rhythm. Some abnormality is almost universal in the first few hours, but only in a small percentage of cases does it seriously interfere with the heart's function.

Traditional Treatment

A strong painkiller such as morphine is given, together with a drug to stop the vomiting that may be induced by the drug. The patient is put to bed for 36–48 hours and his heart is constantly monitored on a screen to which he is attached by wires secured to his chest.

The main purpose of the monitor is to detect any abnormalities of rhythm (arrhythmias) as soon as they occur so that they can be treated. In most cases, treatment consists of lidocaine (a drug that is also used in other circumstances as a local anesthetic) given intravenously through a drip. However, some patients with arrhythmias need the digitalis derivative digoxin and those with abnormally slow heart rates require intravenous atropine. Two percent of patients develop ventricular fibrillation (VF) in which the heart starts to contract in a totally uncoordinated way and therefore fails to pump out blood normally. This is an emergency, with the patient ceasing to breathe and becoming unconscious. However, prompt electric shock treatment to the chest followed by cardiac massage will bring most patients around. Another 6 percent of patients will develop heart block, in which the chambers of the heart that receive blood from the lungs no longer pump in time with the chambers that pump blood out to the body. This results in greatly decreased efficiency and in some cases it may be necessary to implant a pacemaker to ensure that normal function is restored. For some patients, this may only be a temporary measure since the block corrects itself in time.

Heart failure may occur, in which the damaged heart is unable to cope with the demands put on it and fluid accumulates in the lungs (where it causes shortness of breath) and in the ankles (where it causes swelling). In these cases, diuretics (as described in the section on high blood pressure) need to be given, together with digoxin.

Recently a lot of work has been done on the use of a group of drugs known colloquially as "clot busters." The main drug in this group is streptokinase, a protein derived from bacteria that is given soon after a heart attack to dissolve the clots that have formed within the coronary artery and thus it restores the blood flow and limits the damage to the heart muscle. Given intravenously it is effective in up to 60 percent of cases and seems to reduce the death rate in the first weeks after the attack by up to 25 percent. If aspirin is given in addition, the death rate is reduced by over one third. However, the drugs have to be given in the first few hours after the start of the attack. TPA (tissue plasminogen activator) and streptokinase are used regularly. Also, scientists have developed another similar substance, urokinase.

Since arteries unblocked by streptokinase are likely to block up again, it may still be necessary for patients who are treated in this way to have a bypass operation. Long-term therapy may be given in the form of aspirin or beta blockers, both of which seem to reduce the incidence of a second attack and of sudden death.

Complications

Modern coronary care is now so good that the great majority of patients make an uncomplicated recovery and are able to return to work within six weeks of the attack. However, some may continue to be troubled by arrhythmias and this may necessitate long-term medication or the fitting of a pacemaker. Patients who had no chest pain previous to their attack may find that they now suffer from angina.

An uncommon complication is the shoulder–hand syndrome in which the left shoulder becomes stiff and painful and the left hand may swell. Physiotherapy is often helpful, but the condition can take several months to subside.

Patients who earned their living from driving may have problems following a heart attack. The U.S. Department of Transportation has strict guidelines for physicians to follow in qualifying or disqualifying those who have had heart attacks, angina, and/or bypass surgery. Fortunately, a patient who has made a good recovery following infarct or surgery may be requalified.

RECENT ADVANCES

In 1986 surgeons in France used the first coronary stent—a coiled stainless steel spring that when inserted into the coronary artery after angioplasty holds the walls apart and prevents the artery from blocking up again. By early 1988 it had been used to treat seventy-six patients, mainly in Lausanne, and surgeons at the National Heart Hospital in London had started to use it on an experimental basis. Researchers in Dallas are experimenting with absorbable stents that will disappear after a certain period of time. Most stents are usually required temporarily.

Doctors in the United States are using map-guided electrical rejection. An electrode maps out the part of the heart that appears to be causing the rhythm disturbance, then that part is removed. This surgery is usually reserved for people who do not tolerate or respond to antiarrhythmic medication.

New drugs, too, are being developed, including beta blockers, that seem to have fewer side effects than those presently available.

ORGANIZATIONS

American Heart Association
National Center
7320 Greenville Avenue
Dallas, TX 75231
214/373-6300

MENOPAUSE

DEFINITION

The term *menopause* is used loosely to describe the end of a woman's reproductive life and all its associated changes. Strictly speaking, though, the menopause is just the ceasing of the periods. The medical term applied to the period of time over which the body changes and the reproductive organs become nonfunctional is the *climacteric*.

The ovaries, which secrete the hormones that regulate the menstrual cycle, have a limited life span and usually when a woman is in her forties their function begins to decline. Most women have their last period somewhere around the age of forty-nine or fifty, although the menopause may occur in younger or older women (up to the age of about fifty-five). If it occurs before the age of forty it is described as premature and this may often run in families. However, the commonest cause of a premature menopause is surgical removal of the ovaries or their treatment with radiotherapy.

The menopause is considered to have occurred when a woman has not had a period for over six months. Although in some women the periods may just suddenly stop, in many cases the cycle will change in the years leading up to the menopause. The periods may become increasingly scanty or infrequent, or both. Very occasionally there may be no bleeding for several months, followed by an exceptionally heavy period (see section on menstrual problems). Heavy bleeding around the time of the menopause or bleeding occurring more than a year after the last period always requires investigation (usually a D & C or "scrape"), since it may occasionally herald the onset of a malignant condition.

SYMPTOMS AND CHANGES OCCURRING AT THE MENOPAUSE

Fifty percent of women are said to have few symptoms at the menopause except perhaps for the occasional hot flash. Of the remaining 50 percent, one half have symptoms with which they can cope whereas the others have symptoms that interfere with their lives and can become disabling. Smokers are more likely to have problems than other women.

The symptoms that may occur are numerous and include dizziness, palpitations, pain in the chest, shortness of breath, headaches, extreme fatigue, loss of appetite, and digestive upsets. The skin tends to become more fragile and wrinkled and the hair becomes thinner on both the head and body. Hot flashes are the commonest symptom and are experienced by about 85 percent of all women. Lasting for a few seconds or minutes at a time, the woman is aware of a sensation of heat in her chest, neck, and face. Her skin may flush and she may sweat. Twenty-five percent of women have their sleep disrupted by hot flashes and night sweats. Often the flashes are made worse by a hot atmosphere and may be brought on by anxiety or by eating hot food or drinking a hot drink. Thus, they may seriously interfere with a woman's life, making it difficult for her to go shopping in a crowded store, or to eat or even have a cup of tea. For 80 percent of those affected, the flashes persist for at least a year, and 25 percent have to suffer them for over five years.

Other symptoms are associated with changes in the reproductive and urinary tracts, caused by the lack of estrogen in the bloodstream. The muscles supporting the uterus (the pelvic floor) become slack, as do the ligaments that hold the uterus in place, so that prolapse is more likely to occur (see separate section). The wall of the vagina becomes thinner and drier and the vagina itself may contract, becoming shorter and narrower. As a result the vagina may become sore (atrophic vaginitis) and discomfort during intercourse may occur. The increasing fragility of the skin around the entrance to the vagina (the vulva) may result in a persistent itch (pruritis vulvae). The lining of the urinary tract may be affected in a similar way, causing discomfort when passing water; the woman may have to pass water frequently and may also have to get up during the night to empty her bladder. Stress incontinence (the passage of small amounts of urine when laughing, coughing, or sneezing) and urge incontinence (the inability to hold water once the need to urinate has become apparent) may occur, partly because of weakness in the muscles of the pelvic floor (see section on incontinence).

Psychological problems, such as depression, anxiety, irritability, panic attacks, and sleep disturbances, may develop around the time of the menopause. (Insomnia may partly stem from the hot flashes and the need to get up to pass water.) Such problems are more likely to affect women who have previously suffered from psychological problems or from premenstrual tension.

A major cause of ill health after the menopause is osteoporosis (see separate section).

TRADITIONAL TREATMENT

Hormone Replacement Therapy (HRT)
There has been a revolution in the treatment of menopausal symptoms in recent years with the introduction of hormone replacement therapy. However, many specialists are concerned that there are a large number of women who could benefit from this treatment, but who are not yet receiving it.

The hormones used are produced by the ovaries during the reproductive years—estrogen and progestogens. Estrogen stops the hot flashes and the night sweats, reduces vaginal dryness and discomfort, controls the urinary symptoms, and prevents the bone loss that causes osteoporosis. Progestogens also control hot flashes and have some effect on preventing bone loss, although they are not as powerful as estrogen. However, progestogens are less likely to cause side effects than estrogen.

Usually estrogen is used together with a progestogen because on its own it is thought to cause an increased risk of cancer of the womb. However, it is quite safe for a woman who has had a hysterectomy to take estrogen alone. Nevertheless, some experts believe there is still the possible risk of breast cancer with estrogen replacement.

Not all women are suitable for hormone replacement therapy. Surprisingly, an inability to take the contraceptive Pill because of side effects is not necessarily a contraindication to HRT. However, women who have had cancer of the breast, ovaries, or uterus, or have suffered from liver disease, high blood pressure, various tumors or otosclerosis (deafness due to fusion of the tiny bones in the ear) should not have hormone replacement. Some women who have had thrombosis, fibroids, diabetes, gallbladder disease, varicose veins, nonmalignant breast problems, or high levels of blood cholesterol may also be unsuitable.

Once on HRT, the patient may stay on it for many years, since this will give her continued protection against osteoporosis. However, the effect of estrogen and progestogen on the lining of the uterus is the same as if the hormones were being produced naturally and most women on HRT continue to have monthly bleeding, which some find unacceptable.

There are various combinations of estrogen and progestogen, most of which are given for twenty-one days, with a break of seven days between courses. Women with no uterus who can safely be treated with estrogen alone may take this daily. Recently a transdermal patch has been introduced—a sticking patch that when applied below the waist will release a constant flow of estrogen into the skin and thus into the bloodstream. This has the advantage of producing fewer side effects than estrogen taken by mouth, since much smaller doses can be used as the hormone is absorbed directly into the bloodstream. However, some 3–5 percent of women are unable to use the patch because it causes skin irritation. At the time of writing, there is not yet a combined estrogen/progestogen transdermal patch, but one is being developed.

Injections and implants into the skin are other methods that are used to give estrogen, but the implant has the disadvantage that the treatment cannot be stopped quickly should side effects develop. If a woman who still has her uterus is treated in this way, she will need to take a progestogen by mouth in addition.

Side effects of hormone replacement therapy include vaginal discharge, breast tenderness, pain at the time of monthly bleeding, weight gain, fluid retention, and premenstrual syndrome.

Vaginal Estrogen Cream
This may be very helpful in treating vaginal dryness and irritation, especially when these occur in patients who are unable to take HRT. It may also have an effect on the urinary system. At a Scandinavian geriatric center, it was found that the application of a small amount of estrogen to the vagina controlled incontinence to such an extent that the unit's expenditure on incontinence appliances and pads was reduced by 90 percent.

However, if the cream is used over a prolonged period, a certain amount may be absorbed into the bloodstream, so its use must be carefully monitored in those patients for whom HRT is considered unsuitable. Another problem that may occur is the absorption of estrogen by the patient's sexual partner, which may lead to swelling of his breasts. To avoid this, intercourse should not take place until several hours have elapsed after the insertion of the cream.

Nonhormonal Treatment
Clonidine hydrochloride, a drug used in the treatment of high blood pressure, may be helpful in controlling hot flashes when used in low doses.

COMPLEMENTARY TREATMENT

Acupuncture
As in all forms of acupuncture therapy, the aim of treatment is to balance the energy flow whose disruption is causing symptoms. Treatment of menopausal patients will depend on the particular symptoms that the individual is experiencing. There are some points that are specific for the treatment of hot flashes.

Aromatherapy
Geranium, chamomile, cypress, and sage are among the essential oils used.

Bach Flower Remedies
Impatiens, olive, and walnut are the three Bach flower remedies that are likely to be most useful at the time of the menopause. Impatiens is indicated for irritability and tension, olive for severe fatigue, and walnut for people who are going through a major change in their lives.

Herbalism
Herbs such as false unicorn (helonias) root and agnus castus have an effect on the hormonal system and may be used in the treatment of menopausal symptoms. Others, such as hawthorn tops and sage, are effective in controlling hot flashes.

Homeopathy
Pulsatilla may provide relief in a woman who is weepy and in need of reassurance, who suffers from hot flashes, and whose symptoms are

worse for heat and tight clothes and better for gentle exercise and fresh air. Sepia, too, is useful for patients who are weepy and have hot flashes, but those who respond to this remedy are more likely to be anxious, complain of low dragging backache, and be worse for cold and better for vigorous exercise. If hot flashes that are worse for heat and tight clothes are also worse first thing in the morning, and if other symptoms include headache, sweating, dizziness, and tightness in the chest, lachesis may be useful. Several other remedies, too, may be helpful in the treatment of hot flashes. These include glonoinum, belladonna, sanguinaria, amyl nit., strontia carb., aconite, and veratrum viride.

SELF-HELP

Vitamin E can help to relieve hot flashes when taken in doses of 400 i.u. a day. However, people who are suffering from high blood pressure should not start off with this dose as there is a risk that it may push their pressure still higher. They should begin with a dose of 100 i.u. a day and increase it by a further 100 i.u. each month until they are taking the full 400 i.u.

ORGANIZATIONS

National Women's Health Network
224 Seventh Street, SE
Washington, DC 20003
202/543-9222
(Publishes *Network News,* bimonthly, and educational material.)

MENSTRUAL PROBLEMS

TERMINOLOGY

The two commonest menstrual problems are excessively heavy periods and painful periods, the latter being the most prevalent of all gynecological disorders.

Heavy bleeding during periods that occur regularly is known as menorrhagia, and irregular heavy periods are referred to as metrorrhagia. Dysmenorrhea refers to painful periods.

In order to understand how some of these problems occur, it is necessary to understand the basic physiology of the reproductive cycle in women. A diagram of the female reproductive organs is on page 249.

PHYSIOLOGY OF THE REPRODUCTIVE CYCLE

Each month a cell in one of the ovaries develops to form an ovum—an egg, capable of being fertilized and developing into a baby. As this cell develops, the cells surrounding it (the follicular cells) start to secrete estrogen. Some of this estrogen is retained in the fluid around the developing ovum and some is taken up by the blood and circulated around the body. Halfway through the cycle (day 14 of a twenty-eight-day cycle), the follicle surrounding the ovum bursts and the ovum is released. It passes down the Fallopian tube and into the uterus where the lining (endometrium) has become thick under the influence of the secreted estrogen. If the ovum is fertilized, it will implant into this thickened endometrium.

Meanwhile, the part of the ovary that contained the ovum is being replaced by other cells known as the corpus luteum. These cells secrete progesterone and estrogen, which again enter the circulation. If the egg

285

is fertilized and implants into the endometrium, the developing placenta begins to secrete a hormone that stimulates the corpus luteum to continue its production of progesterone so that the pregnancy is maintained. If, however, the egg is not fertilized, this does not occur and toward the twenty-fourth day of the cycle the corpus luteum begins to shrink, producing less progesterone. As a result, the thickened lining of the uterus begins to break down and is shed as the monthly period.

DYSMENORRHEA

Over 50 percent of all menstruating women have some discomfort during their period, but for 10 percent the pain is so severe that they become incapacitated for between one and three days each month. Dysmenorrhea is divided into two types—primary and secondary.

Primary Dysmenorrhea
This condition, which may run in families, usually begins within two or three years of the first period and accounts for 75 percent of all cases of dysmenorrhea. It is unusual for it to occur in the first few periods since these are commonly anovulatory cycles (that is, cycles in which the ovaries do not produce an egg) and primary dysmenorrhea is associated only with ovulatory cycles (those in which an egg is produced). Usually the pain starts as the bleeding begins, although it may come on the day before the onset of the period. It is felt mainly in the lower part of the abdomen, but may also travel to the back and down the front of the thighs. It may last only a few hours or may continue for two or three days. Other symptoms, such as nausea, vomiting, diarrhea, loss of appetite, headache, dizziness, tiredness, and nervousness, may occur in addition to the pain. Usually, after a number of years, primary dysmenorrhea improves, often helped by the birth of the first child.

There have been many theories as to what causes dysmenorrhea, including one that said the pain was "all in the mind." However, in recent years research has shown that its probable cause is an excess of the hormonelike substances, prostaglandins, in the uterus and the bloodstream. Prostaglandins, which were discovered during the 1970s, play a vital role in the control of many essential body functions, but an imbalance of them (as of any hormone) will produce unwanted effects. It is thought that progesterone, which is produced during the second half of the monthly cycle, stimulates the production of prostaglandins, which are released as the lining of the uterus breaks down and is shed as the monthly period. Women who suffer from primary dysmenorrhea seem to have high levels of prostaglandins in the muscle of the uterus, making it abnormally contractile and liable to go into spasm, while prostaglandins that escape into the bloodstream are likely to be responsible for the other symptoms that occur.

Primary dysmenorrhea is more common in women who smoke and who either drink heavily or have done so in the past. The highest incidence is among those between ages fifteen and twenty-four and among women who have had fewer than two children. It also seems commoner among migraine sufferers. The fact that such patients often seem particularly prone to migraine attacks around period time may be due to the increase in circulating prostaglandins.

It has been suggested that anemia, dieting, diabetes, chronic illness, overwork, and emotional problems may be associated with a lowering of the pain threshold and that, therefore, dysmenorrhea may be more likely to occur in patients suffering from these conditions.

Secondary Dysmenorrhea
This begins later in life than primary dysmenorrhea and is due to some other condition affecting the uterus, such as endometriosis, adenomyosis, pelvic venous congestion, pelvic inflammatory disease, or fibroids. Pelvic inflammatory disease (previously known as salpingitis) is a condition in which an infection travels upward through the uterus and into the tubes, which may become blocked as a result. As the disease becomes chronic, all the reproductive organs may become inflamed and, later, scarred. Endometriosis, adenomyosis, and pelvic venous congestion are described later in this section, while fibroids are dealt with in a separate section.

The pain of secondary dysmenorrhea may start a few days before the period begins, gradually increasing in severity; it may continue all through the period and may sometimes persist after it has finished.

MENORRHAGIA

Between 5 and 10 percent of menstruating women suffer from menorrhagia, which is defined as periods that occur more frequently than every twenty-one days, or last longer than seven days, or in which the loss is so heavy that the patient can't cope even if she uses the most absorbent pads. Cigarette smokers are five times more likely to be affected than other women.

Specialists have noticed that there is an increased incidence of anxiety and depression among women suffering from menorrhagia. However, although the condition itself may be partly responsible for this, it is possible that emotional and psychological problems may cause menorrhagia, since they can interfere with the normal functioning of the hormone-producing glands. Other causes may include abnormally high levels of circulating estrogen that are not balanced by progesterone (see metropathia hemorrhagica, below), an increase in prostaglandins production (in which case, the patient will also suffer from dysmenorrhea), pelvic inflammatory disease affecting the ovaries, fibroids, pelvic venous congestion, endometriosis, or polycystic ovaries (a condition in which the ovaries develop cysts that interfere with their function). Sometimes women complain of increasingly heavy periods following a sterilization operation. The exact cause of this is uncertain, but it has been suggested that in some cases it is because the woman has come off the contraceptive Pill on which her periods were lighter and is now experiencing "normal" periods. Very occasionally, what seems to be a rather late and very heavy period is, in fact, a very early miscarriage.

ENDOMETRIOSIS

The endometrium is the lining of the uterus—the section that grows thick each month in response to hormonal stimulus and, if a fertilized egg is not implanted in it, breaks down and is shed as the monthly period. In the condition known as endometriosis, endometrial tissue is found elsewhere in the body, and not just within the uterus. Usually this occurs in the pelvic cavity, around the reproductive organs, the commonest site being on the ovaries. But endometrial tissue is also found in the bowel in up to 35 percent of cases, in the urinary tract in between 10 and 20 percent, and rarely in other parts of the body such as the lungs, where, it is assumed, it must have been carried in the bloodstream. Why and how endometrial tissue is encouraged to grow in abnormal sites is unknown, although the latest theory suggests that affected women may have a deficiency in the immune system, which would normally eradicate such cells.

Like pelvic inflammatory disease, endometriosis tends to cause neighboring structures to stick to each other, resulting, ultimately, in scar tissue involving all the reproductive organs, so that they are locked into abnormal positions.

Endometriosis usually makes its first appearance between the ages of twenty-five and thirty, although it is not unknown in the teens or in postmenopausal women. Some 30–40 percent of affected women are infertile as a result of the disease. In many cases this is probably because it inhibits the normal mobility of the Fallopian tubes, through which the mature egg travels to the uterus, and therefore hinders the egg's passage. However, if it affects the ovaries, it may also prevent ovulation. In addition, the deep internal tenderness associated with endometriosis may lead to less frequent intercourse. Miscarriage, too, is more common.

The main symptoms of endometriosis are dysmenorrhea and pain during intercourse. Menorrhagia may occur but is rarely the first symptom. The endometrial patches, although growing in abnormal positions, still respond to the sex hormones in the same way as the endometrium in the uterus. Therefore, they thicken during the weeks leading up to a period and break down and bleed when the period begins. On the ovary, cysts tend to form, called chocolate cysts because of their color. These may become very large before finally bursting and releasing their contents into the pelvic cavity. Both the monthly bleeding from the endometrial patches and the bursting of a cyst cause pain, and in the latter case the pain may be severe enough to warrant hospital admission.

To begin with, the pain or discomfort is usually confined to one side of the abdomen, but in time it is likely to spread and become more severe. It usually starts before the period and may continue for some days after bleeding has begun. The deep pain felt during intercourse and sometimes for several hours afterward is usually present throughout the month, although it tends to be worse just before the period. Patients may be aware of an increased need to pass water during a period, often associated with some discomfort, and, rarely, may notice blood in the water. They may experience pain when passing stools and may have either diarrhea or constipation just prior to a period. If the bowel is affected by endometriosis, there may be blood in the stools.

ADENOMYOSIS

This is a fairly common condition that may cause both dysmenorrhea and menorrhagia. Like endometriosis, it is caused by endometrium growing in the wrong place, in this case within the muscle (myometrium) of the uterus. As a result the uterus becomes enlarged and occasionally polyps may develop. Anything that grows into the uterine cavity, such as a polyp or a fibroid, may cause dysmenorrhea, since the uterine muscle contracts in an attempt to expel the mass with the menstrual flow.

Adenomyosis tends to affect women in their thirties and forties who have had a least one pregnancy. They suffer from increasingly severe dysmenorrhea together with pain during intercourse and occasionally irregular bleeding.

METROPATHIA HEMORRHAGICA

Although commonest around the time of the menopause, this condition may also affect teenagers. It results from a failure of the follicle containing the mature ovum to burst, so that the ovum is not released and the follicular cells continue to secrete estrogen into the circulation. As a result the endometrium becomes thicker and thicker until eventually it can no longer be controlled by the estrogen and begins to break down. The symptoms are therefore those of heavy bleeding occurring considerably later than the time at which the period was expected.

PELVIC VENOUS CONGESTION

This condition has only been recognized in recent years and is thought by some specialists to account for the many cases in which women suffer from dysmenorrhea, pain during intercourse, lower abdominal pain, and sometimes heavy periods without there being any apparent cause. Doctors at a leading London hospital who have taken a special interest in pelvic venous congestion have estimated that whereas 15 percent of women who suffer from the typical symptoms of secondary dysmenorrhea can be shown to have a cause such as endometriosis, some 72 percent can be shown to have dilated pelvic veins through which the blood moves only very sluggishly.

Patients complain of a dull, aching pain that is worse during exercise and better when lying down and that on occasion may become quite sharp. They suffer from dysmenorrhea, and deep pain during intercourse, which tends to continue afterward. Over half are found to have cysts on their ovaries and it is possible that ovarian dysfunction may contribute to the problem. Another interesting finding has been the apparent association of this condition with emotional and psychological problems. A survey in the United States found that 75 percent of those women observed to have pelvic venous congestion had been sexually abused when children. Similarly, a specialist in Britain has estimated that some 60 percent of patients with this problem have emotional troubles at the time of diagnosis.

TESTS FOR DYSMENORRHEA AND MENORRHAGIA

The type of treatment offered to patients suffering from dysmenorrhea or menorrhagia will vary according to the underlying condition. Therefore, it is very important that the right diagnosis is made. This may require a number of tests to be performed.

Primary dysmenorrhea is usually easily diagnosed from the description of the symptoms and the age of the patient. In the case of secondary dysmenorrhea or menorrhagia, dilation and curettage (D & C or "a scrape") may be necessary in order to make a diagnosis. In this, the neck of the uterus is stretched slightly, under general anesthetic, and the endometrium is scraped, the scrapings being examined under the microscope. Laparoscopy may be performed under the same anesthetic. Here a tiny cut is made in the abdomen, usually just by the navel, and an instrument is inserted through which the gynecologist can see the ovaries, the tubes, the uterus, and the interior of the pelvis. Nowadays, it is possible to do a curettage, or scrape, in an outpatient setting or in the doctor's office, using a small pump or syringe that gently sucks out the endometrium. However, this simplified test is only suitable for older patients since it may cause pain in younger women.

Before carrying out any of these surgical techniques, the gynecologist will have examined the patient through the vagina and sometimes through the rectum in order to feel whether the uterus is bulky or out of position, whether the ovaries feel normal, and whether there seem to be any deposits of endometriosis around the reproductive organs or the bowel. He may take swabs to see whether there is any sign of infection and will usually take a Pap smear if one has not been done recently. Blood may also be taken to see whether the patient is anemic and, in some cases, for hormone estimations, since some imbalances (such as lack of thyroid hormone) may cause heavy periods.

At one center in Britain that specializes in the treatment of pelvic pain, patients are routinely offered screening of the pelvic veins in order to diagnose pelvic venous congestion. This is done in the outpatients' clinic and takes only ten minutes. A long needle is inserted into the uterus through the vagina and an injection of local anesthetic is given into its muscle layer. Then a dye is slowly injected. This is taken up into the pelvic veins and can be followed on an X-ray screen that will show whether the veins are dilated and whether blood flow through them is sluggish.

TRADITIONAL TREATMENT

This, of course, will depend on what is causing the patient's symptoms. Most women with menorrhagia will need supplements of iron and folic acid to prevent them from becoming anemic. If pelvic inflammatory disease is contributing to the problem, a course of antibiotics may be necessary. Because period problems are commoner in obese patients and in those who smoke, weight loss and giving up smoking will be advised where appropriate.

Primary Dysmenorrhea
Since the discovery of the involvement of prostaglandins in primary dysmenorrhea, drugs that reduce the level of these substances in the body have been shown to be very helpful in the control of this condition. These include flurbiprofen, mefenamic acid, naproxen, ibuprofen, and piroxicam. Such antiprostaglandins are effective in 75–90 percent of cases of primary dysmenorrhea provided they are taken in adequate dosage from the moment bleeding starts and for as long as the pain is

likely to occur. Aspirin is also effective, but needs to be started a few days before the period is due since it seems to inhibit the manufacture of prostaglandins rather than having any effect on the formed substance.

Because antiprostaglandin tablets work in slightly different ways, one may sometimes be effective where another has failed, so it is always worth trying at least two before giving up. Unfortunately, they may have side effects, such as diarrhea, stomach upsets, headache, drowsiness, and dizziness. Although they are well tolerated by most women, in those cases where side effects occur or where the tablets are not helpful, or for women who also need a contraceptive, the Pill can be a useful alternative.

Very rarely, in cases where the pain is severe and fails to respond to any of these treatments, an operation may be performed in which the uterine nerves are cut, preventing the pain from being felt.

Menorrhagia

In cases where investigations have failed to reveal anything abnormal, hormonal treatment may be helpful. Very often such excessive bleeding is associated with an anovulatory cycle (in which no egg is produced) so that progesterone is not secreted. Taking tablets of a progestogen (a substance with a similar action to the natural hormone, progesterone) such as norethindrone during the second half of the cycle may relieve the symptoms. However, these can sometimes cause acne and hairiness, so younger women may prefer to take the Pill, which contains a progestogen combined with estrogen. But in a number of cases, curettage itself will solve the problem, so some gynecologists like to observe a patient for a few months following this procedure before prescribing any medication. Menorrhagia may be made worse or even caused by an intrauterine device (IUD, "coil," or "loop") and may settle once the device has been removed.

The prostaglandin-inhibiting drugs described in the section on the treatment of dysmenorrhea may reduce the amount of blood lost but will not make the period any shorter and so they are not helpful for those women whose periods continue for more than seven days. Drugs that actually help to shut down bleeding vessels, such as ethamsylate and tranexamic acid, may sometimes be of value, although the latter may occasionally cause diarrhea, headache, nausea, and weakness. For those patients whose menorrhagia is associated with anovulatory cycles and consequent infertility, clomiphene may not only control the menorrhagia but stimulate ovulation. However, this drug cannot be taken for more than a few months and may produce unpleasant side effects such as depression.

Danazol, which is derived from the male hormone, testosterone, stops the ovaries from functioning and therefore produces a "pseudo-menopause." As a result, in addition to stopping or reducing the periods, it may also cause hot flashes, a reduction in sex drive, a decrease in breast size, and a dry vagina. Its other side effects include acne, hairiness, weight gain, digestive upsets, tremors, cramps, and depression. However, it is well tolerated by most women. But it should never be taken by women who act or sing or whose voices play an important role in their lives, since it may produce an irreversible deepening of the voice.

If all else fails, hysterectomy may have to be considered.

Endometriosis
A progestogen such as norethindrone will reduce the growth of the endometrial deposits and have fewer risks for older patients than the Pill, which may, however, be suitable for the under-thirty-fives. Medroxyprogesterone acetate may also be used either in its oral form or as an injection. Danazol is probably the most effective form of drug treatment, but it has the side effects mentioned above.

Surgical treatment may sometimes be necessary for endometriosis, to remove adhesions (patches of fibrous scar tissue) that are distorting the ovaries or tubes and to restore the uterus to its normal position. If pain is severe, cutting the uterine nerves may be helpful. In some cases, hysterectomy with removal of the ovaries and tubes may be necessary. Some specialists feel that the laser may play an important role in treatment in the future, since it can accurately destroy patches of endometriosis as well as removing adhesions. This form of treatment has been used in an increasing number of centers in both Europe and the United States over the past few years and it is possible that it may, in due course, become the treatment of choice.

The treatment offered to patients with endometriosis will depend on how far advanced the disease is and how severe their symptoms are. In 90 percent of mild cases, drug therapy or simple surgery will be effective. In rather more advanced cases, however, a 50 percent recurrence rate can be expected. Severe cases require radical surgery to remove uterus, ovaries, tubes, and adhesions.

Although pregnancy doesn't cure the disease, it may delay its progression. Seventy-five percent of women with mild endometriosis are able to conceive, but this figure drops to 50 percent of those with more advanced disease, and only 35 percent of those who are severely affected.

Adenomyosis

Sometimes this will respond to curettage alone. In other cases, progestogens may be used or danazol. If drug treatment fails, hysterectomy, in which the ovaries are not removed, may be necessary.

Metropathia Hemorrhagica

The choice of treatment is identical to that for adenomyosis, with 60 percent of patients responding to curettage.

Pelvic Venous Congestion

Since this condition has only been recognized fairly recently, treatment is still in its infancy. However, it seems that medroxyprogesterone acetate is helpful. Hysterectomy seems only to relieve the symptoms if the ovaries are removed as well. Because of the association with emotional problems, psychotherapy can be very effective, but it may be a considerable time before the results are evident.

COMPLEMENTARY TREATMENT

Acupuncture

Dysmenorrhea is said to be due to invasion by cold, which obstructs the flow of energy, or Chi, or to problems in the flow of Chi through the liver. Points are chosen that will eliminate cold, warm the energy channels, and restore the flow of Chi to normal. The liver is strengthened, as is the kidney, whose energy is said to control the function of the reproductive system.

Menorrhagia is said to be due to problems with the spleen, which is involved in the control of blood flow through the body. Treatment is given that will strengthen the spleen and return blood flow to normal.

Aromatherapy

In common with herbalists and homeopaths, aromatherapists find chamomile useful in the treatment of dysmenorrhea. Other oils used include tarragon, cypress, marjoram, sage, and juniper. Cypress, juniper, and geranium are among those used to treat heavy bleeding.

Herbalism

Many herbs are used to treat the various aspects of menstrual disorders. Chamomile is one of the most useful, especially in the treatment of dysmenorrhea. Shepherd's purse is used specifically to reduce heavy bleeding and cramp bark is used to reduce the spasm of the uterine muscle that causes pain. Peppermint, too, is an antispasmodic, as are white deadnettle and thyme. Shepherd's purse and white deadnettle are also used to relieve pelvic congestion.

Homeopathy

Belladonna may be given to a patient who has cramplike pain that begins on the day before the period, a heavy bright red flow, loss of appetite, and pain when passing stools during the period.

Sepia may be appropriate if the period is late and produces fatigue, irritability, and depression together with dragging pains that are eased by crossing the legs.

A very heavy period associated with a tearing pain in the lower abdomen and back, loss of appetite, diarrhea, and a fluctuation in symptoms may be an indication for pulsatilla.

Ipecac is useful when the patient has pain in the umbilical region, dizziness, nausea, and headache. Chamomilla may be chosen for someone with laborlike pains, a flow of brown blood with clots, and a desire to pass water frequently. Very heavy bleeding in obese women may be treated with sabina and very heavy painless bleeding with crocus sativus or, if the patient also has ringing in the ears, with china. Many other remedies are also used for individual variations of symptoms.

Hypnotherapy

This can be very effective in the treatment of dysmenorrhea since not only can it help the patient to relax but it can also teach her how to control the pain when it arises.

Nutrition

Dysmenorrhea may be associated with a calcium deficiency, so a supplement of dolomite (calcium plus magnesium) may be recommended.

SELF-HELP

Since constipation will make dysmenorrhea worse, a high-fiber diet is advisable. Naturopathic recommendations may include a reduction of salt, sugar, and dairy produce in the diet, and a raw food diet for the seven days before the period begins.

A survey of over two thousand women that was carried out in Oxford, England, in 1988 found that women who smoked were more likely to suffer from heavy, prolonged, painful, irregular, or frequent periods than women who were nonsmokers. Giving up smoking might well help to relieve the symptoms of many women with menstrual problems.

ORGANIZATIONS

Endometriosis Association
P.O. Box 92187
Milwaukee, WI 53202
414/962-8972
(Publishes a bimonthly newsletter and educational material.)

MIGRAINE

DEFINITION AND INCIDENCE

The cause of migraine is unknown and the symptoms from which patients suffer may be extremely varied, but the word is used to describe attacks of severe recurrent headaches that do not have any underlying physical cause.

Migraine is said to affect about one person in twenty, with women being affected more often than men (in a ratio of six to four). It usually begins between the ages of fifteen and forty-five, although it may start at any age and 25 percent of patients have had their first attack by the age of ten. Before developing full-blown migraine, some children may suffer from recurrent attacks of vomiting. And some youngsters may grow out of the condition during their teens (one study put the chances of this at between 35 and 50 percent).

The condition tends to run in families, 46 percent of patients having a close relative (often their mother) who also suffers from it. Some may have only one or two migraines a year, whereas others have them far more frequently, the average being between one and four a month. The individual pattern varies and patients may have a number of mild attacks with an occasional severe one, or the occasional mild attack in the midst of a stream of bad ones. In about a quarter of cases, the attack lasts for more than twenty-four hours.

THEORIES ON THE CAUSE OF MIGRAINE

Classical migraine consists of the "aura" (in which the patient may see flashing lights and experience tingling sensations) followed by a severe headache. The traditional theory, first put forward some thirty years ago, is that migraine is caused by a sudden constriction of the blood vessels in the brain (causing the aura), followed by an overdilation (causing the headache). However, Danish doctors have shown recently that the brain may be short of blood for some hours before a migraine attack and that this shortage may continue well into the headache phase when, according to the traditional theory, an excess of blood should be flowing through the brain. Other doctors have come to the conclusion that the primary changes during migraine are concerned with the nervous system and not with the blood vessels at all.

A recent discovery is that an intravenous injection of prostaglandins (the hormonelike substances that are involved in numerous bodily functions including the development of inflammation) will produce many of the symptoms that are associated with migraine. It has therefore been postulated that the primary problem is an overproduction of prostaglandins. Other research has suggested that some migraines are allergic in origin. Levels of 5-hydroxy-tryptamine, a substance involved in the allergic response, are found to be higher than normal in the urine of patients during a migraine attack.

PRECIPITATING FACTORS

Although migraines can occur for no apparent reason, many patients are aware of factors that will bring on an attack. In one study, 81 percent of the patients cited emotional stress as an important factor. Others include excitement, missing a meal, taking the contraceptive Pill, heat, exercise, changes in the weather, and eating certain foods such as cheese, chocolate, onions, peanuts, beer, citrus fruits, monosodium glutamate, and red wine. It is possible that some attacks may be triggered by contact with certain chemicals, such as those used in the production of magazines and newspapers. Women who suffer from migraine tend to be more at risk of an attack during the week leading up to a period, when, it seems, there may be a higher level of prostaglandins in the body.

Doctors are often cautious about giving migraine sufferers the Pill, since this may make them worse. However, occasionally they may improve. Some who have not had migraine before may develop it for the first time when taking the Pill. Unfortunately, when they come off it, they may continue to have migraines.

SYMPTOMS

Migraine is made up of two distinct phases—the early symptoms (known as the prodromal symptoms, or aura) and the headache itself.

Some patients may just have the headache with no previous symptoms and occasionally some may just have the prodromal symptoms that then fizzle out without a headache developing.

The commonest prodromal symptoms are visual. The patient may suddenly be aware of lights flashing across her field of vision or of brilliant shimmering zigzag lines that may be of various colors. Or the symptoms may be less specific, with simply a blurring or a "heat-haze" effect. Gradually it may become more difficult to see, although total blindness never occurs. Very occasionally, the muscles controlling the eyes stop functioning so that the patient develops a temporary squint.

Other symptoms include tingling or numbness that often starts in one hand and spreads slowly up the arm to the face, where it involves the mouth and the tongue. Very occasionally, both arms or the legs are affected. The muscles in the affected area may lose some of their function so that the patient may have difficulty performing fine movements or, rarely, may have problems in speaking. Dizziness or confusion may also occur and in a few cases severe dizziness may be the first symptom. Occasionally there may be changes in mood or behavior. A child may be pale and unusually irritable for several hours before an attack.

Most patients have one or two of these symptoms (usually the same ones each time) and these last for up to twenty minutes, after which the headache begins. In 60 percent of cases, the pain is only on one side of the head, but it may spread to affect the eyes, neck, face, and jaws. With the onset of the headache, most patients prefer to lie in a darkened room, since in 80 percent of cases, the light hurts their eyes and makes the pain worse. Nearly all feel sick and children may complain of abdominal pain. Ten percent of patients vomit and sometimes the headache begins to decrease once they have done so. Occasionally diarrhea may occur. Fluid retention is common during an attack and the end of the migraine may be heralded by a need to pass water. As patients get older, the headache tends to become less severe, although the prodromal symptoms may remain the same.

TRADITIONAL TREATMENT

In the treatment of migraine two types of drugs are used—those that prevent an attack (prophylactic drugs) and those that treat individual attacks when they occur. Prophylactic drugs are not usually recommended unless the patient is having more than two attacks a month. They are thought to work by preventing the abnormal contraction and dilation of blood vessels that are said to cause migraine. However, if one of the other theories of causation proves to be correct, another explanation of how these drugs work will have to be postulated.

Prophylactic Drugs

BETA BLOCKERS
This class of drugs, which includes propranolol, metoprolol, nadolol, and timolol, is also used extensively in the treatment of high blood pressure. Propranolol is the most commonly used to treat migraine, but as explained in the section on blood pressure it is not suitable for asthmatics. More than 50 percent of patients who have moderate or severe attacks more than twice a month will obtain relief by taking beta blockers.

METHYSERGIDE MALEATE
This drug is extremely effective, but unfortunately it may have potentially dangerous side effects. However, used under close medical supervision, it may be the only orthodox answer for patients whose migraine fails to respond to any other drug treatment.

OTHER DRUGS
Other drugs used as prophylactics include cyproheptadine, naproxen (an antiinflammatory, antiprostaglandin drug), and clonidine. Recent research has shown that the calcium-blocking drugs used in the treatment of high blood pressure may also be of value.

Drugs Used During the Migraine Attack
In line with the theory that migraine may be associated with an excess of prostaglandins in the body, drugs that inhibit their production may be very helpful in the treatment of the complaint. These include aspirin and acetaminophen. Certain experts consider aspirin to be the drug of choice in the treatment of migraine, as long as it produces no side effects (such as indigestion). However, the reason why it probably fails to work in many cases is that it is not taken early enough in the attack.

In addition, the stomach is inclined to lose its mobility during a migraine, so that its contents are not passed into the gut to be absorbed. It is suggested, therefore, that patients should take aspirin right at the start of an attack and preferably in a soluble form, which will allow it to be absorbed more easily. Taking a tablet of metoclopramide, which speeds up the emptying of the stomach, followed ten minutes later by three tablets of aspirin or acetaminophen, may be a very effective way of cutting short the attack.

A drug that has perhaps become less popular in recent years for the treatment of migraine is ergotamine. This is believed to act by constricting the overdilated blood vessels of the brain. Here again, if another theory of causation is proved to be correct, a different explanation of how this drug works will have to be put forward. Its effectiveness may be considerably reduced by a failure to absorb it, so it is available in suppository form as Cafergot, in tablets that dissolve under the tongue as Ergostat, and in inhaler form as Medihaler-Ergotamine. It may produce side effects that include nausea, vomiting, abdominal pain, diarrhea, and cramps, and high doses may in fact cause a headache. Like other migraine medication, it should be taken early in the attack. Because there are risks associated with high dosage and with constant use, stated doses should never be exceeded and the drug should never be taken as a prophylactic.

RECENT ADVANCES

Dentists at the Glasgow Dental Hospital, United Kingdom, have shown that in some cases a malalignment of the upper and lower teeth may be instrumental in causing migraine. They found nineteen patients who suffered from migraine attacks every two to three weeks, some of whom had been having attacks for many years and all of whom developed symptoms either upon waking or shortly afterward. Each was fitted with an acrylic splint that was worn at night to bring the teeth into the correct position. During a year in which the patients wore the splints every night, the incidence of migraine attacks fell dramatically. The dentists suggested that the malpositioning of the teeth was putting certain muscles in the jaw into spasm and that this was triggering the migraine.

COMPLEMENTARY TREATMENT

Acupuncture

Very often the pain of migraine is exactly located to the distribution of the Gallbladder channel, which on each side runs from a point next to the eye, back toward the ear, then around the ear to the neck, forward to the forehead, and finally back again, down the neck and, passing under the arm, over the abdomen and down the leg to the little toe. Thus, it is located over the jaw, whose spasm may precipitate migraine, next to the eyes, which are associated with the prodromal symptoms, on the forehead and crown of the head where the pain is often felt, and in the abdomen, which may be affected by nausea. In such cases, the cause of the migraine may be seen as stagnation of energy, or Chi, in the Gallbladder channel, and treatment to restore normal flow of Chi may be very effective in preventing further attacks.

Aromatherapy

In common with the herbalists, aromatherapists find rosemary and lavender useful in the treatment of migraine. Marjoram, basil, melissa, rose, aniseed, chamomile, eucalyptus, and peppermint may also be recommended.

Herbalism

Feverfew has been a popular migraine remedy for many years. However, recently doctors have carried out a scientific trial of feverfew and have proved that it works. Like some of the orthodox drugs used, it dilates constricted blood vessels. Its one drawback is that in a few patients it may cause mouth ulcers. Other herbs used to treat migraine include lemon balm (which relaxes the nervous system), rosemary (which stimulates the circulation and strengthens the functions of the nervous system), motherwort (which is particularly useful when attacks are brought on by nervous tension), and vervain and lavender (which are relaxant and antispasmodic).

Homeopathy

Iris is a commonly used remedy for migraine and is appropriate when the patient complains of a headache associated with diarrhea and preceded by blurred vision.

Silica may be helpful for someone who suffers from recurrent severe headaches that start at the back of the neck, move forward to the eyes, and are associated with nausea and vomiting. When temporary loss of vision heralds a severe throbbing pain often on the top of the head or above the eyes, and is worse for warmth or movement, natrum mur. may be effective. When a right-sided headache is associated with pain in the shoulder, sanguinaria may help. If the pain is on the left, and the patient feels weak and faint and has palpitations, spigelia may be prescribed.

Hypnotherapy

This can be remarkably effective in the treatment of migraine. Under hypnosis, the patient is taught a technique that can be used at the start of an attack to prevent the migraine from developing. This may consist, for example, of a visualization where she pictures the blood vessels in her brain contracting and then, as she clenches and relaxes her fists or as she counts slowly to twenty, she sees them returning to normal. (The fact that this may be physiologically inaccurate doesn't matter at all in a visualization.) She is told that what she pictures will actually occur and that by performing this technique she will be able to control her migraine and prevent the symptoms from developing any further. When patients have used this method for a while and have gained confidence in its effectiveness, they will often find that they are having to use it less often, as the attacks become less frequent.

Manipulation

Patients who suffer from migraine often have excessive muscle tension in their necks and shoulders, which may spark off attacks. Chiropractic or osteopathic manipulation may help to remove this tension and to restore mobility to the neck joints. Manipulation of the jaw to reduce muscle tension caused by faulty bite, together with dental treatment as described above, may also be of value.

Nutrition

Vitamin B_3 in the form of nicotinic acid (niacin) has the effect of dilating blood vessels and, if taken in the early stage of a migraine, can stop or reduce the severity of the attack. The only side effect is flushing of the face. To begin with, 100 mg should be taken, but if this is not fully effective, the dose may be gradually increased to a maximum of 500 mg until the attacks are being controlled.

ORGANIZATIONS

National Headache Foundation
5252 North Western Avenue
Chicago, IL 60625
312/878-5558
(Publishes a quarterly newsletter.)

MONONUCLEOSIS, INFECTIOUS

INCIDENCE AND SYMPTOMS

Infectious mononucleosis, commonly known as "mono," is a very common condition. It can attack people of any age, but usually tends to affect adolescents and young adults. It seems likely that in younger children it takes the form of a slight flulike illness, because there are many people who can be shown to be immune to mono but who have no recollection of ever having had the disease. It is caused by a virus, known as the Epstein-Barr (EB) virus but is not particularly infectious. However, miniepidemics do occur, usually in schools, military barracks, or other institutions where young people live in close proximity to each other. The virus is thought to be transmitted in the saliva and therefore can be passed on by kissing—in fact, it is sometimes referred to as "the kissing disease."

The onset of the illness is usually gradual, with fever, headache, and a general feeling of being unwell. After a few days, the lymph glands swell up, especially those in the neck, armpits, and groins. However, they are not usually tender and unless the swelling is severe it may not be noticed. Between 50 and 80 percent of patients develop a sore throat and in some cases this may be very severe, with badly inflamed and ulcerated tonsils. The fever rarely goes above 40°C (104°F), but it may last up to three weeks.

In 95 percent of cases, the liver is affected and this can be demonstrated by blood tests. However, only 5 percent of patients develop jaundice (although occasionally this may be the first sign of illness) and liver failure is rare. The liver (which is situated under the ribs on the right) is often enlarged, as is the spleen (which is under the ribs on the left). Very rarely, the spleen may rupture—a potentially fatal condition in which the patient develops severe abdominal pain and rapidly becomes pale and sweaty with a thready pulse due to internal bleeding. Urgent hospital treatment is required.

Between 10 and 40 percent of patients develop a generalized red rash. In most cases, the lining of the nose and throat becomes slightly swollen and very rarely this may be severe enough to cause problems with breathing. Other rare complications include meningitis and paralysis, which usually resolve of their own accord, and disorders of the immune system.

However, an almost universal symptom of mono is fatigue. Although full recovery is normal, the patient may continue to suffer from fatigue for a long time after the other symptoms have disappeared.

TESTS

Infectious mononucleosis is diagnosed by a blood test, known as a Paul-Bunnell test. Abnormal white cells (mononuclear cells, which give the disease its name) can be seen when the blood is examined under a microscope.

TRADITIONAL TREATMENT

Treatment consists of bed rest and gradual rehabilitation as the symptoms recede. However, in some cases steroids may be used. Prednisolone given for twelve days in decreasing doses is known to speed recovery and its use seems justifiable in patients who have an important event coming up—for example, those who are about to take final examinations or to get married. Hydrocortisone is used to reduce severe swelling of the lining of the nose and throat and steroids are also given to patients who develop some of the rarer complications such as paralysis.

Patients with mono should not take part in contact sports until they are completely recovered, because of the risk to the spleen. A ruptured spleen requires emergency treatment consisting of blood transfusions and surgery to stop the intraabdominal bleeding.

People whose immune systems are functioning poorly (for example, those taking anticancer drugs) may be given the antiviral agent, acyclovir, for seven to ten days to help them to fight the infection.

Sometimes prolonged symptoms of fatigue may be helped by a two- to three-month course of antidepressants.

COMPLEMENTARY TREATMENT

Aromatherapy
Lavender, eucalyptus, peppermint, or bergamot may be recommended.

Herbalism
Herbs may be given to strengthen the nervous system (such as St. John's wort or vervain), to help to fight the infection (such as echinacea or marigold), to reduce the fever (such as elderflower or yarrow), and to cleanse the lymphatic system (such as wild indigo, poke root, or marigold).

Homeopathy
Carcinosin is usually the remedy of choice for mono. However, in some cases other remedies may be appropriate—for example, phytolacca if the glands remain swollen and sore after the fever has subsided and the patient complains of headaches and generalized pains. For cases where symptoms have been present for a long time, bacillinum, kali iod., calc. iod., or baryta carb. may be prescribed.

MOUTH ULCERS AND BAD BREATH (Halitosis)

MOUTH ULCERS AND BAD BREATH (halitosis) warrant only a few lines in most medical textbooks, but many people find them a considerable problem.

MOUTH ULCERS

Description and Causes

Known medically as aphthous ulcers, these are small, painful erosions of the lining of the mouth that usually appear in groups, last several days, and tend to recur frequently. Attacks often start in adolescence and as the patient gets older they diminish in frequency until finally they stop altogether. The cause is unknown. Patients who suffer from intestinal conditions, such as Crohn's disease, ulcerative colitis, and celiac disease, are more likely to get mouth ulcers than other people, but here again the reason is unknown.

Sometimes mouth ulcers can result from a viral infection and be associated with fever and headache. These ulcers, however, are different than typical aphthous ulcers. Tiny blisters develop in the mouth and throat, which then become ulcers. Usually the infection lasts only a few days and the patient recovers rapidly.

Soreness of the mouth, without ulceration, may be due to poorly fitting dentures or to a vitamin deficiency, particularly of the B complex or folic acid. A doctor's advice should always be sought concerning a painless ulcer or one that fails to heal, since occasionally cancer of the mouth may begin like this. However, there are other reasons why ulcers may not heal, one of which is the constant chewing of gum.

Traditional Treatment

Various preparations are available for the treatment of mouth ulcers. These include carbamide peroxide, local anesthetics such as benzocaine in the form of lozenges or gels, and salicylates (aspirinlike compounds). These are available over the counter. Mouthwashes such as chlorhexidine may also be helpful. In some cases, steroid pastes or lozenges may be prescribed.

Complementary Treatment

Aromatherapy
Myrrh, lemon, tea tree, and geranium may be used.

Herbalism
A number of herbal mouthwashes may be effective in the treatment of ulcers. They include marigold, myrrh, red sage, and thyme, all of which have healing and antiseptic properties.

Homeopathy
For ulcers under the tongue associated with a metallic taste in the mouth, a swollen tongue, and bad breath, merc. sol. may be effective. Borax may be prescribed for ulcers that are worse when acid or salty foods are eaten. Ulcers inside the lower lip associated with cold sores may respond to hydrastis.

Naturopathy
A cleansing program in which the patient takes only fruit, vegetables, and fruit juices for two to three days may be recommended.

Nutrition
Patients who suffer from recurrent mouth ulcers may have an allergy to something in their diet (such as wheat or another grain) or a vitamin A deficiency. A nutrition therapist will inquire for other evidence of vitamin A deficiency and may suggest an elimination diet in order to pinpoint any allergy before recommending treatment—either in the form of a special diet or by vitamin supplements.

Bad Breath (Halitosis)

Human beings are very sensitive creatures and are inclined to think they are smelly when they aren't. This is particularly so among young people. Many people who fear that they have bad breath do not, in fact, smell bad to other people. The best person to consult is the dentist, who is in a very good position to judge while having no reason to tell anything other than the truth. In addition, when bad breath occurs, it is often a dental problem rather than a medical one, being due to decaying teeth or gingivitis (infection of the gums).

Undoubtedly the commonest cause of bad breath is smoking. Other causes include spicy foods, garlic, alcohol, chronic constipation, and overconsumption of meat.

Traditional Treatment

If halitosis is due to infection or decay in the mouth, treatment is the province of the dentist. Once the mouth is healthy again, the smell should disappear.

Complementary Treatment

Aromatherapy
Myrrh and peppermint may be recommended as mouthwashes.

Herbalism
Lavender or vervain mouthwash may be an effective treatment for halitosis. Vervain is also useful for patients undergoing dental treatment as it encourages healing of disease in the teeth and gums.

Homeopathy
If bad breath results from digestive problems, nux vomica or pulsatilla may be helpful. If it is associated with flatulence or infected gums, carbo veg. may be appropriate. Bad breath after eating may respond to chamomilla, and if the breath smells like onions, allium cepa may help.

Self-Help

For smokers, the best remedy is to give up smoking. Changes in the diet may also be helpful. Meat and fats tend to slow down the passage of food through the intestines, so that food spends longer in the stomach. Sometimes, changing to a vegetarian diet with a reduced intake of fat may get rid of halitosis. A diet that includes a lot of natural chlorophyll (in other words, raw green, leafy vegetables) may also be beneficial.

NOSEBLEEDS

CAUSES AND SYMPTOMS

Nosebleeds are common, especially in children, and often entail only a slight loss of blood. However, bleeding may be recurrent and occasionally profuse.

The lining of the nose has many small blood vessels in it and the section covering the front part of the nasal septum (the sheet of cartilage that lies between the nostrils) is particularly rich in vessels. This section is known as Kiesselbach's area and it is from here that most bleeds occur. Perhaps the commonest cause is injury—often from nose picking. Other causes are a broken nose, local infections such as a heavy cold or sinusitis, and general infections including mononucleosis and tuberculosis. Patients with hay fever or chronic rhinitis may suffer from nosebleeds, as may those with high blood pressure, leukemia, and benign or malignant growths within the nose itself. Abnormalities of the blood vessels in the nose or of the clotting mechanism of the blood (such as occur in hemophilia) may also be involved.

Usually some blood trickles down the back of the throat. Heavy bleeding may result in the patient swallowing a lot of blood which, because it irritates the stomach lining, may cause vomiting. Very occasionally, vomiting of blood may be the first sign of a nosebleed.

TESTS

Older patients are usually checked for high blood pressure. When someone has been having heavy nosebleeds, blood tests may be needed to see whether he has become anemic and whether an abnormality of the blood may be to blame. A nose swab will detect any infection that may have caused the bleed.

TRADITIONAL TREATMENT

If the bleeding is coming from Kiesselbach's area, it will often stop if the area is compressed by squeezing the end of the nose between the fingers for about five minutes. If this fails to work, treatment consists of gently opening up the nostril with a small instrument (speculum) and removing any clots. The doctor can then see whether or not the bleeding is coming from Kiesselbach's area. If it is, the insertion into the nose of a small piece of cotton soaked in adrenaline followed by another five minutes of squeezing will often stop it by helping the blood vessels to contract. However, bleeding may begin again once the effect of the adrenaline has worn off, so some doctors like to follow up this procedure by cauterizing the area using, for example, a cotton swab soaked in silver nitrate solution.

Particularly resistant bleeds may require the nose to be packed, although this is not usually necessary. A narrow ribbon gauze that has been lubricated with Vaseline or a similar substance is introduced into each nostril in layers. This produces a firm, constant pressure on the bleeding area. The ends of the gauze are left hanging out of the nostrils and are secured with a safety pin in order to avoid their disappearing back into the nose. Some doctors like to give antibiotics to patients who have nose packs, as, theoretically, they could act as a focus for infection.

Patients who have recurrent bleeds from Kiesselbach's area may need admission to the hospital to have the area cauterized under anesthetic.

Bleeds from the back of the nose are less common than those from the front and are less easy to treat because pressure cannot be exerted on the bleeding point from outside and the point itself cannot be seen. If the bleed doesn't stop of its own accord, the nose has to be packed. However, because the back of the nose is encased in bone, it is only necessary to pack one nostril in order to produce the required pressure. The pack is inserted in the same way as a pack for the front part of the nose and is left for at least twenty-four hours. If bleeding continues after this, it may be necessary to repack the nostril or to insert a postnasal pack. The latter consists of a narrow tube (catheter) with a deflated balloon on its end that is passed through the nose to the back of the throat. The balloon is then inflated until it fits snugly into the back of the nose, blocking it off. The other end of the tube is taped to the patient's face and the nostril is packed with gauze. Some doctors give antibiotics to patients being treated in this way since in theory the blood retained within the nose could promote the growth of bacteria.

Very occasionally, surgery is necessary to stop further bleeding. The artery that supplies blood to the affected area is tied off and this may be done via an incision in the neck, through the maxillary sinus in the upper jaw or through the upper part of the nose itself. In other cases, where there is an underlying cause for the bleeding, such as high blood pressure, this will be treated in the appropriate manner.

All patients who are suffering from nosebleeds should be put to bed and propped up in a sitting position so that blood does not run down the back of the throat. If the nose has been packed, the patient will have to breathe through the mouth and will therefore need frequent mouthwashes and plenty to drink to prevent the mouth from becoming dry. (Patients with packed noses often find it easier to drink through a straw.) Those who have lost a lot of blood may need admission to the hospital for a blood transfusion.

Occasionally drugs are prescribed. For patients who have recurrent nosebleeds and are waiting for admission to the hospital for definitive treatment, a preparation that helps to stop bleeding from small blood vessels, such as tranexamic acid, may be used. Sometimes patients become quite anxious about their recurrent bleeds and, in such a case, phenobarbital or Valium may be prescribed as a sedative.

COMPLEMENTARY TREATMENT

Acupuncture
Nosebleeds are said to be due to an excess of heat in the lung and stomach and a lack of yin (the feminine negative aspect of Chi). The aim of treatment is to eliminate heat, stimulate yin, and restore energy flow to normal.

Aromatherapy
Essence of cypress on a piece of cotton held under the nose may help to stop a bleed.

Herbalism
A piece of cotton soaked in an infusion of St. John's wort or witch hazel may help to stop bleeding if pressed against the nose. Shepherd's purse or yarrow may be prescribed for their antihemorrhagic properties.

Homeopathy

If a nosebleed has resulted from an injury, arnica will be helpful, particularly if the bleeding is heavy. Profuse bleeding that occurs after the nose has been blown vigorously may respond to phosphorus. For the irritable, fearful patient, aconite may be appropriate. Belladonna may be prescribed if the bleed is associated with a throbbing headache, and hamamelis if the blood oozes rather than flows. Many other remedies may be used as well.

Nutrition

For a patient who suffers from recurrent nosebleeds, rutin tablets may be helpful since they will strengthen the blood vessels.

OSTEOPOROSIS

DEFINITION, MECHANISM, AND INCIDENCE

Osteoporosis is a condition in which the bones become thin. It is commonest in postmenopausal women and is not so much a disease as an extreme form of a normal bodily process.

Bones are made up from a framework of living cells impregnated with various minerals to achieve rigidity—primarily calcium phosphate, but also quantities of magnesium and sodium. Like the rest of the body, the bones are continually changing, with cells dying and being replaced. In addition, two types of cells are constantly at work within the bones, one removing bone and the other laying it down again. As a result, a small amount of calcium is lost into the bloodstream each day and fresh calcium is laid down. During childhood and adolescence, the bones become increasingly dense as more minerals are deposited than are lost, and a maximum density is reached during the twenties and thirties. After the age of about thirty-five, more minerals are lost than are replaced and the bones become thinner with advancing age.

In osteoporosis, excessive amounts of minerals are lost and the bones become brittle. The condition probably affects some 24 million people in the United States and is responsible for some 1.3 million fractures a year. It is estimated that 75 percent of all women will develop some degree of osteoporosis and as a result two thirds of these will have at least one major fracture.

CAUSES

Why some people develop osteoporosis and others don't remains a mystery, but there is a tendency for the condition to run in families. Recently a group of "fast calcium losers" has been identified in the population and this natural tendency can be diagnosed by urine and blood tests. These fast losers have a high risk of developing osteoporo-

317

sis, as do people suffering from certain diseases in which calcium loss is increased, such as thyrotoxicosis, diabetes, chronic malnutrition (for example, in alcoholism), inflammatory bowel disease (such as Crohn's disease or ulcerative colitis, in which absorption of calcium may be reduced), hyperparathyroidism (in which the calcium-regulating parathyroid glands are overactive), Cushing's syndrome (in which there is excessive secretion of steroid hormones from the adrenal glands), and rheumatoid arthritis. Certain types of medication also have the effect of promoting calcium loss from the body. These include steroids taken over a long period of time, diuretics (taken, for example, in the treatment of high blood pressure), and thyroid hormones. Some theorize that a high-protein (typical Western) diet facilitates calcium loss.

Osteoporosis is four times as common in women as in men but rarely starts before the menopause. There is no evidence that a lack of female hormones actually causes the condition, but these hormones do seem to promote the retention of calcium within the body so that it is only when their levels drop that osteoporosis will develop in a susceptible patient. Even after the menopause, the ovaries continue to produce a small amount of estrogen, so women who have had their ovaries removed have an increased risk of osteoporosis. So too do women who have an early menopause (before the age of forty to forty-five), because they are likely to spend more years of their lives in a postmenopausal, calcium-losing state. Other women who may be at risk are those whose ovaries functioned imperfectly even before the menopause and who may have had infrequent periods as a result. These women are likely to have thinner bones than normal when they reach the menopause, since their premenopausal hormone levels will have been too low to offer them protection. However, women who have been pregnant or who have taken the contraceptive Pill are likely to have more calcium in their bones than others.

People who have larger bones to begin with have more calcium to lose and therefore are less likely to develop osteoporosis. Normally men's bones are larger than women's and those of black people are larger than those of whites or Asians. Overweight people seem to be less at risk than those who are thin. Men do develop osteoporosis, but it usually occurs at a later age than in women.

Smoking increases the risk of osteoporosis, probably because it breaks down the protective hormones, and heavy smokers are more likely to break bones than other people.

Immobilizing a part of the body can result in considerable loss of calcium from that part and elderly people who remain in bed for periods even as short as a week are likely to start losing calcium at an increased rate from all their bones.

COURSE OF THE DISEASE

Frequently, the first indication that a patient has osteoporosis is when she breaks a bone, perhaps as the result of a fairly trivial injury. Occasionally symptoms of back pain and tiredness may occur soon after the menopause. However, no changes can be seen on an X-ray until about one third of the total bone density has been lost and this may take another ten to fifteen years. Bone loss is most rapid in the first five years after the menopause and then slows to a steady rate. For some reason the skull is very rarely affected, although the jaw, especially the part holding the lower teeth, may become thin.

The commonest fractures that result from osteoporosis are those of the wrist, the hip (upper end of the femur or thigh bone), and the individual bones of the spine (the vertebrae). A vertebra can collapse and lose its shape simply as a result of the weight of the body pressing down on the thinned bone. This is quite common and is known as a compression fracture. Vertebral fractures can also be caused by minor injury or by the strain of heavy lifting. Such fractures affect the shape of the spine and as a result the patient becomes stooped over and loses height.

A compression fracture of a vertebra may cause sudden severe pain in the back that gradually wears off after 4–8 weeks. A patient with osteoporosis may also suffer from a more long-term ache in the back, either in the midline or to either side of the spine. It usually comes on when she has been standing for some time or sitting in one position and it can be relieved by rest. Such a pain may be due to arthritis, which will be made worse by the misshapen vertebrae. The bones themselves are not tender in osteoporosis, except at the site of fractures.

As the patient becomes more stooped over, the movement of her chest becomes limited so that her breathing may become shallower and coughing may be difficult. It is not unknown for the trunk to tip so far forward that the base of the ribs touches the top of the hip bones. Even in less extreme cases, there is often a horizontal crease visible in the skin of the abdomen.

DIAGNOSIS

When a postmenopausal woman breaks a bone, it is usually unnecessary to do a large number of tests in order to diagnose osteoporosis. All that is needed is an X-ray of the spine, which will show thinning of the bone and possibly compression fractures of the vertebrae.

However, if the doctor is uncertain about the diagnosis or if he feels that there may be some underlying condition that needs treatment (such as thyrotoxicosis), he will take some blood or urine tests as well. The level of calcium in the urine is normal in most cases of osteoporosis but may be raised when the condition is due to thyrotoxicosis or to treatment with steroids.

Urine and blood tests may also be helpful in detecting "fast losers" early on, so that osteoporosis may be prevented in these high-risk patients. Therefore, women whose mothers have suffered from severe osteoporosis may be offered tests involving the collection of all the urine passed over twenty-four hours plus a single specimen of blood.

TRADITIONAL TREATMENT

Hormone Replacement Therapy
Although osteoporosis is not caused by a hormone deficiency, taking hormones after the menopause can prevent it from occurring, because estrogen enables the body to retain calcium. Hormone replacement therapy (HRT) starting as soon as possible after the menopause can prevent osteoporosis but, started later, will only stop it from getting worse. Some doctors think all women should be offered HRT postmenopausally and certainly it is advisable for those who are particularly at risk. Its benefits probably last only for as long as it is taken, with bone loss beginning once the treatment has been discontinued. Since some ten to fifteen years of bone loss is usual before fractures occur, it seems sensible for women to continue taking HRT until they are at

least seventy, but in 70 percent of cases this has the drawback that they will continue to have periods.

In 1987, a new form of hormone replacement therapy became available in the United States. Instead of taking tablets, the woman has a patch attached to her skin. The hormones are contained within the patch and are slowly absorbed into the body through the skin. This has the advantage that they travel directly into the bloodstream without having to pass through the digestive system, and therefore are likely to produce fewer side effects than hormones that have to be taken by mouth.

Estrogen, which also controls menopausal symptoms, needs to be taken continuously, but causes a buildup of the lining of the uterus (endometrium), a factor that may predispose the patient to develop cancer of the uterus. To prevent this buildup a progestogen that acts in the same way as the natural hormone progesterone is always given with estrogen unless the patient has had a hysterectomy. The progestogen is given for only twelve days each month. Each time it is stopped, 70 percent of women will have a small withdrawal bleed. However, protection from abnormal endometrial thickening does not depend on the occurrence of bleeding and progestogen is protective in all cases.

Side effects of HRT include breast tenderness, nausea, and swelling of the abdomen, but these frequently disappear after the first few months. If they don't, changing to a different preparation may help. Many believe there is still the possible risk of breast cancer with estrogen replacement. On the plus side, HRT often gives a woman a sense of well-being and may protect the heart and blood vessels against disease.

Although HRT encourages the retention of calcium within the body, it cannot make up for a poor diet and it is essential that the patient has an adequate calcium intake.

Calcium

Many people nowadays seem to eat diets that are deficient in vitamins and minerals. Older women need at least 2 g of calcium a day to try to replace some of that which is being lost. Vitamin D supplements are only necessary if the patient does not absorb enough calcium from the intestines.

Treatment of Fractures

Although the bones are thin, osteoporosis does not prevent fractures from healing normally. However, because they can easily break again, problems may occur when it is necessary to pin the two parts of the bone together or to insert a replacement metal hip bone.

A vertebral compression fracture may need two or three weeks of bed rest. After this, an orthopedic support for the spine may encourage the patient to move around. However, a rigid spinal brace should be used as little as possible because it promotes greater bone loss by restricting movement.

A hard mattress will help to relieve back pain following a fracture, and simple painkillers can be taken.

RECENT ADVANCES

Recently doctors in Denmark, the United States, and New Zealand have been investigating a drug that is used in the treatment of another bone disorder, Paget's disease. Called etidronate disodium, it seems that this drug may have the effect of enabling the patient to build up her bone again. It is taken for two weeks, after which calcium and vitamin D are given for three months and then the cycle is repeated. In the United States, etidronate is currently only indicated for Paget's disease, but it has been approved in Europe for the treatment of osteoporosis in postmenopausal women.

Another drug that is under investigation is the hormone calcitonin. This is very safe and has been shown to be effective when used with estrogen, but until recently it needed to be injected three times a week. It is also expensive. However, a calcitonin nasal spray has been developed that was shown to increase bone mass when it was tried out in Denmark. Similar research has been done in Belgium, where women who were given calcitonin for five days a week, together with calcium, were shown to lose significantly less bone over the course of a year than women who were given only calcium.

Research done recently at King's College Hospital, London, suggests that hormone implants can increase bone density whereas oral

HRT just serves to maintain it. However, this, too, is still in the experimental stage. Other experimental agents include fluoride, parathyroid hormone, and 1,25-dihydroxy-vitamin D_3. All of these need further testing.

PREVENTION

Because immobility promotes bone loss, it is very important that the elderly should stay mobile. It is vital that their homes should be safe so accidents and possible fractures are less likely.

Some doctors believe that exercise in the premenopausal years can be protective against osteoporosis, but this has yet to be proved.

Steroids can counteract the effect of vitamin D, so anyone who has to take these should also take 1500 i.u. vitamin D a day plus a calcium supplement of 1 g a day.

An adequate diet and a good calcium intake is important, especially during the years when the bones are still being built up. An American study showed that women who had less than 405 mg of calcium a day in their diets lost bone density at a significantly faster rate than those who were having over 775 mg.

It has been noticed that osteoporosis occurs less frequently in areas where there is a high fluoride level in the drinking water. However, there is little evidence that fluoride supplements are an effective prevention and indeed the side effects of such supplements would probably outweigh any benefits they conferred.

COMPLEMENTARY TREATMENT

Women who, for reasons of illness or family history, are particularly at risk of developing osteoporosis may find nutrition counseling beneficial. Herbalism, homeopathy, and acupuncture may be indicated for the treatment of diseases such as arthritis or thyroid disease, which predispose patients to osteoporosis (see individual sections), and, by raising the patient's level of health, may reduce the risk of the bones becoming abnormally thin. These therapies may also help to speed the healing of fractures.

ORGANIZATIONS

National Osteoporosis Foundation
1625 Eye Street, NW
Suite 1011
Washington, DC 20006
202/223-2226
(Publishes a quarterly newsletter and educational material.)

PEPTIC ULCER

TYPES OF ULCER AND CAUSE

Peptic ulcers can be divided into two types—the gastric ulcer (situated in the stomach) and the duodenal ulcer (in the first part of the small bowel). Both the stomach and duodenum contain acid that is secreted by cells situated in the stomach lining and is neutralized further down the intestinal tract by bile from the liver and by the alkaline fluids produced by the pancreas (see diagram of the digestive system on page 263). Peptic ulcers are traditionally thought to occur either when excessive amounts of acid are secreted or when the resistance of the stomach and duodenal lining (the mucosa) is reduced, or when both of these happen together. Recently, the discovery that the bacteria *Campylobacter pylori* (abbreviated to *C. pylori*) is commonly present in peptic ulcers has led to theories that it may, in some way, be a factor in their formation. At the time of writing, this has not been proved, but it has been shown that *C. pylori* is present in between 70 and 100 percent of all patients with duodenal ulcers and in two thirds of those with gastric ulcers. Therefore, antibiotic therapy may decrease ulcer recurrence rate.

GASTRIC ULCER (GU)

This may occur in either sex and at any age, although it tends to be more common in the decade between fifty-five and sixty-five. Most patients seem to secrete normal or less than normal amounts of acid, suggesting that the fault lies in the resistance of the stomach lining.

DUODENAL ULCER (DU)

Duodenal ulcer is more common in men than in women and tends to affect younger people than gastric ulcer, having a peak between ages forty-five and fifty-five, although it may also occur in the elderly. It affects some 10 percent of the population, but in recent years the number of cases seems to have been diminishing. One third of patients are found to secrete excessive amounts of acid into the stomach, while the secretions of the rest seem normal. DU seems to run in families and, for a reason as yet unknown, is three times more likely to occur in people with blood group O than in those with other blood groups.

SYMPTOMS

Gastric Ulcer
The commonest symptom is pain, occurring in the upper abdomen, below the V of the ribs. It often occurs after eating and may be associated with pain in the back. It is usually relieved by lying flat and is very seldom felt at night.

Vomiting occurs in over 50 percent of cases and may be self-induced, as it often relieves the pain for a while. Weight loss is common, not because the appetite is affected but because eating (particularly fried foods and spices) causes pain and is therefore avoided. Bloating and nausea may also occur after food consumption. Bleeding from the ulcer occurs in 30 percent of patients and the blood may be vomited or passed in the stools. In the latter case (known as melena) the blood may not be recognizable as such because it has been altered during its passage through the bowel and the stools appear black and sticky.

Attacks, which seem to be commoner in the spring and autumn, usually last between two and six weeks, after which patients are free of symptoms for a few months. However, absence of symptoms does not mean that the ulcer has healed and recurrences are likely to occur if the condition is untreated.

Duodenal Ulcer
In some respects, the symptoms of DU are very similar to those of GU. The pain is felt in the same place in the upper abdomen and may go through to the back. Attacks are commonest in the spring and autumn and last up to six weeks, with symptom-free intervals of up to six months in between. However, there the similarity ends. Unlike gastric ulcer pain, that caused by a duodenal ulcer is eased by food and patients

are inclined to put on weight as a result. Milk and antacids also relieve
the pain and, because patients tend to be woken by the pain in the early
hours of the morning, many will keep milk and antacids beside the
bed. Like patients with GU, those with DU may suffer from bloating,
but vomiting is far less common. They may also experience heartburn,
water brash (a sour, burning fluid rising up from the stomach into the
mouth), and diarrhea or constipation. Duodenal ulcers bleed more
commonly than gastric ulcers so melena and vomiting of blood occur
more often.

COMPLICATIONS

The most common complications of a peptic ulcer are bleeding and
perforation. In the latter, the wall of the stomach or duodenum is
completely pierced by the ulcer so that its contents can enter the
abdominal cavity. This is an emergency requiring immediate medical
care. It is more common in DU than in GU and in men than in
women.

When perforation occurs, the patient experiences severe abdominal
pain that is made worse by movement. Fifty percent also complain of
pain in the shoulder. Usually the pulse is raised, the temperature
drops, the patient appears pale and sweaty, and he may vomit. After
three to six hours he may start to feel better, but this is only a temporary improvement and without treatment the condition is fatal.

Occasionally, hemorrhage may be the first sign that a patient has
developed an ulcer. Although it may settle down of its own accord,
there is a high risk that the ulcer will bleed again and so, like perforation, this requires immediate treatment.

A less common complication is known as gastric outflow obstruction—that is, obstruction to the section of stomach that leads into the
duodenum. Normally the passage of food from the stomach into the
duodenum is controlled by a ring of muscle lying between the two that
opens when the stomach's digestive processes are complete. However,
if an ulcer occurs in this position, it may cause scarring so that the
muscle is no longer able to open fully and the passage of food from the
stomach to the duodenum is obstructed. If this occurs, the patient will
start to vomit and will bring up food that he may have eaten many
hours or days before. He will also be aware of a constant feeling of

fullness or pain, particularly after eating. Vomiting rarely occurs more than two or three times a day, but because very little food gets through to the bowel from which it is normally absorbed, weight loss and constipation are likely to occur.

DIAGNOSIS

The standard method by which an ulcer is diagnosed is X-ray, but in many places this has now been superseded by the use of the endoscope. X-ray diagnosis entails the patient drinking a quantity of fluid containing barium, which is opaque to X-rays (a "barium meal") and pictures are then taken that demonstrate the shape of the stomach and intestines. This method has two drawbacks—first, very small ulcers may be missed and, second, a stomach cancer may, very rarely, look like and be diagnosed as an ulcer. The endoscope is a tube containing a tiny telescope and sometimes a camera; this is passed down the patient's esophagus (gullet) into the stomach and duodenum, and enables the doctor to inspect every part of the stomach and duodenal lining (mucosa), making it far less likely that an ulcer will be missed. In addition, it enables him to take a biopsy from an ulcer in the stomach, which can then be examined to ensure that it is not malignant. The disadvantages of endoscopy are that the patient has to be sedated for the procedure and that it can only be carried out by a specialist.

The patient's stools may be tested to see whether there is any evidence of bleeding and a full blood count may be done to check for anemia.

Although the diagnoses of perforation or hemorrhage are usually fairly obvious, these must be confirmed. In the case of perforation, air passes through the hole in the stomach or intestine and into the abdominal cavity. This can be seen on an X-ray of the abdomen, taken with the patient in an upright position, as black patches under the diaphragm. In the case of hemorrhage, endoscopy will locate the position of the bleeding point. Both these techniques can be used to confirm the diagnosis of gastric outflow obstruction—an X-ray will show a greatly dilated stomach and endoscopy (done after the stomach contents have been aspirated) will show the position of the scarring. A barium meal will demonstrate that stomach contents are retained for more than the normal four hours.

TRADITIONAL TREATMENT

Treatment of peptic ulcers has been revolutionized in the last decade by the development of the group of drugs known as histamine H_2 receptor antagonists. The first of these was cimetidine and others such as ranitidine, famotidine, and nizatidine have been developed. They work by reducing the secretion of gastric acid so that symptoms are relieved very quickly and the ulcer heals in 80 percent of cases. However, once the treatment has been discontinued there may be a relapse—between 50 and 85 percent recur within a year—so that a proportion of patients need either to continue to take a small dose of the medication on a long-term basis or to take repeated courses each time the symptoms recur.

Another medication, bismuth subsalicylate (Pepto-Bismol), has not achieved the popularity of the H_2 receptor antagonists. This is partly because when it was first introduced it was unpleasant to take, although some years ago its formulation was changed so that it is now no more unpleasant than its rivals. In addition, it does not relieve ulcer symptoms quite as rapidly as H_2 receptor antagonists so that patients often need to take antacids as well. However, subsalicylate has recently been shown to wipe out the bacteria *Campylobacter pylori* whose presence, it seems, can promote the recurrence of a healed ulcer. It also increases the healing ability of the mucosa of the stomach and duodenum by stimulating their mucus production. Various studies have shown that, while relapses do occur in patients who are prescribed subsalicylate (usually when *C. pylori* has not been totally eradicated), these are less likely than in patients who are treated with H_2 receptor antagonists. Although more and more specialists are prescribing bismuth chelate, some are still reluctant to use it because the long-term effects of bismuth are as yet unknown, while the action of the H_2 receptor antagonists is fairly thoroughly understood.

Sucralfate is another agent that helps to promote the healing ability of the mucosa. It seems to have no effect on *C. pylori* but still has a low relapse rate.

A new drug, misoprostol, has recently been introduced that works in a different way from those mentioned above, being a prostaglandin derivative. Prostaglandins are hormonelike substances produced by the body that appear to play an important role in inflammatory processes. Misoprostol has the dual effect of reducing gastric acid secretion and protecting the mucosa from erosion. Between 10 and 15 percent of patients who take it develop diarrhea, but this usually clears up in due course, without the patient having to stop the medication.

Despite the efficacy of modern drugs, surgery is sometimes inevitable for the ulcer patient. Nowadays this is usually only performed for patients who fail to respond to medical treatment or for those who have developed complications. For gastric ulcers, it is usual to remove part of the stomach, taking the ulcer together with some of the acid-secreting cells. For duodenal ulcers, the ulcer itself is left intact and the aim of the operation is to reduce the amount of acid secreted by the stomach. This is done by cutting the vagus nerve, one of whose functions is to stimulate the cells lining the stomach. Because the vagus also supplies the muscle that closes off the stomach from the duodenum, cutting it prevents the stomach from emptying efficiently. Therefore, the opening into the duodenum (the pylorus) has to be widened (pyloroplasty) to ensure that there is no obstruction. In recent years, some surgeons have been performing the operation known as highly selective vagotomy, in which only the nerve fibers running to the stomach wall are cut and the rest of the vagus is left intact. However, this is a very difficult operation and has a higher ulcer recurrence rate than does the straightforward vagotomy and pyloroplasty.

Surgery may be required as an emergency when an ulcer bleeds. A few surgeons are now using lasers, introduced into the stomach or duodenum through an endoscope, to seal off bleeding ulcers, but as yet this technique is not generally available.

When a gastric ulcer perforates, the part of the stomach that is involved is removed. However, when it is a duodenal ulcer that has perforated, a patch of membrane taken from inside the abdominal cavity is sewn over the hole, and a vagotomy and pyloroplasty is done at a later date when the patient has recovered from the perforation. In both cases, the abdominal cavity is thoroughly cleaned out and, following the operation, the patient is given antibiotics in order to avoid the risk of infection within the abdomen.

Gastric outlet obstruction is treated in a similar way to a duodenal ulcer, but even if a highly selective vagotomy is performed, additional surgery is necessary to enlarge the outlet from the stomach.

COMPLEMENTARY TREATMENT

Acupuncture
The symptoms associated with peptic ulcer are said to be due to a dysfunction of the spleen, liver, or stomach resulting from either an excess or a deficiency of energy (Chi). Treatment consists of balancing the energy and getting it to flow freely again, while strengthening the affected organs in order to restore their function to normal.

Aromatherapy
Among the oils used are chamomile, geranium, and marjoram.

Herbalism
A number of herbs may be prescribed that promote the healing of ulcers, reduce gastric acidity, and relieve pain. These include comfrey, marshmallow root, meadowsweet, and slippery elm. Licorice is also used. Some years ago licorice derivatives were popular with traditional practitioners for the treatment of peptic ulcers, but these have rather fallen out of favor with the introduction of the H_2 receptor antagonists.

Homeopathy
The choice of remedy will depend, among other things, on when the pain occurs and what makes it better or worse. For example, pain occurring after food consumption may be treated with uranium nitricum, kali bich., or arg. nit. Atropinum and anacardium are both used to treat patients whose pain is relieved by eating.

Hynotherapy
Patients whose lifestyle causes a great deal of stress, which may be preventing the ulcer from healing, can be taught how to relax and to cope more effectively with stress.

Nutrition
The amino acids glutamine and glutamic acid in doses of 50–100 mg a day may be recommended in order to promote the healing of a peptic ulcer.

PREMENSTRUAL SYNDROME

DEFINITION AND INCIDENCE

A syndrome is a condition in which a number of symptoms occur together. It does not necessarily imply that all cases of the syndrome are due to the same cause. In premenstrual syndrome, the actual cause of the symptoms is, as yet, unknown, although a number of theories have been put forward.

Many women become slightly irritable just before a period or experience some breast tenderness. But when these symptoms become severe and are associated with others, a diagnosis of premenstrual syndrome can be made. The condition affects up to 40 percent of all women, 5 percent severely, and is most apparent between the ages of eighteen and thirty-five. Because it is something in the monthly hormonal cycle that brings it about, it is possible for a woman who has had a hysterectomy to continue to suffer from PMS as long as she still has her ovaries. (PMS is sometimes also known as the cyclical ovarian syndrome.)

PMS seems to affect certain types of women more frequently than others. Those suffering from irregular periods are more at risk. So too are those who have sexual or emotional problems, or who are separated or divorced; indeed, it is well known that any kind of stress can make the syndrome worse. Women who take the contraceptive Pill are less likely to have PMS.

SYMPTOMS

Symptoms may begin anywhere between day 15 and day 26 of a twenty-eight-day cycle and usually disappear by the second day of the period. Sometimes they may vanish quite dramatically once the bleeding has started. The commonest symptoms are depression, tension, swelling, and fatigue.

Many of the symptoms seem to be associated with water retention. These include swelling (of the abdomen, legs, ankles, and fingers), a feeling of bloatedness, weight gain (sometimes of several pounds), tender swelling of the breasts (sometimes with increased nodularity or pain), sinus-type headaches, stuffy nose (due to swelling of the lining of the nasal passages), and a reduced output of urine.

Slight swelling of the brain cells as a result of water retention is thought to be the cause of the mental symptoms, which include irritability, anxiety, depression, tension, fits of anger, poor control over the emotions, loss of self-confidence, and problems with concentration and memory. Occasionally these symptoms are very severe and are associated with violence or suicide attempts.

Lethargy and fatigue, added to the mental problems, often mean that the patient is less efficient than at other times of the month.

Other symptoms include tension headaches, clumsiness, muscular pain, cramping pains in the lower abdomen, skin problems, and changes in appetite and sleeping patterns. Patients who suffer from hay fever, asthma, migraine, and epilepsy may find that these conditions are worse premenstrually.

TRADITIONAL TREATMENT

Several treatments have been devised for PMS, all of which seem successful for certain women. Since these treatments work in quite different ways, it is possible that PMS is due to different causes in different patients and that response to a particular treatment therefore depends on whether or not it is the correct one for that individual. This would explain why, for example, despite the great success claimed for progesterone treatment, controlled trials have been unable to show that it has any significant effect.

Because a number of the symptoms seem to be due to water retention, many doctors recommend a reduction in salt intake (since salt encourages water retention) and prescribe diuretics such as spironolactone. These tablets enable the patient to pass more water and so they relieve swelling and some of the other symptoms. Spironolactone, unlike some diuretics, is also able to get through to the brain and it is suggested that the reduction in mental symptoms that it can produce is because it prevents swelling of the brain cells. However, diuretics only treat symptoms and, although helpful in mild cases, may not be the best treatment for patients with more severe problems.

Those doctors who maintain that PMS is due to a relative lack of the hormone progesterone give progesterone supplements in the form of injections or suppositories. These are given for one or two weeks before the period is expected. Some doctors prescribe synthetic derivatives of progesterone, such as norethindrone or dydrogesterone, which can be taken in tablet form. However, others say that the best effects are to be gained only by using natural progesterone. Unfortunately, progesterone and its derivatives may cause side effects such as fatigue, lethargy, and depression. Some patients respond very well to this treatment, but for others it is ineffective. Some women find that taking the contraceptive Pill relieves their symptoms.

In a few cases, PMS appears to be due to excessive secretion of the hormone prolactin by the pituitary gland. For such patients, bromocriptine will be helpful. However, this, too, has side effects including nausea, dizziness, headache, and constipation.

One of the most useful forms of treatment seems to be pyridoxine (vitamin B_6). A series of 630 women with PMS were treated with this at the St. Thomas's group of hospitals (United Kingdom) over a period of eight years and about 80 percent reported a great improvement in mental symptoms, breast problems, and headache. Other symptoms were also helped. There are various reasons for thinking that pyridoxine is needed in PMS. First, it reduces the production of prolactin. Second, it is vital for the production of the chemical serotonin, a deficiency of which may cause depression. Pyridoxine itself is inhibited by estrogen, which is why larger amounts may be necessary at those times of the month when the estrogen level rises. The usual dose is 40 mg twice a day, rising to 75 mg twice a day by gradual steps if necessary, starting three days before symptoms are expected and stopping on the third day of the period. Doses above 100 mg are usually avoided due to the possible development of sensory neuropathies. (The patients at St. Thomas's were actually taking up to 200 mg a day.) A supplement of 10–15 mg of zinc a day should always be taken when one takes pyridoxine because the two substances work together in the body. Large doses of pyridoxine without a zinc "chaser" may produce unpleasant side effects.

The most recent treatment to be acclaimed for PMS is evening primrose oil. This is being used by some doctors and the results seem to be very satisfactory. It is suggested that the true deficiency in PMS is one of the essential fatty acids (EFAs), a component of the diet that is vital for the formation of certain chemical compounds involved in bodily function. Evening primrose oil contains all these EFAs. The recommended dose is 1000 mg three times a day for two months, then 500 mg two or three times a day for as long as necessary. One doctor claims a 90 percent success rate using this regime. It may be beneficial for those who take evening primrose oil to take a supplement of pyridoxine and zinc as well, since this increases the body's efficiency in its use of EFAs.

COMPLEMENTARY TREATMENT

Aromatherapy
Parsley, neroli, or juniper are among the oils that may be prescribed.

Herbalism
Herbs such as agnus castus and false unicorn (helonias) root help to balance the patient's hormones. Motherwort and scullcap are among the herbs that may be prescribed to treat anxiety or stress. Dandelion, parsley, couch grass, and wild carrot are diuretics.

Homeopathy
A patient who has swollen tender breasts, loss of libido, and a bearing-down sensation in her lower abdomen that is relieved by crossing her legs may be helped by sepia. A swollen abdomen associated with swollen tender breasts and irritability may be relieved by natrum mur. Lachesis may be appropriate when the hands swell and the patient complains that her clothes feel tight.

Nutrition
PMS may be aggravated by excessive sugar and coffee, so patients may be advised to reduce their intake of these items. Tension, irritability, anxiety, bloatedness, weight gain, and breast tenderness may be due to a deficiency of B vitamins or magnesium. Magnesium is also necessary

to maintain a normal hormone balance. Therefore, supplements of this mineral and of B complex may be recommended. To ensure that the body uses vitamin B_6 efficiently, zinc will be given as well.

SELF-HELP

The PMT Advisory Service found that its patients were helped by taking a high-dose multivitamin/multimineral tablet and by adjusting their diet, reducing their intake of fat (especially animal fat), sugar, salt, junk food, tea, and coffee, and increasing their intake of fiber, fruit, and vegetables.

ORGANIZATIONS

Premenstrual Syndrome Action
P.O. Box 16292
Irvine, CA 92713
714/854-4407
(Publishes *PMS Connection.*)

PROLAPSE

TYPES OF PROLAPSE, CAUSES, AND SYMPTOMS

The organs in the lower part of the female abdomen are supported by the muscular layer known as the pelvic floor, above which they lie, and by various ligaments and fibrous bands that hold them in place. Damage to, or weakness of, any of these may result in the organs dropping down and bulging into the vagina.

If the anterior (front) part of the vaginal wall becomes weak, the urethra (the tube leading from the bladder, through which urine is passed) or the bladder may sag into it. These conditions are known as a urethrocele and a cystocele respectively. Descent of the rectum into the posterior vaginal wall is known as a rectocele; this is usually due to weakness of the pelvic floor. If the uterus drops down, this is known as uterine prolapse.

There are three degrees of uterine prolapse. In the first, the cervix, or neck, of the womb remains within the vagina. In the second, the cervix protrudes out of the vaginal opening. In the third, the entire uterus, pushing the vaginal lining before it, drops down and out of the vaginal opening. A third-degree prolapse is also know as procidentia.

A few women have an inborn weakness in the muscles and ligaments that hold up the uterus and may develop a minor degree of prolapse. However, the majority of cases are due to injury or acquired weakness affecting these supports. This often occurs as a result of childbirth and is particularly likely in women who have had a number of children. Other causes include conditions such as constipation, recurrent heavy lifting, chronic cough, and obesity that raise the pressure inside the abdomen and therefore put additional strain on the supporting structures. Symptoms may suddenly get worse at the time of the menopause, since the loss of circulating estrogen in the body may lead to a rapid thinning of the uterine ligaments and of the muscles that support the vaginal wall.

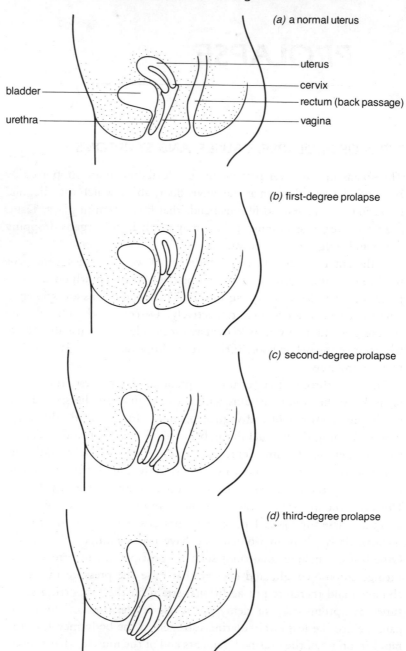

(a) a normal uterus

uterus
cervix
rectum (back passage)
vagina

bladder
urethra

(b) first-degree prolapse

(c) second-degree prolapse

(d) third-degree prolapse

Prolapse of the uterus

The symptoms of prolapse are variable and it is possible to remain symptom-free even with a second-degree uterine prolapse. One of the commonest symptoms is low backache and patients also frequently complain of a sense of fullness in the vagina or a dragging discomfort that is worse after they have been standing for a long time. They may also be aware of a lump that protrudes from the vagina and is worse when they stand or strain, but disappears when they lie down. If the bladder is pulled out of shape, urinary symptoms may occur, such as urgency, stress incontinence, frequency, and pain when passing water. Discomfort or pain may also occur during intercourse. Patients who have second- or third-degree uterine prolapses often have a discharge, which may be blood-stained. Ultimately, ulceration may cause a hemorrhage.

If the angle at which the urethra leaves the bladder is distorted, as may occur in a urethrocele or cystocele, it may be impossible for the patient to empty her bladder completely. As a result she may feel that she wants to pass water again as soon as she has finished doing so (double micturition) and may be troubled by recurrent urinary infections. Patients with rectoceles may have difficulty in passing stools.

TESTS

In most cases, a prolapse is easily identifiable upon examination. The patient lies on her side and a curved metal instrument known as a Sims' speculum is used to hold the walls of the vagina open. She is asked to cough or strain and the doctor can usually see the prolapse coming down. Normally a Pap smear is taken if she has not had one recently and a urine specimen is examined for any indication of infection. In patients with a third-degree prolapse, further tests of the urinary tract (such as an X-ray of the kidneys) may be undertaken, since damage can occur as the result of long-term pressure on the bladder, leading to incomplete emptying.

TRADITIONAL TREATMENT

Because conditions such as obesity, chronic cough, and constipation can weaken the supports of the uterus and vagina, patients are advised to lose weight, stop smoking, or eat a diet with more fiber in it whenever these measures are appropriate.

Minor degrees of prolapse are common immediately after childbirth and usually all that is needed in such cases is a course of special exercises to strengthen the muscles of the pelvic floor. Spontaneous improvement is likely during the six months following childbirth and it is only if the prolapse continues after this period that further treatment will be considered.

For those patients whose prolapse has been exacerbated by the onset of the menopause, hormone replacement therapy may be very helpful.

The use of pessaries, which are pushed into the vagina to hold it in shape, has been standard practice in the treatment of prolapse for many years. However, in recent times, it has become customary to reserve them only for those who are unfit for, are waiting for, or have refused surgery, and for patients who are pregnant or have recently given birth to a child.

The ring pessary consists of a ring of flexible plastic that is pushed high up into the vagina and holds its walls up and apart. The Hodge pessary is similar but more rectangular, and the Gelhorn pessary, which is used for the more severe degrees of prolapse, is shaped like a collar-stud. Long-term use of pessaries may result in ulceration, so patients need to be seen every three or four months and may need to use an antibacterial cream to prevent infection. Postmenopausal patients may also need an estrogen cream to prevent undue thinning of the vaginal tissues.

If the patient is treated surgically, the actual operation used will depend on the form of prolapse from which she is suffering. For a urethrocele or cystocele, the operation is an anterior colporrhaphy in which the sagging part of the vaginal wall is removed and all the tissues are tightened up. A similar technique is used for a rectocele—a posterior colporrhaphy—and, here, the muscles of the pelvic floor will be repaired as well.

The treatment of choice for a uterine prolapse is hysterectomy. However, some women will not want to lose their uterus, and for them a Manchester or Fothergill repair is performed in which part of the cervix is removed and the surrounding tissues are tightened so that the uterus is pulled up into position again.

After a repair, whichever type has been performed, the patient may need to have a catheter draining her bladder for between two and five days, since urinary retention is common. In addition, she may have had a pack of gauze soaked in antiseptic solution placed in her vagina, which will need to be removed after twenty-four hours. This pack helps to prevent bleeding and infection, and stops the raw tissues from sticking to each other.

If a woman who has had a prolapse repair then has another pregnancy, she will need to have a cesarean section, since a normal delivery could easily undo all the surgeon's good work.

COMPLEMENTARY TREATMENT

Treatment by an acupuncturist, homeopath, or herbalist, combined with pelvic-floor exercises, may prevent a mild degree of prolapse from getting any worse and may help to strengthen the supporting tissues.

PROSTATE PROBLEMS

DESCRIPTION

The prostate gland lies just below the base of the male bladder, surrounding the urethra—the tube through which urine is passed—and is responsible for producing some of the fluid which, together with the sperm, makes up the semen (see diagram on page 251). Because of its position, diseases affecting the prostate are likely to cause urinary symptoms. The gland itself has five lobes—anterior, median (or middle), posterior, and two lateral—and the symptoms that occur depend primarily on which lobe is most affected by the disease.

BENIGN ENLARGEMENT (BENIGN HYPERTROPHY)

Incidence

This condition is extremely common, affecting 50 percent of men over age fifty, and increasing to 90 percent of those over age eighty. Why the prostate enlarges no one knows, and why it should do so more in some men than in others is also a mystery. Only about 10 percent of those affected actually need treatment and of these the majority are between the ages of sixty and seventy. European men are more likely to develop benign enlargement than Indian men, in whom the condition, when it occurs, tends to affect a younger age group. In black men it is unusual and in oriental men it is very rare.

Effects of an Enlarged Prostate on the Surrounding Tissues

The prostate may enlarge until it is up to ten times its normal size and it is usually the lateral and median lobes that are primarily affected.

The result is that the urethra, which lies between them, becomes squashed and distorted. In order to pass urine down this flattened, twisting tube, the bladder has to work harder, so the muscular bands in its wall become thicker. However, the areas lying between the thickened muscles may become weaker as a result, and start to bulge, forming little pockets, or diverticula. Urine can collect in these pockets, acting as a focus for infection, or stones may form in the stagnant urine. The increased pressure within the bladder, produced by the thickened muscles, may also cause dilation of the ureters (the tubes that lead from the kidneys into the bladder) and may encourage urine to flow backward toward the kidneys. This makes it easier for any bacteria within the bladder to infect the kidneys and, ultimately, renal failure may occur.

If the middle lobe of the prostate is enlarged, this may add to the stagnation within the bladder, since it pushes up into it and acts as a dam. A small pool of urine is therefore also present in the bladder.

The muscles of the bladder can only enlarge to a certain degree. When the obstruction to the flow of urine becomes too great for them to cope with, they give up and become loose and flaccid, causing total retention of urine.

The enlarged prostate may also press on the veins that run around the base of the bladder, causing congestion within them. Occasionally one of these dilated veins may leak, so that blood is passed in the urine.

Symptoms

Not all men who have enlarged prostates have symptoms and among those who do the severity of the symptoms does not necessarily correlate with the size of the gland. Nor are the symptoms always progressive—it is possible for them to reach a certain stage and then get no worse. Indeed, once the patient has had symptoms for about ten years, it is unusual for them to worsen.

The earliest symptom is usually frequency—the patient finds first that he has to get up during the night to pass water (nocturia) and then that he has to go more often during the day. The band of muscle that controls the exit from the bladder may become stretched as it is distorted by the enlarged prostate and as a result a small amount of urine may leak now and again into the urethra. This automatically causes a desire to urinate so that the patient suffers from urgency—a need to rush to the toilet as soon as he feels that he needs to go.

As the condition worsens, the patient may become aware that his urinary stream is poor. Even when he wants to go, he may have to wait for the stream to start and, when it does so, it is often weak and may stop and start and tend to dribble toward the end. It may take a long time for the patient to empty his bladder and he may be left with the feeling that he has not emptied it completely.

The appearance of a drop of blood either at the beginning or the end of the stream occurs in 20 percent of cases and sometimes may be the only symptom of prostatic enlargement.

Other symptoms include impotence (although, early on, an increase in sex drive may occur), urinary tract infections, stones in the bladder or the kidneys, a feeling of weight in the perineum (the area between the legs), or a feeling of fullness in the rectum.

Retention of urine may be acute or chronic. In the acute condition, the patient feels an urgent need to urinate but finds that he is unable to do so. The bladder is swollen and tender and rapidly becomes extremely painful. Acute retention may be precipitated by the patient having to delay passing water when he feels the need (for example, when driving down a highway or on a long bus journey), by an excess of alcohol (especially when this is combined with going out on a cold night), or by being confined to bed for a few days.

Unlike acute retention, chronic retention is usually painless. Each time the patient passes water, some urine is left behind and the bladder gradually distends. He becomes incontinent because small amounts constantly leak out of the overfull bladder, and kidney failure may occur. Occasionally, a patient suffering from chronic retention may develop acute retention as well.

Kidney failure prevents the body from getting rid of many of its waste products. These toxic materials circulate in the bloodstream and cause drowsiness, headache, and behavioral and intellectual changes. Occasionally, an elderly man who develops what seem to be psychiatric problems may be found to be suffering from renal failure due to an enlarged prostate.

Tests

When a man goes to his GP complaining of a mixture of the symptoms listed above, it is usually quite simple to diagnose that he has a benign enlargement of his prostate. This can usually be confirmed if the GP examines the rectum, through which he will be able to feel the enlarged gland. He may also examine the patient's abdomen and kidneys, looking for signs of retention or of renal failure. A urine test may be taken to see whether it is infected and blood may be taken to check for kidney failure (when this occurs, the level of urea in the blood is higher than normal and the blood cell count may be reduced).

A plain X-ray of the abdomen may be requested if there is any suggestion that the patient has stones in the bladder or the kidneys. And the patient may be given a measuring container and asked to record the number of times that he passes water over a period of seven days, together with the amount passed each time.

If he has noticed blood in his urine, the kidneys may be screened by giving an injection into a vein of a substance that shows up on X-ray when excreted by the kidneys. This test (an intravenous pyelogram or IVP) may also be requested if the doctor suspects that the kidneys have been damaged by back pressure from the bladder or as a result of chronic retention.

If the patient is referred to the hospital as a potential candidate for surgery, other tests may be done. The amount of urine left in the bladder after he has passed water can be measured by ultrasound, and the flow rate may be measured by a special machine into which he urinates. A cystoscopy may be performed in which a special instrument is inserted, under general anesthetic, through the urethra and into the bladder, enabling the surgeon to look for pockets in the bladder wall, stones, or tumors.

Traditional Treatment

If a patient develops acute retention, a catheter is passed into the bladder, allowing the urine to flow out. This will give immediate relief from the severe pain. Catheterization for the relief of chronic retention has to be a more leisurely affair, since bleeding may occur from the kidneys if it is done too quickly. In such cases, the bladder is drained gradually over a few hours.

Early in 1988 it was announced that prazosin, a drug that has been used in the treatment of high blood pressure, had been approved for treating patients with benign prostatic hypertrophy. Trials in Sweden, Italy, and the United Kingdom had shown that 75 percent of patients had a significant improvement in their symptoms when given this drug. In the United States, a similar drug, terazosin, is being tested, but neither it nor prazosin is officially indicated for use in prostate disease. Although surgical removal of the prostate is the only treatment that will permanently and completely relieve the symptoms of benign hypertrophy, prazosin is likely to prove very useful for those patients who have to wait a considerable time before they can have their operation.

For those whose symptoms are disabling, prostatectomy will be recommended. The enlarged inner section of the gland will be removed, leaving behind the outer "false capsule" consisting of normal prostatic tissue that has become compressed by the swollen segments. Prostatectomy is a very safe operation and the results are usually very good, especially if performed before complications such as infection, retention, or renal failure have occurred. There are several ways of doing it, of which transurethral resection (TUR) is the most popular. An instrument is inserted into the prostate through the urethra and the gland is removed piecemeal. Over 90 percent of patients are suitable for this operation, which has the advantage that no skin incision is necessary. However, exceptionally large prostates cannot be treated by TUR and have to be removed in another way. The oldest type of operation is a transvesical prostatectomy, in which an incision is made horizontally, low down on the abdomen, just above the hair line. The prostate is then approached via an incision in the bladder. Nowadays this operation is used mainly for those patients who need some operative treatment on the bladder in addition to prostatectomy, such as the removal of a diverticulum, or pocket. For other patients who are not suitable for TUR, suprapubic prostatectomy can be performed. This is done through the same low abdominal incision as a transvesical prostatectomy, but the bladder is not opened.

Complications of Operation

In 3 percent of cases, the prostate regrows, the symptoms return, and the operation may have to be repeated.

Some 10–14 days after the operation, hemorrhage may occur. This is often associated with an infection. Since clots may form in the bladder, causing an obstruction to the flow of urine, readmission to the hospital is usually necessary so that the bladder can be washed out. Because of the risk of infection, it is usual to do a urine test some two to four weeks after the operation.

Occasionally a patient may be unable to pass urine after the operation, because the muscles of the bladder have become flaccid. However, a short period of catheterization usually resolves this problem.

Two percent of patients develop a stricture (narrowing) in the urethra or at the neck of the bladder in the first year following the operation. This results in an increasingly poor stream of urine but can be treated surgically.

Very occasionally patients complain of impotence following a prostatectomy, although there appears to be no physical reason for this. Incontinence, too, may occur, but this is usually slight and resolves within a short time with the help of special exercises, bladder training and, if necessary, drugs. It is more likely to occur when patients have developed severe symptoms (such as retention) before having the operation.

All these complications, however, are quite uncommon. One that occurs more frequently, especially when a suprapubic prostatectomy has been performed, is retrograde ejaculation. Because one of the two bands of muscle that controls the opening of the bladder is destroyed in this operation, the ejaculate, instead of passing down the urethra, passes up into the bladder. Therefore the patient may not be impotent but is likely to be sterile. Another complication that may occur after a suprapubic prostatectomy is acute epididymitis—infection of the epididymis, the little gland that sits on the top of each testis. In order to reduce the risk of this occurring, some surgeons do a vasectomy before performing the prostatectomy, thus making it harder for infection to reach the epididymis.

ACUTE PROSTATITIS

This is a fairly common condition that usually affects young men. It may be caused by bacteria that have been carried in the bloodstream from another area of infection in the body, such as the tonsils, the teeth, or a crop of boils on the skin. In a few cases, it may be secondary to an infection in the bladder or kidneys.

Symptoms

The onset of the illness is <u>sudden</u>, with the patient complaining of flulike symptoms and a raised temperature. He may develop frequency and dysuria (pain when passing water) and may pass some blood. Pain or discomfort may be experienced in the back, the perineum, the lower abdomen, or the rectum and, if it is severe, retention of urine may occur.

Tests

The doctor may <u>ask the patient to urinate</u>, catching the urine in <u>three containers</u> in turn. The middle specimen is sent for culture while the first is examined for "threads," tiny threadlike structures often associated with prostatitis, although they are not diagnostic of the condition. Very often, the urine has no bacteria in it. A diagnosis is usually made primarily on the patient's symptoms.

Traditional Treatment and Course

Most cases of prostatitis clear up quickly when treated with antibiotics. However, delayed or inadequate treatment may result in the formation of an <u>abscess</u> (this is rare) <u>or</u> the development of <u>chronic prostatitis</u>. If an abscess forms, the pain becomes throbbing and the patient's other symptoms may worsen. However, once the abscess has been drained surgically, it seldom causes any further trouble.

CHRONIC PROSTATITIS

The <u>symptoms</u> of this condition are rather more <u>vague</u> than those of acute prostatitis and are probably due to small areas of chronic infection within the prostate. It tends to affect men between the ages of thirty and fifty but may be a complication of benign hypertrophy of the prostate.

Symptoms

The patient may be aware of a dull ache or a feeling of fullness in the perineum or the rectum that is made worse if he sits on a hard chair. Often he has low back pain that may travel down his legs. Usually he will also have urinary symptoms such as frequency, urgency, and pain when passing water, and he may develop retention. Some patients have a recurrent fever and feel generally unwell. Premature ejaculation or impotence may occur. Some men find that ejaculating relieves their symptoms, whereas for others it makes them worse.

Tests

By inserting a finger into the patient's rectum, the doctor can massage the prostate, causing a few drops of prostatic fluid to run down the urethra. This fluid can be collected and examined for bacterial growth and cells. Often no bacteria can be cultivated, although pus cells are evident. The three-container urine test used for acute prostatitis may also be helpful in diagnosis since, as in the acute condition, the first glass may contain "threads."

Traditional Treatment

Although antibiotics may help to relieve the urinary symptoms, their ability to wipe out an infection deep within the prostate seems to be limited. If the flow of urine becomes obstructed because the urethra is constricted, a prostatectomy may be necessary.

CANCER OF THE PROSTATE

This is the second commonest tumor occurring in men and is the most common in men over the age of sixty-five. About 120,000 new cases are diagnosed in the United Kingdom each year. It is rare before the age of forty and uncommon before fifty, but the incidence rises steeply between the ages of sixty-five and seventy-five. However, many elderly men with prostatic cancer die from other causes—up to 70 percent of men who die in their seventies are found to have the disease upon postmortem, although less than one sixth of them have had any prostatic symptoms.

Symptoms

In 75 percent of cases, the cancer begins in the posterior lobe of the prostate and so, at first, produces none of the symptoms that are associated with benign hypertrophy of the lateral lobes. The first symptom in 20 percent of cases is pain in the hip bones or back, or sciatica, due to the cancer spreading in the blood to the bones. About 50 percent of patients develop urinary symptoms, such as frequency or a poor stream, and retention is not uncommon. Only 10 percent, however, will pass blood in the water. Some patients may have pain in the perineum or in the lower abdomen and some may become anemic.

Tests

The doctor will examine the patient through the rectum. A prostate gland affected by cancer may feel hard and uneven, unlike the smooth outline of a normal gland or of one with benign hypertrophy.

The blood tests that are done are the same as those performed in cases of benign hypertrophy. In addition, blood is taken to measure the enzyme acid phosphatase, which will be raised above normal in 50 percent of cases of cancer of the prostate. A newer test, the PSA (prostate-specific antigen), is also commonly done.

X-rays of the bones, especially those of the pelvis, lower back, thighs, and chest, may indicate whether or not the cancer has spread to other parts of the body. A bone scan is also commonly done in addition to X-rays.

A cystoscopy will enable a biopsy of the prostate to be taken, usually through the rectum, and the specimen will be examined under a microscope.

Traditional Treatment

In many cases, the diagnosis of cancer of the prostate is only made when a TUR (see above) is performed to treat acute or chronic retention. In such cases, if the cancer is small, it may be possible to remove it completely. In the United States, total prostatectomy, in which the entire gland is removed, is performed. The disadvantage of total prostatectomy is that the patient is always impotent and usually incontinent after the operation.

Radiotherapy is a useful treatment, especially for younger patients in whom the cancer shows no evidence of having spread to other parts of the body. It may be given as an external therapy, with an X-ray beam directed at the prostate, or radioactive iodine or gold may be implanted into the prostate during the operation. Radiotherapy is also helpful for those patients whose cancer has spread only to a single site and can often give instant pain relief.

When the cancer has begun to spread, hormone therapy can be very effective, since the cancer seems to need the male hormone, testosterone, in order to survive. The aim of treatment is to remove or suppress the patient's hormone output and this can be done by orchiectomy (removal of the testes), which may produce a dramatic remission in the disease. However, some doctors feel that the psychological problems that may be associated with orchiectomy make this a less valuable therapy and many prefer to treat patients by using female hormones, which suppress the patient's male hormones.

When female hormones are given, it is usually in the form of stilbestrol. This, unfortunately, may have side effects that include enlargement of the breasts, pigmentation of the nipples and scrotum, and shriveling of the testes. It may also cause fluid retention. This is a problem for a patient who has heart disease, because the increased blood volume that the heart has to pump due to the presence of the excess fluid may overtax it and precipitate him into heart failure. Until recently, orchiectomy was the best form of treatment for such patients. However, a new class of drugs has been developed that blocks the production of testosterone by the testes. These are known as LHRH analogues—LHRH standing for luteinizing-hormone releasing hormone. Luteinizing hormone (LH) is the hormone that stimulates the production of testosterone, and LHRH stimulates the production of LH. An LHRH analogue replaces the patient's own LHRH and prevents it from acting—rather like an incorrect key that, although it will not open the lock, will prevent another key from being inserted. At the start of treatment with these drugs, the production of testosterone may be temporarily increased, so the patient is usually given another drug such as flutamide acetate to counteract this. Flutamide is also used in treatment on its own to block the action of the male hormones.

The adrenal glands, too, produce a small quantity of male hormones. This can usually be suppressed by using cyproterone or an LHRH analogue, but sometimes removal of the adrenals may become necessary. This can be very effective for patients who are suffering from pain in the bones due to cancer deposits and whose pain is not relieved by other measures.

PROSTATIC CALCULI (STONES)

Occasionally these may cause symptoms similar to those of chronic prostatitis or benign enlargement, but generally they are symptomless and are discovered on X-ray or at prostatectomy. They usually occur in men over the age of fifty.

If they are small, prostatic massage through the rectum, plus a course of antibiotics, is likely to relieve any symptoms. Otherwise a prostatectomy may be necessary.

RECENT ADVANCES

In Israel, doctors have been using microwaves to treat benign enlargement, prostatitis, and prostatic cancer. The treatment is given via a rod that is inserted into the rectum and that heats the prostate, but not the surrounding tissues, to a higher temperature than normal. For benign enlargement, one or two hour-long sessions of treatment are given a week, up to a maximum of ten. In the treatment of cancer it is used together with radiotherapy. How it works is unknown, but it seems to be effective and to have no side effects. The doctors using it are claiming a success rate of around 60 percent. However, at present, the equipment necessary is very expensive and, at the time of writing, the treatment is not yet available in Britain or the United States, although one London hospital is reported to be considering giving it a trial. If the large-scale studies now under way prove successful, this could be a great step forward in the treatment of prostate problems. Every year over 400,000 prostate operations are performed in the United States, each patient needing up to ten days in the hospital and four weeks off work. Other advances include the use of balloon dilation (analogous to the technique used for coronary artery obstruction), and an experimental medication to shrink benign enlargement or to slow its growth.

COMPLEMENTARY TREATMENT

Aromatherapy
Oils containing essence of onion or pine may be recommended.

Herbalism
Various herbs that act as urinary antiseptics may be helpful in prostatitis. These include horsetail, sea holly (eryngo), and gravel root, all of which also act to reduce inflammation. Herbs with hormonal effects, such as damiana, may be useful in the treatment of benign enlargement. Saw palmetto, horsetail, and couch grass may also help to control symptoms in this condition.

Nutrition
Gamma aminobutyric acid (GABA) may help to reduce an enlarged prostate by stimulating the release of the hormone prolactin from the pituitary.

PSORIASIS

INCIDENCE AND CAUSE

Psoriasis is a fairly common, chronic, scaly condition of the skin that affects about 2 percent of the white European and North American population, but occurs less frequently in black and Japanese people. It tends to run in families and about one third of patients have a blood relative who also has psoriasis. A child who has one parent with psoriasis has a 20–30 percent chance of developing the disease, but if both parents are affected, the risk to the child is nearer 50 percent.

Although psoriasis can cause serious problems for some patients, many have only a few small areas of skin affected at any one time. Some may have a single severe attack that clears up and does not recur, although it is more usual for the disease to come and go throughout the patient's life.

Psoriasis usually makes its first appearance between the ages of fifteen and thirty. It is very rare under the age of five and uncommon between the ages of five and ten. When it does occur in childhood, the attacks are usually mild. There is no upper age limit after which it will not develop, and people have been known to have a first attack in their eighties. The sexes are equally affected, but in men the condition causes fewer cosmetic problems, since the rash can be covered by trousers and the long sleeves of a shirt.

The cause of psoriasis is unknown, but there are probably several factors involved, one of which may be an inherited defect in the skin. Attacks can occur quite suddenly and seem to be precipitated by mental stress, injury to the skin, and some drugs such as the antimalarial chloroquine. They also tend to occur two to three weeks after streptococcal infections.

TYPES OF PSORIASIS

Plaque Psoriasis

Psoriasis may take a number of different forms, the commonest of which is known as plaque, discoid, or scaly psoriasis. In this chronic form the patient has one or more dark red, scaly, circular or oval plaques, raised above the surface of the normal skin. Each plaque has a well-defined border and has the appearance of having been stuck on. The upper surface is covered with silvery or white crumbly-looking scales, although occasionally these are absent. Plaques may be as small as 1 cm across but may grow larger; sometimes smaller plaques merge together to form one large plaque with a scalloped edge.

Although plaques can occur anywhere, the commonest sites are the knees, elbows, lower part of the back, and the scalp, especially behind the ears. They also tend to appear wherever the skin has been injured and so may be precipitated by hard manual work. Affected skin is brittle and therefore prone to injury, which may be a problem for young people whose knees and elbows may get knocked when they are playing sports. The rash can also become worse if it is constantly being rubbed (for example, by a waistband or bra strap).

Sometimes this type of psoriasis can affect skin folds (known as the intertriginous areas)—in the groins, the armpits, under the breasts, between the toes, and around the umbilicus and the anus. In these areas, where the skin tends to be moist and the touching skin surfaces rub each other, the plaques are often smooth and red without any scale on them. Intertriginous psoriasis is more common in older age groups and may cause considerable soreness, which can make it difficult for the patient to move comfortably.

Itching is an unusual symptom in psoriasis but may occur when it affects the intertriginous areas or the scalp.

Guttate Psoriasis

This form usually occurs in children under the age of sixteen and often follows a streptococcal throat infection. The spots, which are small and scattered over the trunk and limbs, are smoother than those of plaque psoriasis, but scratching them will reveal the classic silvery scale. They usually appear suddenly and often clear spontaneously within three months. In most cases the only treatment needed is ultraviolet light (see below) and the majority of patients will be free of the rash within six weeks if treated three times a week. A few, however, will go on to develop chronic plaque psoriasis.

Pustular Psoriasis (von Zumbusch's Disease)

This condition, which is rare, starts suddenly with the appearance of tiny pustules (pus-filled spots) all over the body. The skin may be red and usually the patient has a high temperature, which may precede the appearance of the spots. The pustules themselves are sterile (that is, they do not contain bacteria), but the patient is often quite ill and needs admission to the hospital. Absorption of food from the intestines may become abnormal, making intravenous drip-feeding necessary.

Psoriasis of the Hands and Feet

This has a quite different appearance from plaque psoriasis. The skin may be red, scaly, and cracked, and the affected areas often have a sharp border. The cracks may become inflamed and very painful and may prevent the patient from using his hands normally or from walking.

The hands and feet may also be affected by a localized form of pustula psoriasis, which is sometimes known as persistent palmar and plantar pustulosis or recalcitrant eruption of the palms and soles. Small red scaly areas with sterile pustules develop on the palms and soles and may last for years. Occasionally only one palm or sole is affected, but usually both are involved. However, less than 20 percent of patients affected by this type of psoriasis have plaques on other parts of their bodies.

Psoriasis of the Nails

The nails are commonly involved in cases of chronic plaque psoriasis. The first sign is usually the appearance of tiny pits on the nail surface. The nails may then become discolored, thickened, and distorted and may separate from the underlying nail bed (a condition known as onycholysis) so that the end of the nails looks white. This may interfere with the patient's dexterity, making fine manual work, needlework, and even typing difficult to perform. Bacteria that produce a colored pigment may breed under the detached part of the nail so that it appears green or black.

Psoriasis of the Face and Scalp

One of the few good things about psoriasis is that it rarely affects the face. On the odd occasion that it does so, it produces a rash that looks like seborrheic dermatitis (see the section on eczema). However, the scalp is often involved, occasionally without the rash being apparent anywhere else on the body. It may involve the whole scalp or just small areas, and affected parts feel lumpy and irregular where the scales shed from the surface of the rash have piled up. The shed scales also produce very severe dandruff. Usually the rash stops at the hairline and doesn't spread onto the neck.

Erythrodermic Psoriasis (Erupting Active Psoriasis)

This is a fairly rare complication of chronic psoriasis. The rash suddenly becomes worse, with redness and scaling spreading all over the body, particularly over areas of skin that have been injured or scratched. The increased blood flow to the skin surface causes the patient to lose heat and, particularly in cold weather, hypothermia may result. Fluid can also be lost through the damaged skin. Patients with erythrodermic psoriasis need immediate hospital care.

Diaper Psoriasis

This occurs in babies, starting in the diaper area, and looks somewhat like plaque psoriasis, being a rash of dull red patches with well-defined borders and sometimes large silvery scales. However, experts are uncertain whether this really is a form of psoriasis. It may spread to other parts of the body, but it responds well to simple treatment and does not recur.

MECHANICS OF PSORIASIS

In normal skin the cells of the epidermis are replaced every fifty to sixty days, but in psoriasis the process is enormously speeded up and the

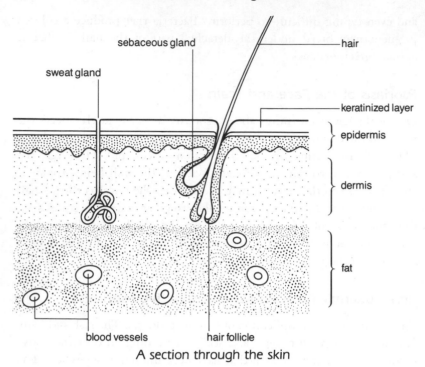

sebaceous gland — hair

sweat gland

keratinized layer

epidermis

dermis

fat

blood vessels   hair follicle

A section through the skin

turnover occurs every five to six days. When the intertriginous areas are affected, the sweat glands may become blocked so that sweating is reduced and heat stroke can occur if the patient works in a hot atmosphere.

Although the skin around the psoriatic plaques usually appears normal, examination under the microscope shows that changes have occurred here too; one of these is a tendency to speed up production of skin cells if the skin becomes injured. Thus, injury can precipitate the production of another plaque.

PROGNOSIS

Most people who have psoriasis will have it for life. However, its course is very variable and sometimes it may disappear spontaneously for periods of months or years. The less severe the condition, the more likely these remissions are to occur. Most patients will be able to find some form of treatment that will either get rid of their rash or will dramatically improve it.

Women usually find that psoriasis improves during pregnancy, probably as a result of the increased hormones that their bodies are producing.

About 5 percent of patients with psoriasis develop an associated arthritis. If their blood serum is tested for the rheumatoid factor found in patients with rheumatoid arthritis, it is negative; this form of arthritis is therefore known as seronegative. It often affects the joints of the hands, knees, and ankles, and may occasionally occur in a patient whose skin is perfectly normal. In such a case, the diagnosis is difficult and may only be made if all other forms of arthritis have been excluded and if the patient has a family history of psoriasis. The treatment of psoriatic arthritis is similar to that of rheumatoid arthritis (see separate section), and the condition usually responds well to antiinflammatory drugs. However, steroids, which are useful in other forms of arthritis, are not recommended because when the dose is reduced the patient's psoriasis may become worse.

DIAGNOSIS

When a patient develops the classic scaly plaques, diagnosis is not difficult. However, sometimes the advice of a skin specialist is necessary before a firm diagnosis can be made.

In some cases the plaques look smooth, but if the doctor gently scrapes one of them with a wooden spatula the typical silvery scales will appear. If he removes all the scale, a red, smooth, slightly moist area will be left with a few tiny bleeding points.

The scaly type of psoriasis that affects the hands and feet may be hard to distinguish from chronic eczema if there is no rash on other parts of the body. And, occasionally, psoriasis affects the nails without there being any skin rash. In such cases it may be very hard to tell it from a fungal infection of the nails. One helpful point is that a fungal infection usually begins in only one nail and rarely affects more than a few, whereas in psoriasis all the nails may be involved. However, in order to make the diagnosis, the doctor will need to take some nail clippings. These will be sent to the laboratory and examined under a microscope. Absence of fungal disease suggests that psoriasis is the cause.

TRADITIONAL TREATMENT

Many cases of psoriasis can be controlled with simple ointments or creams. However, the GP may refer a patient to the hospital if the rash is extensive, if it doesn't respond to simple treatments, or if it is causing problems because of its situation (a rash on the feet, for example). Types of medication available can be divided into topical (applied to the skin) and systemic (taken by mouth or injected). Most of the systemic treatments mentioned below are available only from dermatologists.

Topical Treatment

Emollients
Emollients are used to reduce dryness in the skin. They work by leaving an oily film over the skin surface that allows moisture to build up underneath it. They often come in the form of bath oils or as emulsifying ointments that can be used instead of soap. Unfortunately, the effects start to wear off after three or four hours, so for the best results they need to be applied several times a day.

For patients with just a few small plaques, Vaseline can be useful, rubbed in once or twice a day.

Keratolytics
Keratolytics smooth the skin surface by promoting the shedding of scales. One that is commonly used is salicylic acid (a relative of aspirin) in a dilution of 1–6 percent. However, it is unsafe to use this on large areas of skin since it may be absorbed into the body and produce the same effects as an overdose of aspirin.

Tar
Tar is an end product of the distillation of coal or wood and contains thousands of different organic compounds. It is often helpful in the treatment of psoriasis, although the way in which it acts isn't clear.

The main problem with tar is that the more effective the preparation, the messier it is to use, crude coal tar preparations giving better results than tar-containing creams. Various bath additives and shampoos and a somewhat less messy tar stick are also available. In order to keep messiness and staining of clothes to a minimum, tar preparations should be applied sparingly and should be covered with a light dressing. However, they need only be applied once a day.

Tar is especially useful in the treatment of psoriasis situated in the groin, around the navel, or under the breasts. It is also very helpful for areas where the skin has become thickened or itchy. Its action is improved by ultraviolet light. Used by itself it will usually take three weeks before any improvement is noticeable and may take as long as eight. Unfortunately, some patients are unable to use it because it irritates the skin and occasionally it can produce an acnelike rash.

Steroids
Steroid creams can produce a dramatic improvement in a psoriasis rash, but unfortunately the effect is often short-lived and only lasts for as long as the cream is used. Once it is stopped, the patient relapses and the rash may become worse than it was originally. In addition, it is thought that using steroids on plaque psoriasis may occasionally precipitate an attack of pustular psoriasis.

It is impossible for a patient to continue to use steroid creams long term, in order to prevent relapses, because of the risk of serious side effects. Not only is there a danger that the steroids may be absorbed into the body but they may result in the local area of skin becoming thin. Thin skin may be damaged easily, may bruise readily, and may take several months to return to normal after the steroid cream has been stopped. Stretch marks may also appear in the treated skin and, once formed, these are permanent.

For all these reasons, steroids have only a very limited part to play in the treatment of psoriasis. They can be useful for treating the groin, the navel, and the skin under the breasts, which may be oversensitive to other forms of treatment, and they are also used for patients whose psoriasis has become very active, with new patches appearing rapidly. However, strong steroids should not be used for more than two weeks at a time and there should be an interval of at least two months before they are used again.

No topical treatment has been discovered that will restore the nails to normal. Steroid injections have been tried around the nail beds, but they were found to be painful and relatively ineffective.

Anthralin

Anthralin has two things in common with tar. First, it is a complex organic substance (although it is synthesized in the laboratory rather than being distilled). And, second, the way in which it works in the treatment of psoriasis is not understood. It is useful for plaque psoriasis, but it is not suitable for use on the scalp or the intertriginous areas and should never be used on the face or near the genitalia. Differing concentrations are available, but the strongest are reserved for patients who are receiving treatment in the hospital. Normally anthralin is prescribed only for people whose rash cannot be controlled by tar preparations.

When it is used in the hospital, the patient usually takes a tar bath and is then exposed to ultraviolet light before the preparation is applied to the rash. If this is done five days a week, the plaques will usually disappear within two to three weeks. If anthralin is used without tar and ultraviolet light, it usually takes at least three weeks to produce an improvement and may take up to eight weeks. No benefit has been found from applying it more than once a day.

Anthralin is an irritant and may cause redness or even blistering in some patients. A low concentration is usually prescribed at first, stronger preparations being used later if necessary. It stains the clothes and the skin a brown-violet shade, but once the treatment has stopped, the skin discoloration will peel off within a few days. Treatment must always be stopped as soon as the psoriatic plaques have disappeared in order to avoid irritating normal skin.

Shampoos

Patients whose psoriasis affects the scalp need to wash their hair frequently with a special shampoo. If the scalp is thickly encrusted with scales, it is advisable to use a tar and salicylic acid ointment on the scalp every night and a tar-based shampoo every morning.

Systemic Treatment

Because of their potentially serious side effects, systemic preparations are usually only prescribed by hospital dermatologists. In pregnancy, all systemic therapy must be stopped immediately because of the risk that it may cause malformations in the unborn child.

Cytotoxic (cell-killing) drugs such as methotrexate, which prevent cells from dividing rapidly, are used only for very severe cases that respond to nothing else, and for generalized pustular and erythrodermic psoriasis.

Methotrexate

This drug is usually taken by mouth once a week, although sometimes injections are given. During the course of treatment, all alcohol is forbidden because it can cause severe liver damage when mixed with methotrexate. Even without alcohol, there is a risk to the liver if the drug is taken over a long period. For patients who may be on it for some years, a liver biopsy may be done before the course begins (to ensure that the liver is normal) and then repeated at regular intervals of eighteen months to two years for as long as treatment continues. Any deterioration in the condition of the liver would entail the patient coming off methotrexate immediately.

Other side effects are indigestion, nausea, abdominal pain, and an increased susceptibility to infections. In addition, methotrexate can suppress the production of blood cells in the bone marrow, so regular blood counts are necessary. Other cytotoxic drugs used in the treatment of psoriasis have been shown to affect the liver less, but they are more likely to affect the bone marrow.

Etretinate

This is a derivative of vitamin A that is taken daily by mouth. It takes four to six weeks to work and is always accompanied by side effects such as dry skin, cracked lips, nosebleeds, and sometimes temporary hair loss. It can also cause a rise in the level of fats in the blood, making regular blood tests necessary. It can cause malformation in an unborn baby, so because it stays in the body for a long period it is necessary for women to continue to use contraception for at least a year after stopping treatment. Etretinate is often used to good effect together with PUVA (see below) and is particularly useful in the treatment of generalized pustular psoriasis and erythrodermic psoriasis. The forms affecting the hands and feet also respond well, but in cases of chronic plaque psoriasis the response is often quite poor.

PUVA

PUVA stands for psoralens with ultraviolet light type A. Psoralens are naturally occurring (but now synthetically manufactured) compounds that sensitize the skin to light. In the treatment of psoriasis, the patient takes the preparation by mouth and two hours later is exposed to ultraviolet light from special lamps. Treatment is usually given three or four times a week at first, but once the rash has responded, this may be reduced to maintenance therapy once or twice a week. Most patients become quite tanned during the treatment. There are, however, drawbacks. The lamps are contained in a special cabinet in which the patient has to stand and some people are unable to tolerate this without developing claustrophobia. Also some very overweight patients may be unable to fit into the cabinets safely and comfortably. Occasionally, excessive treatment may burn the skin and fair-skinned people who are known to be sensitive to sunlight may be unsuitable for PUVA.

Because every part of the body, including the eyes, is sensitized to light by psoralens, the patient has to wear special protective glasses from the minute she takes the drug until at least twelve hours have elapsed after treatment. The method of action of PUVA, like the other psoriasis treatments, has not been clearly demonstrated, but it is thought that in the presence of ultraviolet light it acts on the nuclei of the cells to slow down their activity.

Most people need about fifteen treatments in order to clear the rash and after this they will usually have four or five months without relapsing. Even with maintenance therapy, there is a tendency for the rash to return after a period of several months. However, some 90 percent of patients with plaque psoriasis find this form of treatment effective. It is also helpful for localized pustular psoriasis of the palms and soles, where the affected areas can be exposed to the light by putting the hands or feet into a little box containing lamps. PUVA may also be used for some patients with generalized pustular or erythrodermic psoriasis.

PUVA is not generally used on patients under eighteen unless the rash is so severe that the alternative is cytotoxic drugs. And even in older patients it is only used if the rash covers 20 percent or more of the body surface. In patients eighteen to sixty years old, PUVA is usually used only if anthralin has failed to produce results or irritates the patient's skin even in low concentrations.

RECENT ADVANCES

In 1987 a group of Japanese doctors reported that they had treated twenty-two psoriatic patients with a vitamin D compound and had found that the results were almost as good as those that could be expected from using a steroid cream. A trial that used vitamin D preparations taken by mouth and used topically over a period of three months resulted in 76 percent of patients reporting at least a moderate improvement of their psoriasis with practically no side effects.

Doctors at the Royal Hallamshire Hospital in Sheffield (United Kingdom) have found that ten capsules a day of the fish-oil extract Maxepa significantly reduced itching, redness, and scaling in patients with psoriasis.

Meanwhile, some patients have found their condition becoming worse when they have been put on drugs for other complaints. This has resulted in doctors suggesting that the antihistamine terfenadine, the antiinflammatory drug indomethacin, and the blood-lipid-lowering drug gemfibrozil should not be prescribed for those with psoriasis.

COMPLEMENTARY TREATMENT

Aromatherapy
Lavender and bergamot may be prescribed.

Herbalism
Herbalists often equate chronic conditions with toxicity, the accumulation of toxins resulting from and contributing to a malfunction of the tissues affected. The aim of treatment is to cleanse the system and promote normal function in the tissues. Herbs that are often used in toxic skin conditions to cleanse the tissues and restore healthy function are burdock root, red clover, and sarsaparilla.

Homeopathy
The choice of remedy will depend, among other things, on where the rash is worst (for example, behind the ears or on the hands), whether it is itchy, and on the appearance of the rash itself. For example, arsenicum album may be used for a patient whose rash is burning and

itching but whose symptoms are relieved by warmth, while sulphur may be suitable for one whose rash is itchy, sore, and made worse by contact with water.

Hypnosis
For those patients whose psoriasis is made worse by stress or emotional upset, hypnosis is a very valuable therapy. First the patient will be taught how to relax and then how to hypnotize herself. During her sessions of hypnosis with the therapist she will be given the suggestion that as she becomes more relaxed her psoriasis will disappear. She may be given a visualization as well; for example, she may be told to imagine that she is swimming in a clear blue stream and that as she swims her rash is being gently washed away. She can then use the visualization when she practices her self-hypnosis. The improvement in the patient's skin is usually slow but steady and she develops confidence in her own ability to keep the rash under control in stressful situations.

Nutrition Therapy
High-dose vitamin A derivatives are used in orthodox medicine as a treatment for psoriasis, but patients who are not being prescribed this may find a daily supplement of vitamin A helpful, together with zinc, which is important for the maintenance of healthy skin.

SELF-HELP

People with widespread psoriasis, particularly if it affects the intertriginous areas, should avoid working in overheated or badly ventilated places, as their sweating mechanism may be defective.

Humidifiers may be helpful at home, since dry air will make the rash worse.

Baths should be tepid rather than hot and an emulsifying ointment or soap substitute should be used for washing, rather than soap, which has a drying effect on the skin. Once out of the bath, the patient should gently pat her skin dry rather than rubbing vigorously, as damaging the rash may make it worse.

Sunlight often makes the rash better, but an excessive amount may make it worse.

A naturopathic diet may help, in which the patient reduces her intake of meat, refined carbohydrates, dairy products, coffee, tea, and sugar, and increases her intake of nuts, seeds, whole grains, and beans.

ORGANIZATIONS

National Psoriasis Foundation
6443 S.W. Beaverton Highway
Suite 210
Portland, OR 97221
503/297-1545
(Publishes a bimonthly bulletin and educational material.)

RHINITIS

DEFINITION

Rhinitis is defined as a condition in which the patient suffers from sneezing and a running or blocked nose for more than an hour on most days. If it occurs only at certain times of the year it is known as seasonal rhinitis, but if it occurs all year round, it is perennial rhinitis.

SEASONAL RHINITIS (HAY FEVER)

This allergic condition is commonly known as hay fever, although patients are rarely allergic to hay and fever is not one of the symptoms. It is the commonest allergic disease known and most frequently affects boys and girls in their teens—up to one fifth of teenagers will have symptoms during June and July. It can begin at any age, but is rare in children under four. Often, those who develop hay fever will have had eczema when they were younger. Males and females are equally affected, but the condition seems to run in families.

Symptoms include itching in the nose, eyes, and soft palate (the back of the roof of the mouth), sneezing, and a running nose. The eyes, too, may water profusely. Patients may become stuffed up with mucus and lose their sense of taste or smell, and may develop a cough because of the mucus flowing down the back of the throat from the nose (postnasal drip). Occasionally they may have nosebleeds or develop polyps in the nose (see below). Some have sinusitis and about 20 percent (mainly children) have asthma. Children with hay fever frequently have dark rings under their eyes, known as "allergic shiners."

In March, April, and May, hay fever is due to an allergy to pollen from trees. From June to the beginning of August, grass pollen causes symptoms and, overlapping with this, from the end of June to September, hay fever may be due to spores released from molds that grow on a number of cultivated plants and on compost heaps. One of these molds grows around the roots of grass and its spores are released by mowing the lawn. Patients who are allergic to this will find that their symptoms are the same whatever the pollen count, but that they may decrease during wet weather when the lawns remain uncut. The majority of patients with hay fever are allergic to grass pollens, with nearly 80 percent having symptoms during June and nearly 70 percent during July. By comparison, only 15 percent have hay fever during September and less than 10 percent in April.

PERENNIAL RHINITIS

Symptoms
The main symptoms of perennial rhinitis are sneezing and either a running or a blocked nose. The eyes and throat are rarely affected. However, some patients develop sinusitis. The condition is commonest in the teens and twenties, becoming less frequent with age.

Allergic Perennial Rhinitis
The commonest cause is an allergy to the droppings of house dust mites, tiny insects invisible to the naked eye, that live in their thousands in dust, especially in older, damper buildings. The next commonest cause is an allergy to domestic pets, especially cats. Molds, fungi, industrial dust, and fumes can also cause symptoms, and affected patients are likely to be particularly sensitive to things such as cigarette smoke, strong perfumes, and traffic fumes, although these, in themselves, cannot set up the allergy.

Nonallergic Perennial Rhinitis
Some patients have symptoms without any cause being apparent. This is sometimes known as vasomotor rhinitis, although the abnormality of the nasal blood vessels implied in the word *vasomotor* has not been proved. However, in some cases, symptoms may be due to a hormonal imbalance and are seen in pregnant women or at the menopause or in some patients on the contraceptive Pill. When symptoms occur in pregnancy they usually disappear within a few hours of the baby being born.

NASAL POLYPS

Polyps are round, smooth, soft, fleshy structures that grow out of the lining of the nose and are attached to it by a thin stalk. They may occur in association with any type of rhinitis and, by blocking the nose, may result in loss of taste and smell and may make breathing through the nose difficult.

TESTS

Many patients can work out for themselves what it is that causes their allergy. A skin-prick test is sometimes used to test for allergies, but this may be misleading because 20 percent of people without symptoms will have positive tests. Sometimes a nasal swab can be helpful in differentiating between allergic and nonallergic rhinitis since, in the former, white cells involved in allergic reactions (eosinophils) will be found in the nasal mucus.

TRADITIONAL TREATMENT

For allergic patients, antihistamines are particularly effective in controlling sneezing, itching, and watering of the eyes. They are less effective in stopping the nose from running and do little to relieve blockage caused by mucus. Many of them cause drowsiness, although the newer ones such a astemizole and terfenadine are free from this effect. Antihistamines can also be used as eyedrops for those patients in whom the eyes are badly affected.

Topical decongestants are useful in the acute attack, but must never be used for more than a few days because otherwise they can produce a "rebound" congestion, so that the symptoms are worse at the end than they were to begin with. Such substances include ephedrine, phenylephrine, oxymetazoline, and a number of preparations that are available over the counter.

Antiallergic drugs such as cromolyn sodium are very effective since they prevent the nasal lining from reacting to the allergen (the substance causing the allergy). Eighty percent of patients with allergic rhinitis find them helpful, as well as a smaller number with nonspecific rhinitis. Cromolyn sodium is also available in the form of eyedrops.

A steroid spray such as beclomethasone is very effective in all forms of rhinitis. Only small amounts are used so it is not absorbed into the bloodstream and harmful side effects are therefore avoided. In very severe cases of rhinitis, another steroid, prednisolone, may be given by mouth for very short periods. Continued use of a steroid nasal spray may prevent nasal polyps from recurring after they have been surgically removed.

Desensitizing injections are used only for patients who are known to be allergic to grass pollen or to the house dust mite. Increasingly larger amounts of the allergen are injected over a period of time, until the patient can tolerate contact with quite large amounts without developing symptoms. Because of the possibility of a severe allergic reaction (anaphylaxis) the patient must be monitored in the doctor's office for thirty minutes after the injection. An injection of adrenaline can counter anaphylaxis.

COMPLEMENTARY TREATMENT

Acupuncture
Chronic rhinitis is said to be due to a deficiency of Chi in the lung. Acute rhinitis is said to be caused by invasion by wind and cold. Depending on the individual symptoms, treatment will consist of using points to stimulate Chi in the lung or to eliminate wind and cold. In either case, points will also be used that will restore the flow of energy to normal.

Aromatherapy
Eucalyptus, peppermint, and hyssop are among the oils that may be useful as an inhalation.

Herbalism
Many herbs have an antimucus effect. These include elderflower, eyebright, golden rod, garlic, yarrow, and agrimony. Chamomile and eyebright may also be used by patients with hay fever, to bathe the eyes.

Homeopathy
Arsenicum alb. may be useful if the patient's eyes are running and feel hot, if he has a profuse burning discharge from his nose, sneezes a great

deal, and feels worse after midnight. A patient whose nasal discharge is worse during the day and whose nose becomes blocked at night, whose eyes feel gritty, and who has a headache may respond to euphrasia. When chronic thick mucus and loss of taste and smell are the symptoms, becoming worse in a warm room and better out of doors in the evening, pulsatilla may be appropriate. Patients whose symptoms are worse in the early hours of the morning and who suffer from chronic mucus, loss of smell, sore throat, and bad breath may be given kali bich. For someone whose symptoms include a running nose, sore upper lip, itching eyes, tickling cough, and sneezing whenever he enters a warm room, allium cepa may be the remedy of choice.

Manipulation
Massage and manipulation of the neck may help to drain the sinuses and produce some relief in cases of chronic rhinitis.

Nutrition
Dairy products are mucus-promoting and should be avoided by patients with mucus. Dolomite (calcium and magnesium) helps to stabilize the levels of histamine, which is involved in allergic reactions, and may therefore be helpful in cases of hay fever. Allergies may also respond to 5000 mg of vitamin C or to supplements of vitamin B_6 and zinc.

SELF-HELP

Patients should try to avoid whatever it is they are allergic to, although in some cases this is difficult, if not impossible. However, finding another home for domestic pets and avoiding industrial fumes may relieve the condition entirely in some cases. For those who are allergic to pollens, it may be helpful to wear sunglasses, keep the car windows shut when driving, avoid walking in the country, especially in the late afternoon when the air may be thick with pollen, and keep the bedroom window shut at night. Patients often find they are better when at the seaside, since sea breezes tend to blow pollen inland.

The house dust mite is impossible to eradicate. However, putting plastic covers on the mattress and pillows, removing carpets, and keeping floors scrupulously clean may help reduce the count considerably. A powder called Acarosun, available from the Fisons Drug Company, 755 Jefferson Road, Rochester, NY 14623, is sprinkled onto carpeting, binds the excrement of the dust mite, then is vacuumed away (the excrement is supposedly the allergenic property).

RINGWORM

DEFINITION

Ringworm is the name given to a group of fungal infections that affect the skin. The medical term for this condition is tinea—a Latin word meaning "gnawing worm." In actual fact, the infection itself is usually a great deal less unpleasant than the names given to it.

There are various types of fungus that can affect the skin and, depending on which type is involved and which part of the body is affected, the symptoms will differ. The fungi can be divided into those that affect only human beings and those that can also affect (and can therefore be caught from) animals. On the whole, the human-only types tend to produce chronic low-grade infections whereas those that can affect animals tend to cause more intense and shorter-lived infections. Apart from one type of ringworm of the scalp, these fungal infections are not particularly contagious—indeed, it is well known that a man with ringworm of the feet can share a double bed with his wife for many years and never transfer the infection to her. It seems likely that those people who do develop the infections have some sort of inbuilt susceptibility.

Although ringworm can be uncomfortable at times or even painful, and can look very unsightly, it is not capable of doing any real harm to its host because it infects only dead cells. It lives in the uppermost layer of the skin, which is made up of cells that have died and in which keratin, a hornlike substance, has been laid down. It also lives in the hair and the nails, which are composed mainly of keratin. The fungus secretes a chemical that enables it to break down and digest the keratin in these structures. If, as occasionally happens, the body reacts to the infection and inflammation occurs, this may cure the infection, since the upper layer of the skin may be shed rapidly, getting rid of much of the fungus while that which remains is unable to survive in cells that contain little or no keratin.

Ringworm infections are usually divided into categories, according

374

to which part of the body is affected. The feet and the groins are the two commonest sites, probably because the fungus grows more readily in moist areas.

RINGWORM OF THE FEET (TINEA PEDIS)

This is the commonest ringworm infection and accounts for a large number of cases of "athlete's foot" (which may also be due to other types of infection or just to poor foot care). It occurs mainly in young and middle-age adults, more often in men than in women, and is rare in children.

Tinea pedis usually begins with peeling and slight maceration of the skin between the toes. Maceration occurs, for example, when a patch has been left on too long and the skin becomes waterlogged, white, and soggy. Usually a fungal infection begins between the fourth and fifth toes and may extend to the other spaces, although it is rarely found between the first and second toes. Between the toes the only symptom may be slight irritation and the infection may never spread any further. However, in some cases it extends to the undersurface of the toes and to the sole and sides of the foot.

Depending on which fungus is causing the infection, the rash may be dry and scaly with thickening and hardening of the affected skin, or it may produce blisters and painful cracks. Sometimes it can be very itchy. A sudden flare-up may occur, with the formation of blisters filled with yellowish fluid, and splits in the skin, associated with itching and pain. In such cases, a bacterial infection may take hold on the inflamed skin, causing further complications.

RINGWORM OF THE GROIN (TINEA CRURIS)

This is the second commonest site for ringworm to occur and like tinea pedis it is commoner in men than in women. It tends to occur more frequently in warm weather and may appear in patients who already have tinea pedis.

It usually begins with redness and slight maceration in the skin fold of one groin. The infection extends outward, developing a raised red border that may have tiny blisters on it. The whole area is scaly and usually slightly itchy and it may, in the long term, become darker than the surrounding normal skin. Sometimes the infection remains confined to one groin, but it may spread to affect not only the other groin but the genitalia, the buttocks, the thighs, and the abdomen. Other "satellite" patches may develop elsewhere on the trunk, the feet, or the hands.

RINGWORM OF THE BODY (TINEA CORPORIS)

This usually starts as one or more little red spots that extend outward over the course of the following week or two to form a round or oval plaque that may have tiny blisters and a paler center with a raised, red border. The pale center is due to the fact that the skin tends to heal as the infection spreads outward and away from it. Sometimes, however, the entire area remains red, raised, and scaly.

The commonest sites for tinea corporis to occur are the face, neck, arms, and legs. Usually the patches remain relatively small, although extensive infections are quite common in tropical climates.

Sometimes a lump will form in the skin, known as a tinea granuloma, which may be associated with little pus-filled spots.

RINGWORM OF THE SCALP (TINEA CAPITIS)

This is the most infectious form of ringworm and can cause outbreaks in schools. Although adults can develop tinea capitis, the most commonly involved fungi tend to attack only children.

The affected area is usually an oval or round patch on which the skin has become scaly and the hairs have broken off, their remnants looking like small black dots. The fungus digests the keratin in the hair, making it brittle, but hair loss is not uniform and usually some can still be seen growing from the infected skin. Most of the scalp may become involved and in many cases the patient has patches on the neck, just below the hairline, as well.

Sometimes acute inflammation occurs and the area becomes red and swollen and oozes pus. Although this may look very alarming, it is thought to be due to an immune reaction occurring in the skin. If left untreated, it will heal after about six to eight weeks, usually without any scarring or permanent hair loss.

RINGWORM OF THE HANDS

Ringworm seldom affects the hands. When it does so, it causes slight redness and scaling of the palms. Inflammation with blistering and scaling may occur, but this is rare in temperate climates.

RINGWORM OF THE NAILS (TINEA UNGUIUM)

Some patients may have tinea pedis for many years without infection of the nails. Similarly, infection of the hands does not necessarily involve the nails. Other patients, however, may have signs of infection in both the skin and nails. Why the nails become infected in some people but not others is not known.

The first parts of the nail to become infected are usually the sides and the tip, which become yellow and thickened. As the fungus spreads, the whole nail may become distorted. Although eventually all the nails may be involved, it is usual for the infection to be confined to one or two at first.

TESTS

In many cases the diagnosis of ringworm may be obvious simply from its appearance. However, particularly when it occurs on the feet, it may be hard to distinguish from eczema or psoriasis. Nails that are affected by psoriasis, eczema, or the thrush organism, monilia, may look very similar to those infected by a fungus.

The tests necessary for a diagnosis of ringworm are quite straightforward, although it may take some time before the results are available. Normally, when the skin is affected, it is gently scraped and the resulting flakes are sent to the laboratory for examination or are immediately examined under a microscope. If the nails are involved, a small piece is cut off for examination.

Two of the fungi that cause tinea capitis have the peculiar quality of fluorescing when put under a particular type of ultraviolet light known as Wood's light. This is an easy way not only of diagnosing the infection but also of screening classes of schoolchildren who may have become infected. However, tinea capitis can be caused by a fungus that does not fluoresce, so absence of fluorescence does not necessarily rule out the diagnosis, particularly in adults, in whom the condition is usually caused by the nonfluorescent variety.

TRADITIONAL TREATMENT

There are numerous products available nowadays for the treatment of fungal infections, but griseofulvin has proved to be outstandingly useful. It is taken by mouth and is deposited in the skin cells and the growing hair and nail. However, it cannot penetrate the dead keratinized cells, but has to wait until the cells that it enters become keratinized in their turn. Thus, it takes a long time to work—up to a month for skin infections, two to three months for hair infections, and up to two years for infections of the toenails. Because of this, and because there are a number of effective ointments, creams, and paints available, only those patients with particularly troublesome skin infections are offered griseofulvin. However, it is invaluable in the treatment of tinea capitis and tinea unguium, since topically applied preparations cannot penetrate the hair or the nails. It has the advantage of having few side effects, although occasionally it may cause nausea, headaches, or rashes. Ringworm of the skin responds well, although that occurring between the toes tends to relapse. The relapse rate is also high for the toenails, but there is a much greater chance of a permanent cure when treating the fingernails. Patients with tinea capitis should trim down any remaining hair in the area after two to three weeks on griseofulvin, to remove a potential source of reinfection. Because tinea capitis is quite infectious, it is usually advisable for children to stay away from school after the diagnosis has been made. They can return three or four weeks after they have started to take griseofulvin.

Topical agents come as creams, ointments, lotions, and paints. One of the oldest is Whitfield's ointment, which has the advantage of being cheap and effective and the disadvantage of being greasy so that it may be unpleasant to use. Equally effective but more pleasant and more expensive are substances such as clotrimazole, econazole, miconazole, and sulconazole, all of which come as creams. Econazole is also available as a lotion, which is useful in the treatment of a rash that has become moist, blistered, or weepy. Another antifungal agent is salicylic acid, which is available in a cream or a paint, the latter having the property of drying up moist skin, although it cannot be used on areas that are cracked. For skin that has become particularly inflamed and weepy, potassium permanganate soaks are helpful in the early stages of treatment.

Although several of these preparations are available over the counter, it is advisable to have the condition correctly diagnosed before trying to treat it yourself. It is also important that the treatment is continued for several weeks after the infection seems to have disappeared completely in order to prevent a relapse. Medicated dusting powders should be avoided as these may irritate the skin. Griseofulvin is only available by prescription.

COMPLEMENTARY TREATMENT

Herbs can be used in the treatment of ringworm, particularly marigold and myrrh, both of which have a healing action on the skin. Aromatherapists may recommend a tea tree for tinea pedis and other forms of athlete's foot. Homeopathy may also be helpful.

SELF-HELP

Because tinea cruris and tinea pedis prefer moist conditions, avoiding tight underwear and close-fitting unventilated shoes will help to speed recovery. After bathing, it is very important to dry carefully between the toes.

Patients who are being treated for tinea capitis would be well advised to throw away their brushes, combs, and hats, or else to clean them very thoroughly before using them again.

SCHIZOPHRENIA

DEFINITION AND INCIDENCE

Although, nowadays, mental illness is no longer a taboo subject, being openly discussed in the press and on television and radio, there is still confusion in the minds of many people as to what constitutes schizophrenia. The old, incorrect notion that it is a condition in which the mind is "split" and in which the patient exhibits multiple personalities is still fairly widely accepted. In fact, the condition of multiple personalities is extremely rare, whereas schizophrenia, which is characterized by bizarre delusions, hallucinations, illogical thinking, and, often, inappropriate emotions, is not uncommon.

Schizophrenia affects between two and four people in every thousand. The majority of cases begin between the ages of fifteen and twenty-five, and it is unusual for the condition to develop in people over the age of forty. It tends to run in families—the brother or sister of a patient is sixteen times more likely to develop schizophrenia than the average person, the son or daughter of a patient is nineteen times more likely, and the grandchild of a patient is four times more likely. In the case of identical twins, if one develops schizophrenia, the other is also likely to be affected in between 50 and 90 percent of cases.

SYMPTOMS

Patients who develop schizophrenia have often had strange personality traits before any indication of illness becomes apparent. They may have been introspective and unsociable, cold and aloof—although, of course, by no means all people with this so-called "schizoid" personality develop schizophrenia. A little while before the onset of overt symptoms, the patient may have been inclined to have headaches or attacks of anxiety or depression, and may have lost his appetite or become absentminded. The onset may occur soon after an infection or an operation, or at a time when the patient is worried about something, such as important examinations.

Most specialists now agree that there is an organic basis to schizophrenia—in other words, that it is caused by a disturbance in the chemicals of the brain. However, the exact mechanism has not been discovered and it seems likely that it is not a single disease but a number of conditions in which the symptoms are similar. Although it has been customary to divide schizophrenia into certain fairly well-defined types, these may overlap in the individual patient.

There are some common symptoms to several of these types, such as an inability to relate to the real world, a lack of insight into what is happening (although occasionally a schizophrenic patient may realize that he is ill, particularly at the start of an attack), a reduction in emotional response, and thought disorder.

Thought disorder comprises a number of symptoms. The patient is not confused, but his thought processes become irrational. He may jump from subject to subject in conversation, use words of his own invention, and be unable to concentrate, even on what he himself is saying. He may be unable to think in abstract terms and may exhibit "concrete thinking"—for example, if asked to explain a proverb, such as "half a loaf is better than no bread," he may say it means that if the baker has run out of large loaves, you have to buy a small one.

The patient may complain that he has lost control over his thinking and that thoughts that are not his own suddenly appear in his mind. Or he might say that his thoughts are broadcast to other people or that they are removed, so that his mind goes blank. He may attribute these effects to hypnosis or telepathy on the part of others or to the use of radio, television, or electronic instruments.

Delusions are defined as false unshakable beliefs. First of all, the patient may become convinced that an everyday event has a special meaning specifically for him. For example, he may believe that there is a message coded into how many people get on and off a bus at each stop. This "message" is then elaborated on, forming a basis for further delusions. Hypochondriacal delusions, in which the patient believes that part of his body is withering away or is grossly diseased, may sometimes be present for some years before there is any other evidence of schizophrenia or may appear once the disease has become established. The patient may also come to believe that people are talking about him and doing certain things specifically to annoy him or, at the other extreme, that he does not exist, or that the world around him does not exist. Paranoid delusions may occur in which he believes himself to be very important and thinks that he is being persecuted by those who are jealous of his success.

Hallucinations are defined as false perceptions—in other words, the patient sees, hears, tastes, smells, or feels something that is not there. When they occur in schizophrenia, they usually take the form of voices (auditory hallucinations). Some patients hear them only when they are relaxing, but for others they are there all the time, to the extent that they are unable to concentrate on even the simplest task. They may believe that the voices are being transmitted by machines or are being sent out by other people around them. Occasionally patients see visual hallucinations, but they are usually aware that these are unreal and they may refer to them as visions. They may also have hallucinations of taste and smell and of bodily sensations such as pain or pressure.

Emotional abnormalities may occur, particularly at the start of the illness. The patient may begin to hate someone whom he has previously loved and may have outbursts of anxiety, rage, or misery. Or his emotions may appear shallow and may fluctuate rapidly.

TYPES OF SCHIZOPHRENIA

Paranoid Schizophrenia

This form of the disease is more likely to occur in someone who is over the age of thirty when he becomes schizophrenic. His first symptom is often fear, which is associated with a delusion that he is being persecuted. This may be reinforced by auditory hallucinations. As time goes on, although he still believes that "people are after him," the patient exhibits far less anxiety about it and may appear quite complacent. However, he may become aggressive and attack anyone whom he believes to be his enemy. In some cases there is a religious element to the delusion—the patient believing that he has a special relationship with God and so constitutes a threat to people of a certain religion who are "out to get him."

Catatonic Schizophrenia

Catatonic schizophrenia affects not just the mind but also the body and is most common in teenagers and young adults. Patients may develop a stiff, rigid way of walking and may have periods during which they lie totally immobile and uncommunicative. If allowed to, they may sit or stand in one position for hours on end. They don't eat, drink, or voluntarily empty their bladders or bowels, and they may be incontinent as a result. If someone tries to move them, they may resist, and if they are asked to do something, they may do the opposite. They may also develop the strange condition known as waxy flexibility in which they allow their limbs to be moved into positions that they then hold for minutes at a time. As well as these attacks of stupor, patients may have episodes of overexcitement in which they suffer from delusions and hallucinations.

Rapid recovery from attacks is not unusual and patients may remain free from symptoms for several years. In some cases, after one attack, the condition never recurs.

Hebephrenia

This is the least common form of schizophrenia. It affects teenagers and young adults, usually developing slowly and taking a chronic course. The patient has delusions and hallucinations and his thinking is disturbed. His emotional response to situations is shallow and inappropriate—for example, he may laugh or remain unmoved when told of some disaster or of the death of a near relative—and he behaves in a silly way. The disease may progress steadily or may be interspersed with periods of excitement that can result in a sharp deterioration in the patient's condition.

Simple Schizophrenia

In this type, there is a general deterioration of the patient's personality, with blunting of the emotions and disorders of thinking but no delusions or hallucinations. The patient becomes apathetic and withdraws from social contact with other people. The condition often begins in adolescence and may develop insidiously.

Chronic Schizophrenia

Eventually, after many years, the patient ceases to have acute attacks and is left dull and apathetic, with hallucinations, delusions, and sometimes disorders of thinking. He is unable to look after himself and may become anxious about his health and the world around him.

Paraphrenia

This is a condition in which a patient in his forties or fifties develops paranoid delusions and hallucinations but none of the other symptoms of schizophrenia.

COURSE OF THE DISEASE

In the past a diagnosis of schizophrenia usually meant that the patient would be shut up in a mental institution for life. Just before the Second World War, two thirds of all schizophrenics who were admitted to the hospital would stay there for two years or more. Nowadays, thanks to modern medication, only 10 percent of schizophrenic patients need long-term hospital care. Forty percent have frequent relapses, but 30 percent are able to adapt to life in the community. The final 20 percent recover completely after a single attack.

In some cases the progress of the disease is a steady downhill course. In others, new symptoms appear in acute attacks; they then die down after some months, leaving the patient worse than he was before. Those who suffer from hallucinations are more likely to become chronically ill, and hebephrenia, on the whole, has a poor outlook.

Patients who are depressed or excited and who do not demonstrate emotional blunting have a better chance of recovery. Early diagnosis and treatment also improves the prognosis. Other factors associated with a good prognosis are a sudden onset, a previously normal personality, above-average intelligence, a stable home environment, a good work record, and a short first attack. Patients who have no family history of schizophrenia, who were under stress at the time of the first attack, who are married, and are over the age of thirty are also likely to do better, as are those whose symptoms are mainly catatonic.

Poor prognosis is associated with an insidious onset, a previously unsociable (schizoid) personality, an absence of precipitating events (such as stress), blunting of the emotions, onset at an early age, and a family history of schizophrenia.

TRADITIONAL TREATMENT

Strong sedatives are used to reduce the symptoms of an acute attack. These include chlorpromazine, thioridazine, trifluoperazine, and haloperidol. Trifluoperazine is usually the drug of choice for the more apathetic patient since it also has stimulant properties. All of these drugs have some side effects, such as drowsiness and dryness of the mouth. They can also produce disturbances of the nervous system so that symptoms similar to the tremor and muscle rigidity of Parkinson's disease may occur, although these can be controlled by using drugs such as procyclidine, benzhexol, benztropine, or orphenadrine in addition. Patients who relapse after recovering from a first attack are usually put on long-term treatment that may consist of one of the drugs mentioned above or a long-acting injection, such as fluphenazine, which needs only to be repeated every two to three weeks. It is usual to give an anti-Parkinson's drug as well.

Most patients respond well to drug treatment, but occasionally ECT (electroconvulsive therapy) may be required for someone who is severely depressed or who cannot be roused from a catatonic stupor. Very rarely it may be necessary to operate on a chronically ill patient who fails to respond to other forms of treatment. The operation, known as a lobotomy, consists of making a tiny cut in the brain, and can produce a considerable improvement in the patient's symptoms.

All patients need to be followed up for life. As well as medication, they need support, which will help them to adjust to living in the community, and family psychotherapy may be helpful.

COMPLEMENTARY TREATMENT

Treatment by an herbalist or homeopath may help to stabilize the patient's condition so that less medication is needed.

However, some of the most important work on schizophrenia that has been done recently is in the field of nutrition. Dr. Carl Pfeiffer of the Brain Bio Center in Princeton, New Jersey, has found that most patients with psychoses (severe mental illness in which insight is lost) have either high or low levels of histamine in their bodies. Histamine is usually thought of as the body chemical involved in allergic reactions, but it also plays an important role in the functioning of the nervous system. Patients who are severely histapenic (that is, low in histamine) tend to have disorders of thinking, hallucinations, and paranoia. They are also inclined to have a lot of fillings in their teeth, few colds, and few allergies. Associated with the lack of histamine is an excess of copper and a deficiency of zinc. Dr. Pfeiffer and his colleagues have found that treating schizophrenic patients with supplements of zinc and manganese (to raise the zinc levels and bring down the copper), vitamin C (to prevent the uptake of more copper), and the amino acid methionine (to detoxify the excessive histamine in the brain) can have remarkable results.

ORGANIZATIONS

American Schizophrenia Association
900 North Federal Highway, #330
Boca Raton, FL 33432
305/393-6167

Schizophrenia Research Branch
National Institute of Mental Health
5600 Fishers Lane
Room 10C-6
Rockville, MD 20857
301/443-4707

SHINGLES
(Herpes Zoster)

CAUSE

Shingles and chicken pox are caused by the same virus—the varicella/zoster virus or VZV. But whereas chicken pox is caught from someone else who has the disease, shingles is due to a reemergence of the virus that has lain dormant in the patient's body, sometimes for many years, since she had chicken pox. If her resistance to infection is lowered, the virus may become active again, producing an attack of shingles. This is why shingles is most common in the elderly population, whose resistance is often less than robust, and rare in children, many of whom have not yet had chicken pox.

The virus seems to lie dormant in the nervous system. Inside the spinal column, or backbone, is the spinal cord from which all the nerves that supply the body originate. The backbone itself is made up of a series of bones called vertebrae and between each pair of vertebrae a pair of spinal nerves runs to each side of the body. Clumps of nerve cells known as the root ganglia are situated on the nerves soon after they leave the spinal cord and it is here that the dormant VZV seems to lie. Because the virus is usually activated only in one root ganglion, the area affected is normally confined to one side of the body and to skin supplied by a single spinal nerve (this area is known as a dermatome). Sometimes shingles involves areas of the head and neck supplied by the cranial nerves that run directly from the brain. Here, too, the rash is confined to the area supplied by a single nerve.

SYMPTOMS

Shingles often begins with pain, a bruised feeling, or itching over the area of skin where the rash will develop. The patient may also feel unwell and have a slight fever. After two or three days a crop of blisters

387

appears, usually with some redness of the surrounding skin. The blisters are often in groups and new groups may continue to appear over the next few days. As the disease progresses, the blisters may become purplish due to the presence of blood in them. Eventually they crust over and the rash usually clears up within two weeks, although occasionally it may last twice that time. It can be both painful and itchy, and these symptoms sometimes continue after the rash itself has gone. Because the rash contains the virus, it is possible for someone who has not had chicken pox to catch it by coming into close contact with a patient suffering from shingles.

The most usual area of the body to be affected is the chest, with the rash extending in a sweep from the spine around to the center of the chest in the front. If the arm is involved, there may be weakness and wasting of the muscles, which may persist after the infection is over.

Shingles affecting the lower spinal nerves that supply the bowel and bladder may cause problems with emptying the bowels or with passing water. Such complications usually resolve completely within four months.

Involvement of the facial nerve causes paralysis of the facial muscles that it supplies. Fifty percent of patients recover fully from this and another 39 percent have a good, if not complete, recovery, but it may take over a year. In the Ramsay Hunt syndrome, facial paralysis is associated with a shingles rash on the ear and in the throat and sometimes deafness may occur.

Perhaps the most troublesome form of shingles is that affecting the ophthalmic nerve, in which the rash can affect the eye. Conjunctivitis, ulceration, and inflammation of the whole eye can occur. Scarring may result in reduced vision or blindness. In about a third of patients, the muscles that move the eye become paralyzed, but this usually resolves within three months.

Occasionally a patient whose immunity is greatly reduced (such as the very elderly or someone suffering from another serious disease) may develop generalized shingles in which the rash covers the entire body.

While the patient has the rash, there is a risk of secondary bacterial infection that may need treatment with antibiotics. Once the rash has subsided, the greatest problem is postherpetic neuralgia, a condition that affects about 10 percent of patients, being commonest in those over the age of sixty-five and those who had a rash involving the ophthalmic nerve. The patient has a burning, continuous pain that does not respond well to painkillers. Usually it disappears after a period of weeks or months and most patients have recovered after about two years, but in some cases it continues indefinitely.

TRADITIONAL TREATMENT

Many cases of shingles can be treated simply with painkillers and rest. Because of the distressing nature of the pain, some patients need mild tranquilizers. Antihistamine tablets may be useful to reduce the itching, but these can make the patient drowsy.

In recent years the discovery of antiviral agents has made possible the treatment of shingles on more than just a symptomatic level. Dressings soaked in idoxuridine applied to the rash for the first three or four days of the illness help to reduce pain and accelerate healing. However, acyclovir (ACV) seems to be emerging as the treatment of choice. Given orally five times a day for seven days, it has the effect of reducing the severity of the attack and promoting healing. If the eye is involved, ACV ointment can be used in addition. Patients with generalized shingles or serious complications may need to be given ACV intravenously.

ACV does not seem to reduce the risk of postherpetic neuralgia. However, the steroid prednisolone, given in gradually decreasing doses over a period of three weeks, may prevent this complication in patients over sixty if given early enough in the illness. A new topical cream, Capsaicin, is now available for postherpetic neuralgia.

COMPLEMENTARY TREATMENT

Acupuncture
A red rash with blistering is said to be due to heat in the channel it overlies. The aim of treatment is to eliminate heat and restore energy flow to normal.

Aromatherapy
Clary sage, eucalyptus, geranium, and lavender are among the oils that may be beneficial.

Herbalism

A preparation of oats may be used, as this is a nervous restorative that will strengthen the nervous system as a whole. Scullcap works in a similar way and marigold is used to promote healing of the rash.

Homeopathy

If the patient has large blisters and the skin is red, swollen, burning, and feels better if something cold is put on it, apis may be helpful. If, however, the symptoms are relieved by a warm application and itching is severe, arsenicum alb. may be the remedy of choice. For a patient who has a hot itchy rash of small blisters that is better for warmth, rhus tox. may be appropriate.

Hypnotherapy

Hypnosis may be useful in some cases of postherpetic neuralgia to teach patients how to control their pain.

SINUSITIS

THE SINUSES

Sinus means a hollow or cavity, and when referring to the sinuses, doctors mean the cavities within the bones of the skull. They are also known as the paranasal sinuses, because they lie alongside and communicate with the nasal passages. Whether they have any function other than that of making the skull lighter and the voice more resonant is doubtful.

The two maxillary sinuses lie in the cheekbones, the two frontal sinuses in the forehead, and the two sphenoidal sinuses behind the nose. The ethmoidal sinuses vary in number and may consist of as few as three large cavities or as many as eighteen small ones situated between the eyes. These are the only sinuses to be fully developed at birth; the others grow during childhood, the maxillary sinuses becoming evident after the age of eighteen months and the frontal and sphenoidal sinuses after the age of ten. For this reason, infection of the frontal and sphenoidal sinuses is rare in children.

The sinuses are lined with mucous membrane, similar to what lines the nose. The individual cells of this lining have tiny projections (cilia) that sweep the mucus secreted within the sinus out into the nasal passages.

ACUTE SINUSITIS

Inflammation of the lining of the sinuses usually occurs as the result of a heavy cold. The exits of the sinuses, through which mucus drains, become blocked and there is a buildup of fluid that may become infected with bacteria. Other circumstances that can bring on sinusitis include foreign bodies in the nose (which also prevent adequate drainage), injury to the sinus involved, infection of the teeth, and jumping into cold water without first holding the nose.

When, as is usual, sinusitis is preceded by a cold, the patient will

391

find that on the third or fourth day, just when the symptoms should be getting better, they suddenly get worse. The nose is more blocked and any nasal discharge becomes heavier. The patient loses his sense of smell, is feverish, and may feel quite unwell. A heavy feeling in the face and head is made worse by bending forward and the patient may awake in the morning with a headache that takes some time to wear off.

The exact location of the pain depends on which sinuses are inflamed. Usually the maxillary sinuses are involved, resulting in pain and tenderness in the cheekbones. The ethmoidal sinuses, too, are frequently affected, producing pain between and behind the eyes. There may be swelling of the overlying skin, particularly in children.

Inflammation of the frontal sinuses may be one-sided and often produces a severe headache over one eye that is there when the patient wakes in the morning and lasts until late afternoon. It may also cause pain around the eye and, if severe, swelling of the eyelids. Specific infection of the sphenoidal sinuses is hard to diagnose, but it may produce pain in the center of the head, which radiates to the temples and may occasionally be mistaken for earache. There may be a thick green discharge from the nose, but the patient doesn't usually complain of a blocked nose.

Very occasionally, the maxillary sinuses become infected as a result of an infection in the teeth. In such cases, the nasal discharge is likely to be very foul-smelling.

Tests

The diagnosis is often clear from the history, but a nasal culture is usually taken to try to determine which bacteria are involved in the infection. An X-ray of the skull may show clouding in the normally clear sinuses, an indication that fluid has accumulated there. A full blood count may also be taken and later repeated, the number of white cells reflecting the course of the infection.

Traditional Treatment

The patient needs to be put to bed in a room that has an even temperature and even humidity. The nasal lining contains a network of blood vessels whose job is to warm the inhaled air, while its cells secrete mucus to moisten the air before it enters the lungs. By keeping the temperature and humidity constant, the nasal lining is allowed to rest as it does not have to keep adapting to changes.

The patient should drink plenty of fluids, which not only allows the mouth to remain moist and helps to combat the fever but also helps to prevent the nasal mucus from becoming too sticky.

Painkillers are usually prescribed together with antibiotics that should be taken until at least forty-eight hours after the symptoms have subsided. For adults, steam inhalations may be very helpful, but because there may be a risk of scalding, these are not recommended for children. Menthol or Friars Balsam in the steaming water may help to clear the nasal passages.

Usually the condition settles quite quickly if treated in this way. However, occasionally the symptoms may persist and in such cases it may be necessary to wash out the appropriate sinuses. Depending on the sinuses involved, it may be possible to do this through the nose under a local anesthetic, or a larger operation may be necessary.

Complications

It is essential that acute sinusitis be treated promptly and cleared up completely since there are a number of complications that can occur. Not least of these is progression to chronic sinusitis.

Other complications are uncommon. They include a spread of the infection to the eye socket, causing swelling of the eyelid and eye and resulting in double vision. Failure to treat at this stage may result in blindness. Antibiotics and draining of the collected pus from both the eye socket and the infected sinus will usually resolve the condition.

Infection may also spread to the bone of the forehead from the frontal sinuses. This usually occurs in children and young adults (more often boys) and there may be a history of injury to the area. The patient is quite ill and often drowsy, although initially the only symptoms may be swelling of the eyelid and of the forehead. Urgent treatment is required to prevent the infection from spreading to the brain. An X-ray will usually confirm the diagnosis by showing a "moth-eaten" appearance of the bones of the forehead, and a blood culture will enable the doctor to determine the bacteria involved. The patient is admitted to the hospital and is given large doses of antibiotics. If abscesses form, these will need to be drained.

The bone of the upper jaw may become infected, particularly if maxillary sinusitis is the result of a dental infection. This is a rare condition, usually occurring in children. The patient is quite ill, with extensive swelling of the cheek. Urgent treatment is necessary to prevent damage to the jaw and teeth. The infection usually responds rapidly to large doses of antibiotics and drainage of any abscesses. Once the patient has recovered, it may be necessary to wash out the sinuses.

Infection spreading to the brain causes drowsiness, headache, seizures, vomiting, and weakness. After X-rays and blood cultures, treatment consists of large doses of antibiotics and drainage of abscesses.

CHRONIC SINUSITIS

Although many cases of chronic sinusitis seem to result from acute sinusitis that has not completely resolved, other factors may be important. Allergies, such as hay fever, that cause swelling of the lining of the nasal passages may reduce the drainage from the sinuses and encourage stagnation of mucus within them. Smoking may act in the same way, as may living in a polluted atmosphere and the consumption of large amounts of alcohol. Dental infection is often associated with chronic sinusitis, but it is often not clear which condition came first.

The patient suffers from discomfort in the nose and face, mucus production, headache, and a poor sense of taste and smell. The nose may be blocked or constantly running. The nasal discharge is often green-yellow or brown. Sudden onset of pain suggests that an acute infection has taken hold on top of the chronic condition. Some patients have recurrent attacks of tonsillitis, sore throat, and laryngitis.

Tests

A nose culture will show whether bacteria are contributing to the problem. An X-ray of the skull will often show that the lining of the sinuses has become thickened.

Traditional Treatment

Adequate treatment will help to prevent attacks of acute sinusitis from occurring and will prevent the condition from getting any worse. It is difficult to resolve chronic sinusitis completely, however.

Lifestyle is an important part of the treatment, so the patient may be advised to stop smoking, eat a more nutritious diet, avoid alcohol, and have regular dental checkups. If an active infection is detected, antibiotics will be given. Steam inhalations are very helpful. However, the use of decongestants may be counterproductive since, although these will help to clear the nasal passages initially, they usually cause a "rebound" congestion if used for more than two or three days and in the long term they make the condition worse. For those patients in whom there seems to be an allergic component, a steroid nasal spray may be prescribed.

For those patients in whom chronic sinusitis causes intolerable long-term symptoms, surgery may be necessary. This usually consists of opening up the exit from the sinus into the nose or forming a new one so that the mucus from the sinus can drain away more readily.

COMPLEMENTARY TREATMENT

Acupuncture
Sinusitis is said to be due to a deficiency of Chi in the lung that leads to the accumulation of harmful factors in the respiratory system. Points are chosen that have the specific properties of eliminating these harmful factors, strengthening the Chi of the lung, and promoting normal flow of Chi through the system.

Aromatherapy
Niaouli, eucalyptus, pine, or thyme may be recommended as inhalants.

Herbalism
Herbs such as elderflower, eyebright, marshmallow, and golden rod are used to combat excessive mucus production. The last two also have

antiinflammatory properties. Echinacea may be prescribed for patients with chronic sinusitis, since it increases resistance to infection and is valuable in the treatment of chronic infections.

Homeopathy
Patients with frontal sinusitis may benefit from kali bich., natrum mur., or pulsatilla. Other remedies that may be prescribed for sinusitis include hepar sulph. and silica.

SELF-HELP

A naturopathic cleansing diet consisting of fresh fruit and fruit juice for a few days followed by a further few days on a restricted diet of mainly salads and vegetables with a reduced quantity of starch may be helpful.

STYES

DEFINITION, CAUSES, AND SYMPTOMS

A stye (or hordeolum) is a type of boil that occurs on the upper or lower eyelid. It is caused by an infection in the root of one of the eyelashes and produces a firm, painful, red swelling that usually lasts several days before finally bursting and then subsiding.

The infection itself is caused by bacteria called staphylococci that are fairly widespread and are responsible for a number of skin diseases, such as impetigo and boils. However, it is possible for them to live on the human body without causing illness and 30–40 percent of normal people are nasal carriers, having staphylococci living in their noses without it doing them any harm. But it may be only in the nose that this harmony between humans and bacteria can be maintained. If carriers blow, pick, or rub their noses and then rub their eyes, they run the risk of transferring the bug to the eyelids where it may cause an infection.

Although most styes are fairly short-lived affairs, some persist, gradually becoming smaller, without bursting. This type is known as an internal stye and is caused by an infection of one of the tiny meibomian glands situated in the eyelids. The glands have tough walls, so pus from an infection remains contained within them and is not discharged to the surface. Once the infection has died down, the stye may disappear completely or it may leave a small cyst behind.

TRADITIONAL TREATMENT

Styes clear up by themselves, so normally no treatment is necessary. However, a doctor may prescribe an antibiotic cream to be applied to the eyelid. This will not speed healing but will prevent the bacteria contained in the discharging pus from infecting another eyelash root.

If a patient has recurrent styes, a nasal culture will show whether or not the nose is harboring staphylococci. If the culture is positive, an antibiotic cream inserted into the nostrils for a few days may clear the bacteria and thus stop them from spreading to the eyelids.

A meibomian cyst resulting from an internal stye can be cut open under anesthetic and its sticky contents removed, after which it is likely to heal very well.

COMPLEMENTARY TREATMENT

Acupuncture
Traditional Chinese medicine ascribes boils of any kind to an invasion by heat. In an acute attack needles are inserted into points that have the specific function of dissipating heat. One of these, which is situated on the side of the nose, is particularly appropriate for conditions affecting the region of the eye. If the patient has recurrent styes, this suggests that the protective body energy, or Chi, is deficient, so points are used to stimulate this energy in order to increase the body's resistance.

Herbalism
Burdock is used for toxic conditions that affect the skin and may be prescribed for a patient with styes. A lotion of eyebright may help to reduce pain and inflammation.

Homeopathy
Remedies need to be taken early in the development of the stye if any benefit is going to be felt. They may prevent an internal stye from turning into a cyst.

The choice of remedy will depend on the position of the stye, the symptoms, and whether or not the condition is recurrent. Recurrent styes on the upper lids associated with redness of the eyes may need sulphur, whereas phosphorus or staphysagria might be used for styes on the lower lids. If the eyelids are swollen, itchy, burning, and sticky, and the whole eye seems inflamed, pulsatilla may be prescribed. Often this is the first remedy to be tried. Aconite may be given to a feverish patient with a very painful stye.

Nutrition
Healthy skin depends on vitamins A and C, so patients with recurrent styes may be advised to take supplements of these.

During the attack itself (and, indeed, during a bacterial infection of any kind) extra vitamin B should be avoided since bacteria thrive on this.

SELF-HELP

Sometimes, when the stye seems ready to burst, pulling out the eyelash in whose root it has formed will help the discharge of pus. Before this, bathing the eyelid with warm water can relieve some of the pain.

The naturopathic treatment of recurrent styes may include a cleansing regime—either a fast or a diet of raw foods only. Fasts should only be undertaken if prescribed by a qualified naturopath, but a raw diet is quite safe to follow without supervision. Nothing but raw fruit and vegetables, yogurt, fruit juices, mineral water, and herb teas are taken for up to a week. A diet of this sort undertaken at regular intervals may prevent styes from recurring.

THRUSH

DEFINITION AND OCCURRENCE

Thrush is caused by a yeastlike organism called monilia or candida that often lives in the mouth and intestines of perfectly healthy people. Usually symptoms only arise when excessive amounts of monilia appear or when it starts to grow in a situation in which it does not normally occur.

Like the fungi that cause ringworm infections, monilia likes moist places. It also seems to thrive on sugar. This is thought to be the reason why it is more likely to affect patients with diabetes, whose blood and urine may contain excessive amounts of sugar. It tends to grow in the vagina of pregnant women, possibly because the cells lining the vagina have a high glycogen content during pregnancy. (Glycogen is the form in which glucose is stored within the body.) Other patients who are at risk of getting monilial infections are the very young and the very old, debilitated patients (especially those suffering from leukemia and some forms of cancer), those whose parathyroid glands (which control calcium metabolism) function inadequately, those with iron-deficiency anemia, patients taking steroids or the oral contraceptive Pill, and anyone who takes antibiotics. One of the side effects of antibiotics is to kill off the useful bacteria that normally inhabit the large bowel. Since monilia is kept in check by these bacteria, their destruction may allow monilia to multiply to such a degree that it begins to cause problems.

ORAL THRUSH

Babies, especially if they are premature, are prone to develop thrush in the mouth. The infection can be seen as white patches that look rather like milk curds, usually on the tongue, the palate, the gums, the inside of the cheeks, and the back of the throat. It may be confined to a small area of the mouth or may be quite widespread and cause the infant to go off its feed. If the patches are rubbed off, they come away quite easily, leaving a red, raw area. Sometimes the infection spreads down the esophagus (the gullet) and can cause vomiting, which may be blood-stained. Because monilia can travel through the digestive system and be passed in the feces, oral thrush is often associated with a monilial skin infection around the anus.

It has been suggested that infants pick up monilia from the mother's birth canal while being born or that it is a contaminant of feeding bottles. Whatever the reason, babies who are completely breast-fed are less likely to be affected than those who have bottle feedings.

Oral thrush can also affect adults, particularly those who have been on antibiotics. Here it may cause a smooth, painful, red tongue ("antibiotic tongue"), sometimes associated with inflamed lips and cracks at the angles of the mouth (cheilosis). Occasionally thrush may affect denture wearers, causing redness of the palate against which the denture lies. Usually this is symptomless, but some patients develop cheilosis.

VAGINAL THRUSH

This common condition affects some 15–20 percent of all pregnant women and a considerable number of those who take the contraceptive Pill. Women who have recurrent infections find that they seem to occur just before a period is due.

Monilia is not normally found in the vagina and, once there, can cause a thick white discharge with intense irritation and soreness. Intercourse may become painful and the infection may spread to the surrounding skin, making it red and sore. Occasionally, however, a monilial infection in the vagina causes no symptoms and is discovered by chance when the patient has a cervical smear.

INFECTIONS OF THE HANDS

Unlike ringworm, monilial infections of the hands are far more common than infections of the feet. Occasionally there may be redness, peeling, and maceration (soggy white skin) between two fingers, but more commonly monilia infects the nails. The commonest infection of the hands is a paronychia—infection of the nail fold, the area from which the nail grows. This tends to occur in people who spend a lot of time with their hands in water and in children who are thumb-suckers, the infection probably getting in through a damaged cuticle.

At first there is pain and swelling of the nail fold, which may become red and exude a small amount of pus. Later, the condition tends to become chronic, with the nail fold remaining swollen and slightly red, but not painful, and the cuticle disappearing. If the nail itself is infected, it may turn brown-green and become distorted. Ultimately all the nails may be involved.

INFECTION OF THE SKIN FOLDS (INTERTRIGO)

This is more common in women than in men. Because the skin folds tend to be moist places, monilia is more likely to take hold in the groins, between the buttocks, around the vagina, and below the breasts. From here the infection may spread outward. The rash often looks shiny and pink, has an irregular scaly edge that may show tiny blisters, and tends to itch or burn. The skin fold itself may be macerated and the skin may be cracked. Satellite patches often occur around the original rash, starting as small pimples that burst, leaving red areas.

In babies, a monilial infection of the bowel may be associated with a monilial diaper rash that is red, often macerated, and slightly swollen and weeping. Often it takes advantage of skin that is already affected by eczema.

INFECTION OF THE URETHRA (URETHRITIS)

Monilia may invade the urinary tract, but this is much commoner in men than in women. It may cause an acute infection with a profuse green-white discharge that may contain some blood. The opening of the urethra at the end of the penis becomes red, itchy, and swollen, and passing water may cause pain. Sometimes the infection is subacute, in which case the patient is aware only of a very small amount of discharge, usually early in the day, associated with itching at the opening of the urethra and a burning sensation when passing urine first thing in the morning.

BALANITIS

This is an infection of the end of the penis and the foreskin. When due to monilia it occurs mainly in young men, although it may affect boys and older men. Red patches with blisters appear, often associated with intense burning and itching. The area where the foreskin is attached to the penis may become swollen and the infection may spread to the surrounding skin.

TESTS

A culture will usually be taken of the affected area and this will be examined under a microscope and cultured in the hospital laboratory. However, some 5 percent of vaginal infections may produce negative cultures. If the doctor strongly suspects that monilia is present despite a normal culture result, he may wish to repeat the test. He may also take a blood test to check that the patient is not developing diabetes, since occasionally a monilial infection may be the first sign of this.

TRADITIONAL TREATMENT

There are several substances that are useful in the treatment of monilia. Nystatin is one of the oldest, but some strains of monilia have now become resistant to it. More recently discovered drugs are the imidazole derivatives including clotrimazole, ketoconazole, econazole, and miconazole. A recently introduced medication, flucanazole, produced a 93 percent success rate in trials where it was used to treat vaginal thrush. Normally, suspensions or gels are used for mouth infections, pessaries and creams for vaginal infections, and creams for skin infections. Ketoconazole, if taken orally, is absorbed into the bloodstream and is sometimes used for resistant infections that are not responding to topical treatment. Nystatin is not absorbed when taken orally and is therefore useful for treating infections of the large bowel, since it passes straight through.

In some resistant cases of vaginal thrush a gentian violet paint can be useful, but it stains the underwear. This, too, is a disadvantage of nystatin pessaries, which leave a yellowish stain.

Unfortunately, vaginal thrush can become recurrent and can seriously disrupt the patient's life. Sometimes, it appears that a woman is being reinfected by her partner and in such cases treating both together may be helpful. However, for those who continue to have attacks, recent research has shown promising results. At the Royal West Sussex Hospital in Chichester, United Kingdom, it was found that giving the patient clotrimazole a week before her period and again two weeks later and then repeating this every month prevented recurrence in 81 percent of the patients treated over the course of a year; in the control group not offered this treatment regime, 76 percent of patients had a recurrence within three months. Another trial at St. Mary's Hospital, Portsmouth, United Kingdom, gave 100 women who had suffered from recurrent thrush a course of two pessaries of miconazole a day for a week followed by one twice a week for three months and then one a week for a further three months. While on this treatment, not one of the patients had a repeat attack. Studies at Wayne State University Medical School in Detroit have shown some benefit in treating recurrent vaginal thrush (candidiasis) using clotrimazole and ketoconazole. However, the effect may be lost once the medicines are stopped.

COMPLEMENTARY TREATMENT

Aromatherapy
Tea tree or thyme may be recommended.

Herbalism
Marigold and myrrh are among the herbs that may be used to treat thrush, since their action is to heal inflamed and infected tissues. Thyme may be used as a douche for vaginal thrush.

Homeopathy
A patient who has an inflamed mouth, a red tongue, and bad breath as a result of a monilial infection may respond to arsenicum alb. A sore mouth in a child, associated with blisters inside the cheek and bad breath, may call for merc. sol. If the tongue is white and associated with blisters in the mouth, and if the patient complains of excessive salivation and a foul taste, sulphur may be appropriate. Other remedies may be prescribed for vaginal thrush and monilial skin infections.

Naturopathy

In order to restore balance to a bowel that has become overgrown with monilia, it is essential to replace the bacteria that usually keep it in control. This can be done by eating live yogurt or taking capsules of acidophilus or superdophilus (the bacterial element in live yogurt). These bacteria will also help to eliminate monilia in other sites, and live yogurt or acidophilus may be used as a douche in cases of vaginal thrush. Garlic is also a valuable antimonilial agent. If a needle is used to insert a piece of thread through a clove of garlic, it can be used as a tampon. Changed for a fresh clove twice a day, it can have a dramatic effect on vaginal thrush. However, some patients may be sensitive to garlic and if it seems to be causing inflammation the treatment should be stopped immediately.

A naturopath may also recommend a special antimonilial diet.

SELF-HELP

Because monilia likes moisture, it is important to keep affected areas as dry as possible. Patients with a skin infection or vaginal thrush should avoid tight underwear, especially if it is made of nylon, while those with infections of the hands should wear a pair of cotton gloves inside rubber gloves for all household chores.

THYROID DISEASE

FUNCTION OF THE THYROID GLAND

The thyroid is a butterfly-shaped gland that lies in the front of the neck and is responsible for controlling the body's rate of metabolism—that is, the rate at which it uses up energy. It does this by secreting two hormones, thyroxine or T_4 and tri-iodothyronine or T_3, both of which contain iodine as an essential ingredient. The rate of secretion of T_4 and T_3 is controlled by another hormone, thyroid-stimulating hormone or TSH, which is produced by the pituitary gland in the brain. Thyroid problems can therefore be due to a dietary deficiency of iodine (found in seafood, vegetables, milk, and meat) or to disorders of the pituitary gland. However, the vast majority of cases are due to disease within the gland itself.

In many cases of thyroid disease, the gland becomes swollen and this may be accompanied by a disruption of its function. In some cases the patient may develop hypothyroidism—a lack of thyroid hormones; in others hyperthyroidism or thyrotoxicosis—an excess of thyroid hormones—may develop.

TESTS FOR THYROID DISEASE

If a doctor suspects that a patient is suffering from some form of thyroid disease, he will usually begin by taking a blood sample to measure the levels of T_4, T_3, and TSH. Some thyroid diseases are autoimmune conditions in which the body manufactures antibodies against itself and in such cases these antibodies can be detected in the blood.

Although the thyroid is usually situated in the neck, in a few people it is lower down and part or all of it is retrosternal—that is, lying behind the sternum or breastbone. An X-ray may show whether or not a retrosternal gland is enlarged. Sometimes the patient is asked to swallow some liquid containing barium (such as is used in X-rays of the intestines to diagnose peptic ulcers). This outlines the esophagus, or gullet, and shows whether the thyroid is pressing into it.

Ultrasound is sometimes used to assess whether a lump in the thyroid is a cyst or a solid mass. When a sample of thyroid tissue is needed in order to diagnose the cause of a lump or swelling, this is usually taken from the anesthetized patient with a fine needle.

Because the thyroid takes up iodine from the bloodstream, if the patient is given radioactive iodine (or "radioiodine"), this will be absorbed into the functioning parts of the gland. A scan can then determine whether any part of the thyroid is either underactive or overactive by its concentration of radioiodine.

SMOOTH NONTOXIC GOITER (COLLOID GOITER)

This condition occurs when there is inadequate iodine available to the thyroid, either as a result of a deficiency of iodine in the diet or because the patient is taking something that prevents the thyroid from using iodine correctly. Some drugs may occasionally do this, as may an excess of a natural chemical that is found in vegetables of the cabbage family.

The output of thyroid hormones is reduced, and this results, by a feedback mechanism, in more TSH being secreted by the pituitary. This, in turn, causes a swelling of the thyroid that in mild cases will manage to produce enough hormone to keep the patient healthy. However, in severe cases of deficiency the patient may become hypothyroid.

Smooth nontoxic goiter is, like most thyroid conditions, much commoner in women than men. It usually develops between puberty and the age of thirty. The gland is smooth and sometimes large enough to cause symptoms such as shortness of breath when the patient lies in a certain position (due to pressure on the trachea, or windpipe), or redness of the face, dizziness, or fainting (due to pressure on the jugular veins). Rarely, it may cause hoarseness because is presses on the nerves that run down the neck to the larynx (voice-box). Occasionally, bleeding may occur into part of the gland, causing a sudden increase in size.

Treatment consists of ensuring that the patient is receiving adequate iodine in the diet and if necessary giving T_4 to stop the excessive secretion of TSH. Surgery is only rarely necessary.

PHYSIOLOGICAL GOITER

Some adolescents (nearly always girls) develop a soft swelling of the thyroid around the time of puberty. This usually disappears of its own accord by the age of twenty or twenty-two and no treatment is necessary.

THYROIDITIS

The suffix -itis usually implies an inflammation of the organ concerned. There are several forms of thyroiditis.

Hashimoto's Thyroiditis

This is an autoimmune disease and is the commonest form of thyroiditis. Antibodies that attack the thyroid are found in the blood of about 90 percent of patients. Within five years, a quarter of those affected have developed hypothyroidism. Eventually, 90 percent become hypothyroid.

The disease mainly affects women, who are usually between the ages of thirty and sixty. However, it can occur in younger patients and even in children. The thyroid becomes swollen and feels firm and rubbery; distinct lobules can sometimes be detected or the gland may feel smooth. The swelling may only be slight and often the first symptoms are those of hypothyroidism.

Treatment consists of giving T_4, which will reduce the size of the gland and remedy the hypothyroidism.

De Quervain's Thyroiditis

This mainly affects middle-age women and seems to be due to a viral infection. It often follows a head cold or sore throat and may come on suddenly or may be preceded by a few days in which the patient feels unwell and has a slight fever and headache. The symptoms include swelling and tenderness of the thyroid with pain radiating up into the jaw or the ears, together with fever, generalized aching, and headache. For four to six weeks, the patient may become hyperthyroid because of an excess of hormones leaking into the bloodstream from the inflamed gland. After that, she may develop hypothyroidism, which gradually recovers after a period of weeks or months. Less than 10 percent of patients remain hypothyroid. Episodes of inflammation may recur, but each time these are less severe and eventually they peter out.

Treatment consists of rest and antiinflammatory drugs such as aspirin or NSAIDs (nonsteroidal antiinflammatory drugs). In severe cases steroids may be given to reduce the inflammation. Hypothyroidism is treated with T_4.

Postpartum Thyroiditis

Some specialists claim this condition affects up to 9 percent of women after pregnancy. Symptoms are those of mild hyperthyroidism, occurring between two and four months after the birth of the baby. Up to three quarters of those affected have a swelling of the thyroid. One quarter have a close relative who has suffered from thyroid disease. Usually the condition subsides of its own accord, although in a few cases, hypothyroidism may result.

HYPOTHYROIDISM

Myxedema

This is the adult form of hypothyroidism that affects between 0.5 and 2 percent of all patients who seek medical care. Women are affected almost ten times more than men. The commonest cause is an autoimmune condition, either so-called idiopathic atrophy or, less often, Hashimoto's thyroiditis. It may also occur in patients who have previously been treated for hyperthyroidism with surgery or radioiodine. Idiopathic atrophy usually affects women between the ages of thirty and fifty, particularly around the time of the menopause. Antibodies against the thyroid are found in over 80 percent of patients.

The condition may come on very gradually so that neither the patient nor her relatives are aware that she is ill until quite a late stage.

The symptoms are very varied and a patient may have a few or many. Often they are vague, particularly at first. The patient may feel unusually tired and may notice that she gets cold very easily. She is likely to put on weight and may become constipated. She may complain of aching muscles, stiffness, deafness, chest pains, unsteadiness when walking, and shortness of breath upon exertion. Other symptoms include heavy or prolonged periods, infertility, a constantly running or blocked nose, and swelling of the ankles.

The patient's appearance also changes. Her face becomes heavy and expressionless and develops a yellowish tinge, with a flush over the cheekbones. Her eyelids become puffy and her skin is dry and rough. Her hair becomes thin and dry and often the outer section of the eyebrows is lost.

Her speech becomes hoarse and slurred because the larynx and the tongue are swollen. Her thinking processes slow down and her memory is poor. In severe cases, she may become very confused. Depression is quite common, as is headache.

Upon examination, the doctor will find that the patient's pulse is slow. In a quarter of cases, the blood pressure will be raised. An X-ray may show that the heart is enlarged because of fluid that has accumulated in the sac (the pericardium) that surrounds it. Blood tests may reveal a mild anemia that resolves when the myxedema is treated or an iron-deficiency anemia resulting from increasingly heavy periods. In 12 percent of cases, the patient has pernicious anemia, another autoimmune disease, which has to be treated with regular injections of vitamin B_{12}.

There are two serious complications of myxedema that are rare. One is so-called "myxedema madness," in which the patient may develop schizophrenia-like symptoms, sometimes shortly after starting treatment. This is usually confined to elderly patients with severe hypothyroidism. The other is myxedema coma that may be precipitated by a sudden stress such as infection, trauma, or coldness, and is fatal in some 50 percent of cases.

Cretinism

Rarely, about once in every 3500 births, a baby develops hypothyroidism as soon as it is born. This is usually because the thyroid gland has failed to develop. U.S. newborns are routinely screened for this disease. The condition affects boys and girls equally and in some cases may be mild, only becoming apparent after a few months of life.

In mild cases symptoms may include failure to develop at the normal rate, floppiness, constipation, and a hoarse cry. The skin may seem coarse, cool, and dry, and the tongue is large and may protrude from the mouth.

In more severe cases, jaundice is often the first symptom. It is not uncommon for newborn babies to be jaundiced, but in the hypothyroid baby this lasts much longer than the usual few days. The symptoms observed in mild cases are soon apparent and the baby's large tongue may interfere with feeding and may make the breathing sound noisy. The face is characteristic, with a low hairline, wrinkled forehead, and broad flat nose, and the eyes are set well apart. The neck is short and thick, and the limbs are short with broad hands and feet. The baby may be overweight, has a large abdomen, often with a bulge at the umbilicus caused by a hernia, and tends to lie very still. The danger of cretinism is that it can lead to severe mental retardation. However, if treated early, this can usually be avoided. Treatment will also reverse most of the physical symptoms of the condition.

Traditional Treatment of Hypothyroidism

The treatment simply consists of replacing the missing hormone, T_4 (thyroxine), in tablet form. However, T_3 (triiodothyronine) is usually given to patients who have angina, since it has a shorter duration of action than T_4 and hence allows greater flexibility should the drug make their angina worse. Once the patient is no longer hypothyroid, it is quite safe to change to T_4.

HYPERTHYROIDISM (THYROTOXICOSIS)

Like hypothyroidism, this can be produced by several different conditions and the symptoms vary somewhat according to the cause, but the overall picture will be outlined here before the individual diseases are described. It affects between 2 and 5 women in every 100 but only 2 men in 1000.

The first symptom is often extreme fatigue. The patient may lose a considerable amount of weight, despite the fact that her appetite is increased. She becomes intolerant of heat and sweats a lot.

Anxiety, restlessness, and irritability are common and the periods may become scanty. The patient may complain of loss of strength, palpitations, shortness of breath, and swollen ankles. Upon examination, the doctor may find that she has a fine tremor of her outstretched hands and of her tongue, and that her movements are jerky and clumsy. Her skin appears warm, pink, and moist and may have a velvety texture, and her hair is fine and silky. A fast pulse rate (over 90 per minute) is common and in older patients there may be an irregular heartbeat. Sometimes this irregularity may be the only sign of hyperthyroidism in the elderly.

When hyperthyroidism is due to Graves' disease, the eye condition known as exophthalmos is not uncommon. In mild cases, the upper eyelids become retracted and the eyes bulge slightly, making the patient look as though she is staring. The bulging is due to swelling within the eye itself and to an increase in the bulk of the fat and muscles within the eye socket. In more severe cases, the conjunctiva may become thickened and the eyes may water a lot, especially in the morning. Sometimes one eye may seem to bulge more than the other. The muscles that move the eyes may become weak, resulting in double vision or even a noticeable squint. Occasionally the eye symptoms may become temporarily worse after treatment for hyperthyroidism has been started. Rarely, a progressive condition may occur in which the surface of the eye becomes ulcerated, the whole eyeball becomes inflamed, and the patient's eyesight is threatened.

Seventy percent of patients find that their eyes return more or less to normal after they start treatment for hyperthyroidism. In a further 20 percent the eyes remain unchanged, and in 10 percent of cases the symptoms may get somewhat worse.

Graves' Disease (Smooth Toxic Goiter)

This is the commonest cause of hyperthyroidism. It tends to run in families and may occur at any age but mainly in women between the ages of twenty and forty. Like Hashimoto's thyroiditis and idiopathic thyroid atrophy, it is an autoimmune disease. However, in this case the antibodies stimulate the thyroid to produce more hormones, rather than depressing its secretory function.

Usually the thyroid is enlarged, smooth, and firm. Eye problems are common, as are anxiety, trembling, and other symptoms affecting the nervous system. It is not unusual for symptoms to come and go and in about 40 percent of patients they disappear completely and do not return.

Blood tests will show raised levels of hormones and antibodies.

Solitary Toxic Nodule (Adenoma)

This only accounts for some 5 percent of cases of hyperthyroidism. A little nodule of hyperactive tissue forms within the thyroid and secretes large amounts of hormone, while squashing the normal thyroid tissue around it. The amount of hormone circulating in the blood will prevent the pituitary from secreting TSH (via the feedback mechanism), so that the rest of the thyroid may stop functioning while the nodule, which is independent of TSH, carries on secreting.

This condition occurs mainly in women and at any age over ten. The patient may complain of a swelling in the gland that may be large enough to cause shortness of breath (from pressure on the trachea) or hoarseness (from pressure on the nerves leading to the larynx). Sometimes a cyst forms within the nodule and bleeding may occur into the cyst cavity, causing sudden pain and an increase in swelling.

Tests that can be used include a needle biopsy and also a radioiodine scan, in which the injected substance will be shown concentrated within the nodule.

Multinodular Goiter

Patients who develop this condition are usually over fifty and have had a nontoxic goiter for some time. Sometimes multinodular goiter runs in families. More women are affected than men, but the ratio is not as great as in Graves' disease.

The thyroid is enlarged and individual smooth, rounded swellings can be felt within it. In some patients the gland grows faster than in others and may press on the trachea, esophagus, laryngeal nerves, or the jugular veins, causing a cough, breathing difficulties, discomfort when swallowing, hoarseness, or faintness.

Not all patients become hyperthyroid, but in those that do the symptoms are more likely to be associated with the heart than with the nervous system. An irregular heartbeat is common and heart failure may occur, so that the patient may complain of severe shortness of breath, palpitations, fatigue, and swollen ankles.

Traditional Treatment of Hyperthyroidism

Exophthalmos

In mild cases, treatment consists of diuretics to reduce water retention within the eyeball and socket plus glasses to protect the overexposed eyes from foreign bodies and the drying effect of wind. In more severe cases, steroids may be necessary to reduce the swelling. In progressive cases, where there is a danger that the optic nerve may be damaged by swelling or that the surface of the eyeball may become ulcerated, operative treatment may be necessary. This consists of reducing the pressure within the eye and socket and partially sewing the eyelids together. Sometimes this is combined with radiotherapy, which may be helpful. Occasionally, surgery is also necessary to improve a squint.

Graves' Disease

Although drugs are very effective in controlling 95 percent of cases, up to 60 percent recur and then need other treatment. The drugs available are carbimazole, propylthiouracil, and methimazole. All have side effects and patients who cannot tolerate one are usually switched to another. Carbimazole is generally tried first. It reduces the production of thyroid hormone and in most cases symptoms begin to disappear within two to three weeks. It is customary to prescribe it for a period of 12–18 months, but after this period relapses are common, usually within two years of the treatment ending. Side effects of carbimazole include rashes, joint pain, and a sudden drop in the numbers of white blood cells produced by the bone marrow. The last of these is very serious, since white blood cells are responsible for the body's immunity. It is always accompanied by a sore throat, so patients are warned that at the first sign of soreness they must stop the treatment and report to their doctor immediately.

Beta blockers, which are described more fully in the section on high blood pressure, may be used in the early stages of treatment to control symptoms associated with the heart and circulatory system while the patient is waiting for surgery or before the full effect of carbimazole or propylthiouracil has been felt.

Radioiodine, as well as being used as a diagnostic tool, can be used in treatment. The patient drinks a glass of water containing the substance, which is then absorbed into the bloodstream and taken up by the overacting parts of the thyroid gland, where it suppresses the excessive secretion of hormones. It usually takes two to three months before the effect is felt, so drug treatment may be necessary in the interim. Sometimes it may cause discomfort in the neck and a worsening of symptoms in the early stages of treatment. The ultimate success rate is 75 percent, but it is not suitable for all patients. Normally, it is not offered to women who are under forty, or perhaps forty-five, since there is a risk that it might affect an infant's thyroid were the patient to become pregnant. Unfortunately, it often produces hypothyroidism, affecting some 30 percent of those treated within ten years. These patients then have to have supplements of T_4 for the rest of their lives.

Surgery is used for patients who have failed to respond to drugs, who have relapsed more than once or twice on drug treatment, who have large goiters, or who for one reason or another are not suitable for radioiodine treatment. Complications are rare, although 20 percent of those treated will eventually become hypothyroid. Propylthiouracil is given first of all, until the patient is no longer hyperthyroid. Then this is stopped and potassium iodide is given for 10–14 days. This has the effect of making the gland less active and reducing the amount of blood flowing through it. Finally, an operation is performed in which a large section, but not all, of the thyroid is removed. In 5 percent, the operation doesn't control the condition and the patient relapses. In such cases radioiodine is very effective as a follow-up treatment.

Toxic Nodule
Usually the nodule itself is removed and TSH is given to stimulate the rest of the gland back to normal function. Drugs and radioiodine are less effective.

Multinodular Goiter
In elderly patients, in whom the diagnosis is clear that there is no evidence of hyperthyroidism and the patient has no symptoms, it is

customary to do nothing. However, if the gland is causing symptoms through pressure on surrounding structures, part of it is surgically removed. In younger patients, a partial thyroidectomy is usually done, whether or not there are symptoms, because there is a danger that hyperthyroidism will occur or the bleeding may occur into the gland, and a small risk that one of the nodules may become malignant.

THYROID NODULES

The vast majority (85 percent) of single nodules are adenomas or toxic nodules. The rest are malignant growths.

Cancer of the Thyroid

This is a rare condition that is two to three times more common in women than in men. Many patients have had goiters for several years. There are five main types of thyroid cancer, known as papillary, follicular, medullary and anaplastic carcinomas, and lymphoma.

Usually the first sign is a nodule in the thyroid or an enlargement of the gland, which feels firm or hard. There may be a sudden increase in size over a matter of days or weeks, with the patient complaining of a choking sensation or a tightness in the throat. Hoarseness and difficulty in breathing or swallowing may also occur.

Each type of cancer is treated slightly differently from the others, but because most thyroid tumors are under the control of TSH secreted by the pituitary, supplements of T_4, which suppress the production of TSH, can cause regression of the tumor. Therefore, T_4 is given to most patients who are diagnosed as having thyroid cancer.

Papillary Carcinoma
This accounts for 70 percent of cases and is commonest in children and young adults. It usually takes the form of a single hard nodule in a previously normal gland. The outlook is excellent, since the cancer is very slow growing.

Treatment consists of removing all the thyroid on the affected side and part of it on the other side. The patient will then have to take T_4 supplements for the rest of her life. If the cancer seems to have spread, the whole of the thyroid will be removed, together with the lymph glands in the neck. This is followed up, if necessary, with radioiodine treatment.

Follicular Carcinoma
This accounts for 20 percent of cases and it, too, has a good outlook if caught early enough. It mainly affects young and middle-age adults. Treatment is the same as for papillary carcinoma.

Medullary Carcinoma
This affects patients of any age, men equally with women, and forms 5 percent of all cases of thyroid cancer. It may run in families and may be associated with growths in other glands. The outlook is not as good as for papillary and follicular carcinoma, but, even so, 60 percent of patients are still alive five years after the diagnosis was first made.

Treatment usually consists of removal of the entire thyroid gland and the lymph glands of the neck.

Lymphoma
This is rare and is usually treated with a combination of surgery, radiotherapy, and chemotherapy.

Anaplastic Carcinoma
This, too, is rare, mainly affecting older patients. Treatment is by surgery and radiotherapy, but the outlook is poor.

COMPLEMENTARY TREATMENT

Acupuncture
Goiter is said to be due to obstruction of the flow of blood and of energy (Chi) and to accumulation of phlegm in the neck. Treatment uses points that will relieve the obstruction, disperse the phlegm, and restore normal flow.

Herbalism
For those patients who need extra iodine, kelp may be prescribed. This may also help to regulate the function of the thyroid.

Homeopathy

Patients with exophthalmic toxic goiter and weight loss may benefit from thyroidinum or natrum mur. Calc. iod. and calc. carb. may be used for simple nontoxic goiter, and iodium and spongia may be helpful in the treatment of either condition.

Nutrition

Since vitamins C, B_3, and B_5, and the minerals manganese, calcium, and zinc are especially important for the normal function of the pituitary gland and the thyroid, supplements of these may be prescribed.

URINARY TRACT INFECTIONS

CAUSE OF INFECTIONS

The urinary tract, which comprises the kidneys, ureters, bladder, and urethra, is the commonest site of bacterial infection in the human body. (See diagram of the urinary tract on page 222.) Normally, although the end of the urethra closest to the exterior may contain bacteria, these are prevented from spreading further by the antibacterial properties of the lining of the urethra and by the fact that the urinary tract is repeatedly being flushed out by sterile urine. Urinary tract infection (UTI) occurs much more frequently in women than in men because the female urethra is comparatively short, wide, and straight, making it easier for bacteria to travel along it.

Although many cases of infection occur in otherwise healthy women, there are certain abnormalities that can predispose patients to UTI. These include obstruction of the urinary tract, which causes pooling of urine (incomplete emptying of the bladder) and encourages the growth of bacteria, stones (which can act as a focus for infection), and diseases, such as diabetes, in which the patient's resistance to infection is lowered. Pregnant women have an increased risk of developing UTIs because the pressure of the fetus on the bladder can lead to pooling of urine. In addition, the high level of progesterone found in the bloodstream during pregnancy causes dilation of the ureters, which allows this stagnant urine to flow backward toward the kidneys. Patients who have disorders of the nervous system and are unable to empty the bladder completely are also more prone to infection. Vigorous sexual intercourse is quite a common cause of UTI in women (sometimes known as "honeymoon cystitis"). It is thought that this results either from injury to the urethra or from bacteria being forced up the urethra and into the bladder.

Vesicoureteric reflux is a condition in which the one-way valve that

419

leads from the ureter into the bladder ceases to function correctly and, as the bladder contracts, forcing urine out, it also forces some back up the ureters. When the bladder relaxes, this urine flows in again, so that the patient never has a completely empty bladder. When seen in children, it is thought to be associated with the development of chronic pyelonephritis (see below).

ACUTE CYSTITIS

Cystitis, or inflammation of the bladder, is very common, affecting about 50 percent of all women at some time in their lives. Most have only one or two attacks, but a few go on to have frequent recurrences. This is especially likely if there is a predisposing cause.

The attack comes on suddenly, the patient developing pain, tenderness in the bladder area, and an urgency to pass urine. Passing water causes pain (dysuria), but she feels that she wants to go very frequently (frequency). The urine is likely to be smelly and may be blood-stained (hematuria). Sometimes patients develop abdominal pain, fever, or hematuria without frequency or dysuria. In children, especially, the symptoms may be vague and may include fever, abdominal pain, bed-wetting, and a general sense of being unwell.

About 5 percent of school-age girls have UTI at some time and of these 80 percent will have more than one attack. Thirty-five percent of affected children are found to have vesicoureteric reflux—a much higher proportion than in the population as a whole.

CHRONIC CYSTITIS

This is always associated with a predisposing cause and if that can be successfully treated (for example, removal of a kidney stone) the condition may well be curable. The symptoms are those of frequency and dysuria occurring over a prolonged period of time, sometimes clearing up but never for more than a week.

The symptoms of chronic cystitis can also be caused by other conditions than bacterial infection. Most of these are rare and include tuberculosis (which is always secondary to TB elsewhere in the body, usually the lungs), Hunner's ulcer or interstitial cystitis (ulceration of the lining of the bladder, which tends to affect middle-age women), and cystitis cystica (in which little glands in the bladder lining enlarge to form nodules or polyps). In men, prostatitis can also cause urinary symptoms.

Fifty percent or so of women who suffer from persistent or oft-repeated attacks of frequency and dysuria have no bacteria in their urine. The term *urethral syndrome* is used to cover this group, but it is probable that there are a number of causes for their symptoms. In some cases, it seems to be due to an attack of thrush and in postmenopausal patients it may be associated with a lack of estrogen, which also causes drying of the lining of the vagina (atrophic vaginitis).

ACUTE PYELONEPHRITIS

If an infection travels up the urinary tract to the kidneys, it can cause acute pyelonephritis, a potentially serious disease that affects women in nine out of ten cases. There is a sudden onset, the patient becoming feverish and ill, shivering and vomiting, and complaining of pain and tenderness around the kidney area, in the back just below the ribs. Unlike acute cystitis, the urinary symptoms of dysuria and frequency may be only slight or absent altogether. If the infection is untreated, it may spread to the bloodstream, causing septicemia, in which case the patient becomes very ill with a high fever.

CHRONIC, OR ATROPHIC, PYELONEPHRITIS (REFLUX NEPHROPATHY)

This is a condition in which the kidneys become scarred and eventually cease to function effectively. The patient develops high blood pressure (see section on secondary hypertension) and this may be followed by renal failure. Unlike the other forms of UTI, chronic pyelonephritis affects as many men as women.

It is thought to originate in childhood in patients who have vesicoureteric reflux due to the incompetent valve mechanism. The constant pool of stale urine in the bladder predisposes the patient to infection and the bacteria may be swept up to the kidneys in the refluxed urine. Usually reflux stops around puberty, as the bladder becomes stronger, but by this time the damage may have been done.

Thirty percent of those children with reflux who suffer from UTI are at risk of developing scarring of the kidneys. About 10 percent go on to develop high blood pressure and renal failure. Because vesicoureteric reflux may run in families, some doctors now recommend screening the children of parents with chronic pyelonephritis, since early detection and treatment can prevent damage to the kidneys.

TESTS

Many U.S. women with typical UTI symptoms are treated without urine cultures. However, any patient who is thought to have a recurring UTI will be asked to provide a midstream urine specimen, or MSU. A swab is used to clean the area around the urethra. The patient starts to pass water into the toilet, and then introduces a receptacle to catch some of the urine before finishing into the toilet. Thus, any bacteria that just happen to be in the urethra, but not in the urine itself, will be flushed out and will not contaminate the specimen. If TB of the urinary tract is suspected, however, the patient will be asked for a specimen of the first urine of the morning (early-morning urine or EMU), since this is the most concentrated and is best able to show up the presence of TB.

Only if a patient has recurrent infections, or if there is reason to believe there may be an underlying abnormality, will further investigations be performed. Men and children are always investigated, since they are far more likely than women to have a predisposing cause. An intravenous pyelogram (IVP) consists of an injection of dye into a vein followed by a series of X-rays of the kidneys and bladder as the dye is excreted in the urine. It will show up any stones in the urinary system, scarring of the kidneys, and other abnormalities. The patient is asked to pass water and as he does so it is possible to detect any vesicoureteric reflux and to see whether the bladder is emptied completely. Ultrasound investigation can also be used to detect some abnormalities.

Cystoscopy (inspection of the inside of the bladder under general anesthetic, using a special telescope) is rarely used in the investigation of UTI. However, it may be considered necessary in some cases of hematuria or if a condition such as Hunner's ulcer is suspected.

TRADITIONAL TREATMENT

In all cases in which there is an underlying cause, such as stones or diabetes, treatment will be directed at this as well as at the infection itself.

Acute cystitis is treated with antibiotics and an increased fluid intake. If necessary, a preparation such as potassium citrate may be prescribed to make the urine less acidic and therefore reduce the burning. Although potassium citrate can be bought over the counter, it is vital that patients do not rely solely on such symptomatic treatment, but see their doctors in order to have the infection correctly treated. Potassium citrate should be used sparingly since prolonged or excessive use can lead to a dangerous rise of potassium levels in the body. If a patient has a history of thrush infections, she may need to be given some antithrush treatment (such as nystatin) to take together with her antibiotics, in order to prevent a recurrence.

Usually antibiotics are given for one to two weeks, but recently it has been discovered that short courses (one to three days) of certain antibiotics are as successful and have few side effects. Some specialists, however, are still not entirely convinced about the value of short courses and continue to prescribe antibiotics for a longer period. It is very important, because of the way in which antibiotics work, that whatever length the course, all the tablets are taken.

If a first attack does not respond to antibiotic treatment, a longer course, for up to six weeks, may be necessary. For patients who have repeated attacks, a low-dose course of antibiotics given for between six months and a year is often successful in producing a cure.

Acute pyelonephritis, too, is treated with antibacterial drugs (sulphonamides are usually preferred to the newer antibiotics, since 90 percent of cases will respond to these).

Vesicoureteric reflux is sometimes treated surgically, the ureters being reimplanted into the bladder in such a way that reflux is less likely to occur. Prompt treatment of UTI in children will also help to prevent scarring of the kidneys. However, a badly damaged nonfunctioning kidney needs to be removed and, if possible, replaced with a healthy transplant.

Tuberculosis of the bladder is treated with anti-TB drugs given for a period of a year. Sometimes surgery is necessary to relieve constrictions caused by scarring. Surgery may also be helpful in the treatment of Hunner's ulcer. Dilation of the bladder under general anesthetic will relieve the symptoms for up to six months, and this treatment can be repeated whenever necessary. In severe cases, removal of that part of the bladder affected by the ulcer may be required.

Urethral syndrome may respond to painkillers, antispasmodic drugs, or dilation of the urethra. In postmenopausal patients in whom it is associated with atrophic vaginitis, an estrogen cream applied to the vagina may be helpful.

PREVENTION

Patients who are susceptible to UTI should drink at least five pints of fluid a day—more if they are in a hot climate. They should try to avoid constipation, since this may cause pressure on the bladder and prevent complete emptying. They should pass water at least every three hours and should always do so before going to bed.

A woman in whom UTI seems to occur after sexual intercourse should pass water immediately after having sex, thus flushing out any bacteria that may have been forced up into the bladder. Because bath additives—such as bath salts and foam baths—may predispose susceptible patients to UTI, these should be avoided by women who have recurrent attacks. No one should ever use disinfectants in the bath, as these can cause damage to the lining of both the urethra and the vagina.

For children in whom vesicoureteric reflux is a factor and for other patients in whom bladder emptying is incomplete, a technique known as double micturition is helpful. (Micturition simply means passing water.) The patient passes water, walks around for a few minutes, and then tries to go again. This helps to avoid pooling of stale urine in the bladder.

COMPLEMENTARY TREATMENT

Acupuncture
Treatment will consist of strengthening the kidney and its energy flow.

Aromatherapy

Sandalwood, pine, and juniper are among the oils that may be helpful.

Herbalism

Various herbs have the effect of increasing urinary flow, thus flushing out bacteria from the bladder. Some have an antiseptic action and relieve inflammation and spasm within the bladder. Such herbs include bearberry and buchu (both potent antiseptics), cornsilk, marshmallow, and horsetail.

Homeopathy

Cantharis may be helpful if the symptoms are made worse by standing or walking and if passing water is slow and painful. If the urine is dark and bloody and associated with burning pain and spasm, merc. cor. may be prescribed. Abdominal pain with severe dysuria and a few drops of blood in the urine may indicate a need for sarsaparilla. Aconite is particularly useful for treating children and staphysagria for "honeymoon cystitis." Other remedies may also be appropriate in individual cases.

SELF-HELP

During an attack of cystitis it is advisable to drink plenty of fluid in order to flush out the urinary system frequently. Cranberry juice, garlic (taken in capsule form), and barley water will all help this flushing out, by increasing the kidneys' output, and they all have a soothing action on inflammation within the bladder and urethra.

Naturopathic advice may include a reduction in intake of animal protein and citrus fruits and avoidance of acidic foods such as tomatoes, rhubarb, gooseberries, and pickles.

VAGINAL DISCHARGE

CAUSES OF DISCHARGE

Large numbers of women suffer from a vaginal discharge at one time or another and many are uncertain whether or not this is abnormal. The normal vagina and cervix (neck of the uterus) are covered with fine mucus membrane—very similar to the lining of the mouth—which has cells in it that secrete fluid. This fluid is necessary to keep the vagina lubricated, and the cells that produce it are under the control of the female sex hormones, the amount they secrete being influenced by the hormone levels in the bloodstream. More may be secreted in midcycle (halfway between two periods) and by women who are on the contraceptive Pill, but after the menopause the vagina may become dry as the cells cease to function. The cells also respond to sexual stimulation, so that the vagina is well-lubricated for intercourse. A slight discharge after intercourse, consisting of vaginal fluid and some of the male ejaculate, is not uncommon.

However, a discharge that occurs regularly and either wets or stains the underwear or that is smelly or irritating is never normal and needs investigation and treatment. There are a number of organisms that may produce a vaginal discharge. One of the commonest is monilia, which causes thrush. This is dealt with in a separate section.

TRICHOMONAS

This relatively common organism causes a profuse discharge that is often frothy and smelly, may be grayish, yellow, or green, and is usually worse after intercourse and following a period. It causes itching and soreness, and intercourse may become very uncomfortable or even painful. In about one quarter of cases the infection spreads to the urinary tract and causes discomfort when passing water and frequency. Occasionally the organism is found on a Pap smear in a woman who has no symptoms. Infected men are often asymptomatic, although they may have some discomfort when they urinate.

To diagnose trichomonas, samples of the discharge are examined under a microscope and are sometimes cultured in the laboratory.

Several drugs can be used in treatment, of which the commonest is metronidazole. Side effects include nausea, vomiting, and a metallic taste in the mouth, but these can all be minimized by taking the tablets during or immediately after a meal. Drinking alcohol tends to make the side effects worse, so it is advisable to remain teetotal while having treatment. It is important that the patient's partner is treated as well, even if he or she has no symptoms, since otherwise the couple are likely to keep passing the infection back and forth to each other. About 90 percent of patients are cured by a single course of tablets and those who fail to respond will usually do so if given a larger dose over a longer period of time.

CHLAMYDIA

This is a common cause of discharge from the penis in men and they may pass the infection on to their sexual partners. In women it may cause few symptoms. However, a watery or purulent discharge can occur and if this is untreated the infection may spread to the tubes and ultimately cause a chronic pelvic infection with resulting infertility.

A vaginal culture is necessary for diagnosis and the infection can be treated with the antibiotics tetracycline, trimethoprin-sulfamethoxazole, or erythromycin.

GARDNERELLA

This organism is often found in the vagina and there is debate among specialists as to whether it does in fact cause an infection or whether it is one of the several nonharmful bacteria that normally live there.

However, it does seem in many cases to be associated with a vaginal discharge that is often gray-white and profuse and has a distinctly cheesy smell. The discharge is often worse around the time of a period. Other symptoms may include itching, discomfort or pain during intercourse, bleeding after intercourse, pain when passing water, and frequency.

Like trichomonas, gardnerella can be treated with metronidazole.

GONORRHEA

This is a relatively common disease, although it is to be hoped that the precautions recommended to reduce the spread of AIDS (fewer sexual partners and the use of condoms) will also help to reduce the spread of gonorrhea.

It is very contagious, so someone who has sex with an infected partner can expect to be infected themselves within a month. Unfortunately, although over 95 percent of infected men have symptoms, up to half of all infected women may be symptom-free. Not realizing that they have the disease, they do not request treatment and therefore may spread it still further. This is why anyone who is diagnosed as having gonorrhea will be asked about his or her sexual contacts within the past month or so, so that others who may be infected can be diagnosed and treated.

Men who have gonorrhea usually have a purulent discharge from the penis, swelling around the end of the urethra, frequency, and pain when passing urine. In women, however, the discharge may only be slight. It may be any color between white and green and is sometimes brown or blood-strained. If it is profuse, it is usually because the patient has a trichomonas infection as well—in fact, over half the women who are diagnosed as having gonorrhea are also infected with trichomonas. There may be urinary symptoms—frequency and discomfort—and pain and swelling in the vulval area caused by infection of the Bartholin's glands, which are situated there. The infection frequently spreads to the anus and rectum, but although discomfort may occur, this is often symptomless.

If gonorrhea is untreated, it is likely to spread and cause a chronic pelvic infection that may produce constant lower abdominal pain and may result in the tubes becoming blocked, with subsequent infertility. Patients may also experience heavy, painful periods and pain during intercourse.

Testing of both sexes consists of cultures taken from the urethra and the rectum and, in female patients, additional cultures from the neck of the uterus and the vagina. Blood tests are also taken to test for syphilis, which may occur together with gonorrhea.

There are several antibiotics that can be used to treat gonorrhea, the choice often depending on whether or not the patient has another infection (such as syphilis or chlamydia) as well. Treatment for chlamydia is routinely given with gonorrhea treatment. After the treatment is finished, further cultures will be taken to ensure that the infection has been eradicated.

COMPLEMENTARY TREATMENT

If there is any chance that a patient with a discharge is suffering from gonorrhea, she must see a doctor to ensure that a correct diagnosis is made, since this infection must be treated with antibiotics.

However, combined with orthodox medicine, complementary treatment may be used for any form of vaginal discharge to speed recovery. In those cases where the patient continues to have a discharge despite negative cultures and traditional treatment, complementary therapies may be particularly helpful.

Acupuncture
A white discharge is said to be due to a lack of energy (Chi) and the presence of damp in the reproductive system. A yellow discharge is said to be due to damp heat. Specific points are chosen to restore Chi to normal levels, to eliminate damp and, where appropriate, heat, and to strengthen the kidney, one of whose functions is said to be control of the reproductive system.

Aromatherapy
Bergamot may be recommended to treat an irritating discharge; among other oils used are eucalyptus, thyme, geranium, hyssop, and juniper.

Herbalism
Various herbal preparations may be prescribed that will help to reduce inflammation and discharge when inserted into the vagina. These include marigold, myrrh, beth root, and arbor-vitae.

Homeopathy

A patient who has a smelly yellow discharge that is associated with burning and severe itching and that is worse after a period may benefit from kreosotum, while someone with a smelly brownish discharge, itching, and a prickly pain may be helped by nit. ac. Pulsatilla may be appropriate for a woman who has a thick, burning, yellow-green discharge and sepia for someone whose discharge is white or yellow and jellylike.

SELF-HELP

Some people recommend using a tampon soaked in yogurt and changed several times a day as an additional treatment for gardnerella. It seems that by itself it is not very effective, but in combination with orthodox drug treatment, it may help to clear up the condition more rapidly. It does this by making the secretions of the vagina more acidic and thus less suitable for gardnerella to live in, and by helping to restore the normal bacteria of the vagina, which will themselves overpower the invaders.

VARICOSE VEINS

DEFINITION AND CAUSES

Animals who walk on four legs don't suffer from varicose veins. However, as soon as man pulled himself upright and started to walk on his two hind legs, he started to put much greater pressure on the veins in those legs. The arteries, through which blood is distributed to the body, have a layer of muscle and a layer of elastic tissue in their walls, and are thus able to respond to the rhythmic pumping of the heart (as felt in the pulses). But once the blood has flowed through the tissues in the tiny capillaries and has been gathered together again into the much thinner-walled veins, the pumping action has been lost. This is why blood spurts from a cut artery but flows from a cut vein.

The blood returns to the heart through a system of veins, assisted by the movement of the surrounding muscles that helps to push it along. To prevent the blood from pooling, the veins contain a series of valves that stop it from flowing backward. Normal blood flow in the leg runs from superficial to deeper veins through small communicating vessels known as perforators, and these connections are also controlled by valves. The pressure of blood on the valves in the leg veins is much greater than elsewhere in the body because of their position below the heart and because of the effect of gravity. If one valve gives way under the pressure, then the pressure on the valves beneath it will become even greater and they, in turn, will be more likely to give way. Where the valves are no longer functioning, the vein swells up, forming varices.

Varicose veins can be divided into primary and secondary, with 80 percent of patients falling into the first category. In these cases, there is probably an inborn defect in the valves and this may run in families. Women are affected more frequently than men. Although the varices may enlarge considerably in time, the chances of ulceration of the leg (see below) are small.

Secondary varicose veins occur as the result of increased pressure

431

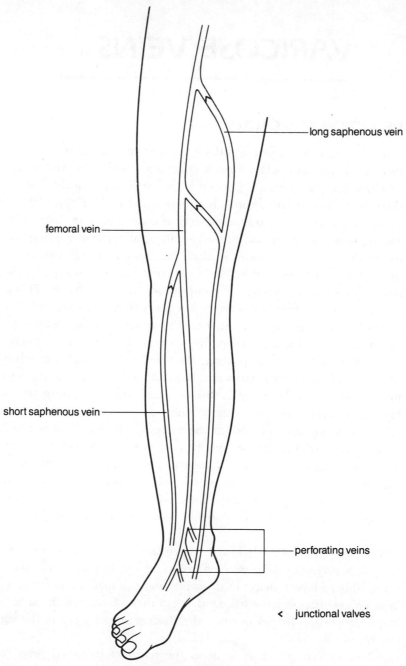

long saphenous vein

femoral vein

short saphenous vein

perforating veins

<   junctional valves

The veins of the leg

within the abdomen, which makes it harder for the blood in the legs to flow "uphill." The increased pressure may be due to a tumor (benign or malignant), chronic constipation, or pregnancy, and, indeed, any of these conditions may make primary varicose veins worse. Secondary varicose veins may also be due to destruction of the valves by a deep venous thrombosis (blood clot in the leg). Ulceration is more likely to occur with this type of varicosity and treatment is aimed at preventing this. Some specialists suggest that support stockings should be worn by all pregnant women and by anyone who has ever had a deep venous thrombosis (DVT).

SYMPTOMS

Symptoms are caused by the blood trying to flow backward through the vein and include a tired, aching sensation in the whole of the lower leg, especially the calf, that is worst at the end of the day and when the patient has been standing. Patients who have large varices in the thighs may experience sharp pains there. Some patients suffer from swelling of the ankles, especially after standing. Other symptoms include itching in the skin of the ankle and cramps in the calf soon after going to bed.

Very large varices may form, particularly at points where the valves between superficial and deep veins are no longer functioning. These are sometimes referred to as "blowouts."

If the valves between the superficial and deep veins at the ankle become incompetent, the tiny blood vessels in the skin become more prominent and may form a fan-shaped flare over the ankle bone. This may be associated with an abnormal firmness and a darkening of the skin, the three signs together being known as lipodermatosclerosis. This is a danger sign that an ulcer is likely to form.

COMPLICATIONS

A minor injury to a varicose vein may cause hemorrhage, which may be very profuse and frightening because of the high back pressure within that vein, although it is easily treated (see below).

Sometimes phlebitis occurs, in which the blood in a varicose vein clots. The vein becomes very tender and hard, the overlying skin is inflamed, and the patient may have a fever and be quite unwell. Very occasionally, this occurs as the result of treatment of the veins by injection.

Ulceration is the most worrying complication of varicose veins, since once ulcers have formed, although they heal easily, they tend to recur. They are particularly associated with incompetent valves in the deep veins of the leg, frequently occurring as the result of a DVT. They usually develop around the ankle rather than on the foot itself. Why this should be so is unclear and the actual mechanism of their development is not fully understood. However, it is suggested that fibrinogen, a substance involved with the clotting of blood, leaks out of the veins as a result of the very high pressure within them and forms a barrier in the surrounding tissues. This barrier prevents oxygen and nutrients from getting through to the tissues, which therefore start to die. Very rarely, the edge of a longstanding varicose ulcer may become malignant—this is known as Marjolin's ulcer.

TESTS

Varicose veins can be diagnosed simply by looking at them, but some tests are necessary to determine which method of treatment will be best.

One method is to tie a rubber tube around the patient's leg while she is lying down (and the veins are comparatively empty), in order to prevent blood from flowing backward. If the tube is applied around the thigh and when the patient stands up the lower varices do not fill rapidly, this suggests that it is only the valves in the upper part of the leg that are incompetent and that the Trendelenburg operation described below will give a good result. If, however, the lower varices do fill rapidly, this suggests that there are incompetent valves in the perforating veins lower down the leg. Further experiments in tying the tube at different levels will demonstrate which these are. Just before treatment, these points will be marked so that the perforators can either be injected or tied off.

A large varicosity in the thigh (called a saphena varix) may sometimes be difficult to differentiate from a hernia. In order to make the diagnosis, the doctor will keep one finger on the varix and will tap gently on the dilated veins lower down the leg. If the swelling is indeed a saphena varix, he will feel a vibration.

Patients with ulcers are usually assessed initially in the hospital. A Doppler machine uses sound to measure the blood flow and pressure in the veins around the ankle. Sometimes phlebography (venography) is performed, in which a dye is injected into the veins and an X-ray is then taken that will show their outlines.

TRADITIONAL TREATMENT

Elastic Stockings
Elastic stockings are used to prevent minor varicosities from getting worse and to prevent the development of varicose veins in pregnant women and people who have had a DVT. They are especially valuable for patients who because of age or frailty are unsuited to other forms of treatment.

People who have established varicose veins should put their elastic stockings on before they get out of bed in the morning, thus preventing any back pressure on the valves, and they should take them off last thing at night. Patients are measured very carefully for their stockings but sometimes complain that they feel tight. This, however, is not due to poor fitting but to swelling of the leg under the stocking. It is an indication to the patient to do some gentle exercise (such as walking) in order to reduce the swelling. The only patients for whom elastic stockings are not suitable are those who have hardening of the arteries in the legs, resulting in inadequate amounts of blood reaching the lower legs and feet. In such a case, the compression produced by elastic stockings could make the problem worse.

Drugs
Some doctors prescribe over-the-counter pain relievers that may relieve the aching and swelling resulting from varicose veins.

Injection
Patients with minor varices can be treated with injections, although these are not suitable if the varices are in the upper part of the thigh. The points at which the varicosities connect with the deep veins of the leg are determined and a sclerosing solution is injected into them. This has the effect of closing off the vein at these points. Once the injections

have been given, the leg is bandaged firmly with an elastic bandage and this is kept on for two weeks. Injections are getting more popular in the United States.

Surgery

For more advanced varicose veins, surgery is usually necessary. In the Trendelenburg procedure, the saphenous vein is disconnected from the femoral vein (see diagram) and the individual branches of the saphenous vein are tied off. This may be combined with stripping (complete removal) of the vein. This is often done if there are large varicosities in the thigh. Between 60 and 70 percent of patients have a good long-term result from surgery.

Treatment of Complications

The treatment of hemorrhage is to lie the patient down, raise the leg that is bleeding, and apply a pressure bandage over the bleeding point (a thick layer of folded handkerchiefs tied firmly in place with a scarf will do as a first-aid measure). It is most important that a pressure bandage is used and not a tourniquet, which will cut off all the blood supply to the leg. Bleeding will stop quite quickly with this treatment, but the doctor should be called to inspect the injury and the patient will later need either injection or operative treatment for the varicose veins.

Phlebitis is treated with bed rest, the foot of the bed being raised. A bandage is applied to the leg, which flattens out the superficial veins and increases blood flow through the deep veins. In severe cases, an anticoagulant (blood-thinning drug) may be necessary in order to relieve pain and prevent the thrombosis from spreading.

There are two main methods of treating varicose ulcers. The first is to put the patient to bed, with the foot of the bed raised, and keep the ulcer clean until it has healed. In severe cases, an elastic bandage may be needed in addition. Although this is an effective treatment, it may entail the patient remaining in bed for some weeks, which may be inconvenient for a younger patient and inadvisable for an older one. In such cases, the patient may be treated simply by tight elastic bandaging and regular dressing of the ulcer itself. Sometimes zinc-impregnated bandages are used since zinc helps to promote skin healing.

Over the past few years, some hospitals have been using dressings derived from seaweed in the treatment of ulcers. These have two great advantages over traditional gauze dressings. First, they form a gel that absorbs fluid from the ulcer, reducing the risk of infection. Second, they are very easy to remove, as they can just be washed away. Thus, not only is their removal painless but there is also no risk that delicate healing tissue will be damaged when the dressing is changed.

Some patients with varicose ulcers need skin grafting. This may be done by removing a slice of skin from another part of the body (such as the thigh) or by a "pinch graft" in which a number of tiny pieces of skin are used. Done under a local anesthetic, pinch grafting can dramatically reduce the time needed to heal a bad ulcer.

Once an ulcer has healed, the patient must continue to wear elastic stockings in order to reduce the risk of a recurrence. Some patients with ulcers are not suitable for injection or operation, but in other cases one of these may be necessary.

COMPLEMENTARY TREATMENT

Aromatherapy
Cypress, lemon, lavender, and rosemary are among the oils that may be recommended.

Herbalism
Various lotions such as marigold, witch hazel, or horse chestnut may be prescribed for patients with varicose veins or ulcers. Marigold has a healing action on local tissues, both witch hazel and horse chestnut are astringent and help to prevent bleeding, and horse chestnut has additional antiinflammatory properties. Lime blossom, too, is antiinflammatory, aids circulation, and has a healing effect on the walls of the blood vessels.

Homeopathy
Carbo veg. may be suitable for patients whose legs tend to be blue from poor circulation and whose feet and legs are always cold. For those whose legs are constantly painful and tired, and who have purple blotches on the skin of the legs, hamamelis may be appropriate. Pul-

satilla is useful for patients with painful inflamed veins whose symptoms are relieved by walking in cool air.

Nutrition
Rutin tablets help to strengthen the walls of blood vessels and may be recommended. In addition, supplements of vitamin C and E, which are essential for the health of the skin and blood vessels, may prevent varicose veins from getting any worse.

VERTIGO AND TINNITUS

THESE TWO CONDITIONS commonly arise as the result of disorders affecting the ear and may occur together.

VERTIGO (DIZZINESS)

This word is often used by laypeople to mean fear of heights. However, the medical term for fear of heights is acrophobia. Vertigo is, in fact, a sensation of abnormal movement in which the patient feels that either he or his surroundings are going around and around or rocking to and fro. The sensation is often accompanied by vomiting, sweating, and faintness. Frequently the patient will have other symptoms of ear disease, although vertigo can occur in someone with perfectly normal ears—after whirling around and around or after drinking a lot of alcohol, for example.

Although vertigo is usually the result of diseases of the ear (such as acute or chronic infections, injury, Ménière's disease, or labyrinthitis), it may also be due to conditions affecting the brain (such as stroke or migraine) or the blood supply to the ear (such as hardening of the arteries).

Labyrinthitis

The labyrinth is the section of the inner ear concerned with the maintenance of balance. Acute labyrinthitis or vestibular neuronitis is sometimes known as viral labyrinthitis, although there is no firm evidence that it is caused by a virus. However, some experts think this is likely because the condition often occurs in little epidemics. It usually affects patients between the ages of thirty and fifty and may follow a feverish illness. It often starts with severe vertigo that is made worse by move-

439

ment or by putting the head in certain positions. Recovery is rapid over a period of two or three days and there are no aftereffects. Some patients have repeated attacks, but these become less frequent and less severe over time and have usually disappeared within twelve to eighteen months. Occasionally, if labyrinthitis has followed an attack of mumps, the patient may be left with some degree of deafness.

Labyrinthitis may also occur as a complication of chronic suppurative otitis media (described fully in the section on ear infections). The patient may have had a discharging ear for many years but has not seen his doctor about it because he has not experienced any pain. Suddenly he develops severe vertigo and vomiting that is made worse by moving his head and sometimes by pressing on the diseased ear. This is associated with headache and fever, and the patient feels very unwell.

Ménière's Disease

This is a relatively uncommon condition that tends to affect middle-age men and women. The cause is unknown, although it seems to be associated with an increased amount of fluid in the inner ear (the part housing the balance mechanisms and the nerve endings that transmit sound to the brain).

The first symptoms are usually deafness and tinnitus (a buzzing or ringing sound) in one ear. Then the patient starts to have attacks of severe vertigo that may come on very suddenly but are usually preceded by a worsening of the tinnitus. The dizziness is made worse by movement and is often accompanied by vomiting and sometimes by diarrhea. The patient is pale and clammy and cannot hear with the affected ear. However, once the attack has subsided, after a period of between fifteen minutes and two hours, the hearing starts to return. If an attack is severe, it may be several hours or even days before the patient feels quite well again. But attacks may be quite mild and may consist simply of a slight degree of vertigo upon waking in the morning that gradually wears off after about an hour. Sometimes they are brought on by a sudden movement, coughing, or sneezing, but this is the exception rather than the rule. Patients who are under stress seem more liable to frequent attacks, but as time goes on most patients find that they become less frequent and less severe, although this improvement may be associated with gradually increasing deafness. If the inner ear is completely destroyed by the condition, the attacks will cease altogether, but the patient will be profoundly deaf in that ear. Occasionally, in severe cases, both ears may become affected.

Traumatic Vertigo

This may follow a head injury or an ear operation. Usually the patient recovers completely, although a fracture of the base of the skull may damage the labyrinth to such an extent that the problem becomes a long-term one.

Positional Vertigo

In this condition, the patient complains of fleeting episodes of vertigo brought on by moving the head or by bending down. What causes these attacks, which last only a few seconds, is unknown, but most patients recover after a period of two or three months. In some cases, positional vertigo may be associated with arthritis of the spine, in which case the wearing of a cervical collar may considerably relieve the symptoms.

Tests

The doctor will first need to determine whether the patient is suffering from vertigo (due to a problem in the ears) or from another disorder of balance, which may be associated with eye problems or with an abnormality in the balance-sensing mechanism, which is made up of special nerve endings (proprioceptors) situated in the feet and legs and the major posture-maintaining muscles of the body. If the diagnosis seems to be one of vertigo, then the ears will need to be tested. Often such a diagnosis can be made from the history alone (such as in Ménière's disease) and tests are necessary just to determine the cause.

The doctor will examine the patient's eyes and may test his sense of balance and coordination. Blood tests may be done, including one for blood sugar, since proprioceptor abnormalities may occur in diabetes.

The ears will be inspected through an otoscope and a hearing test will be performed. Sometimes, it may be necessary to X-ray the skull to determine whether there is any infection of the mastoids. A caloric test, in which cold water and then warm water is run into one ear, helps the doctor to assess the normality of the balance mechanism in that ear. The test provokes nystagmus—a rhythmic movement of the eyes—which is due to irritation of the labyrinth. (Patients with labyrinthitis may develop nystagmus as part of their illness.) In a patient with Ménière's disease, where the labyrinth has been destroyed, the caloric test may fail to provoke nystagmus.

Traditional Treatment

The treatment of vertigo depends to a certain extent on its cause. Acute labyrinthitis needs nothing more than a few days of bed rest and, if necessary, a mild antivertigo drug. Labyrinthitis resulting from chronic suppurative otitis media, however, requires outpatient treatment, antibiotics, and, as soon as possible, a radical mastoid operation (see the section on ear infections). Antivertigo drugs are also given, such as meclizine, cyclizine, dimenhydrinate, prochlorperazine, promethazine, thiethylperazine, or scopolamine.

Various treatments have been tried for Ménière's disease and although none has proved outstanding each is helpful in a number of cases. During the acute attack of vertigo, the patient needs bed rest and an antivertigo drug. Relief of stress, reducing salt intake, and stopping smoking may result in fewer and less severe attacks. If the ear has become very deaf but vertigo continues, an operation to destroy the remaining labyrinth (which will also destroy any remaining hearing in that ear) will halt the attacks. Some specialists advocate the insertion of a grommet into the ear in cases where blockage of the eustachian tube seems to be contributing to the problem. The eustachian tube, running from the ear to the throat, ensures that air pressure on both sides of the eardrum is equal (see the section on ear infections). A grommet is a tiny plastic tube inserted through the eardrum and thus provides the same service. This may produce a considerable improvement in the patient's condition. The grommet is removed after a period of at least three months.

TINNITUS (RINGING IN THE EARS)

Tinnitus, or "ringing in the ears" is a fairly common condition among elderly people. It affects about 15 percent of the adult population and may be mild or severe. Usually the sound takes the form of a high-pitched hiss or a noise similar to that of running water. Rarely, tinnitus is caused by an abnormality in the blood flow to the ear and in such cases the noise may pulsate. The intensity of the sound may change from day to day, but usually the patient is most aware of it when in quiet surroundings, especially when in bed at night.

Although tinnitus is usually associated with some degree of hearing loss, many patients have nothing else wrong with their ears. The sound is thought to be caused by damage to the nerve cells that transmit hearing to the brain, so that they send abnormal "messages." However, why the cells become damaged is unknown. Occasionally tinnitus may occur as the result of taking certain drugs such as quinine or aspirin. In such cases, the symptom usually disappears when the drug is stopped.

Traditional Treatment

For some patients in whom tinnitus is combined with deafness, a hearing aid may be useful, since by amplifying the background noise of their surroundings it makes them less aware of the noise being generated in their ears. However, the standard treatment is to use a masker. This device, which is suitable for about two thirds of patients with tinnitus, is fitted into the ear in the same way as a hearing aid and produces a constant soothing noise. Unlike the sound of tinnitus, it doesn't fluctuate in any way and so is not distracting. Although it may take two or three months for a patient to adjust to a masker, in most cases it is very successful. It is not uncommon for patients to find that the effect lasts for some time after they have removed the masker and in some cases they may eventually be able to do without the device altogether.

COMPLEMENTARY TREATMENT

Acupuncture
Vertigo is said to be due to overactive yang (the positive, masculine aspect of Chi) in the liver, retention of phlegm, and damp within the body obstructing the flow of Chi, or a deficiency of Chi and of blood. Treatment consists of balancing the Chi of the liver, dispelling the

phlegm and damp, or stimulating the Chi and blood, and, in all cases, restoring the normal flow of Chi and of blood.

Tinnitus is said to be caused by a disturbance in the flow of Chi through the ear—there being either an excess or a deficiency. Points around the ear are used to restore the flow to normal.

Because the kidney is associated with the regulation of hearing in the Chinese theory of energy flow, points may also be chosen that will stimulate kidney function.

Alexander Technique and Manipulation

Because vertigo may sometimes be caused by postural problems in the neck cutting off the blood supply to the ear, postural training by the Alexander system may be very effective in some cases. Similarly, osteopathic or chiropractic manipulation may be very beneficial by loosening the neck and restoring full movement.

Aromatherapy

Onion may be recommended for tinnitus and a number of oils for vertigo, including caraway, aniseed, fennel, and lavender.

Herbalism

Balm, hawthorn, mistletoe, and betony are among the herbs used to treat dizziness. Hawthorn and mistletoe are also used for patients with tinnitus. Balm has a relaxant effect on the nervous system as a whole, while betony, as well as acting as a relaxant, stimulates the blood supply to the brain and head.

Homeopathy

For patients who hear a roaring or humming sound when they are in bed at night, who are chronically dizzy with a tendency to fall to one side, and who have a chronic ear infection, sulphur may be effective. If the patient becomes dizzy when getting up after lying down, if this is associated with nausea, and if he is very sensitive to noise of any kind, aconite may be prescribed. In case of Ménière's disease when vertigo is brought on by sudden movement and the patient has a tendency to fall backward, bryonia may be appropriate. Nux vomica is also used for patients who tend to fall backward, when the dizziness comes on during or after a meal. Many other remedies are available to treat both tinnitus and vertigo.

Hypnotherapy

This can be very effective in the treatment of tinnitus, but the subject must be capable of going into a moderately deep trance. By using hypnosis, it is possible to make a patient have positive or negative hallucinations—that is, believe that something is there when it isn't or that it isn't there when it is. For patients with tinnitus, a negative hallucination is induced in which they are made to believe that they cannot hear the noise in their ears—after which it ceases to trouble them. Various techniques may be used, one of which is to suggest to the patient that he can see a dial that controls the tinnitus and that it is possible for him to use this to turn the sound off. The patient is taught self-hypnosis so that he can practice the technique at home and after a while he should find that he can "turn off" his tinnitus for hours or days at a time.

SELF-HELP

Alcohol, smoking, and strong tea or coffee may make tinnitus worse and should be avoided when this is found to be the case.

ORGANIZATIONS

American Tinnitus Association
P.O. Box 5
Portland, OR 97207
503/248-9985
(Publishes a quarterly newsletter.)

WARTS

DESCRIPTION AND CAUSE

Warts are extremely common. They are caused by a virus, known as the human papilloma virus, or HPV, which causes localized excessive growth of the skin cells together with overproduction of keratin, the substance that gives hardness to skin, nails, and hair. They affect between 7 and 10 percent of the population at any one time and are especially likely to affect children and young adults. No treatment has been discovered that can guarantee a cure; at the same time that some warts are being cured, others may appear on the neighboring skin. About one fifth of all warts will disappear spontaneously within six months and two thirds within two years. However, some may take much longer.

TYPES OF WARTS

The main sites of warts are the hands, face and neck, feet, genitalia, and the skin around the anus. Those affecting the hands, face, and neck usually fall into one of two categories—common warts or plane warts. The latter are fairly flat, often brownish, and usually 2–3 mm in diameter. Common warts are raised, rough nodules that may appear in groups and that most frequently affect the fingers. Spread may be caused by injury—nail biters may get warts around their nails and thumb-suckers may spread them from their hands to their mouths. A man may spread warts across his face while shaving. Apart from warts on the feet (plantar warts) and those around the nails, both of which may be painful, most warts remain painless unless they become infected by bacteria.

A plantar wart is often known as a verruca (although this is actually the medical term for any sort of wart). It may become painful because the pressure put on it when the patient stands or walks drives the wart into the flesh of the sole, pressing on nerve endings. Groups of warts (known as mosaic warts) may form, spread being encouraged by dampness. Most warts are only slightly contagious, but the exception is anal and genital warts, which are easily spread by sexual contact. Growth in this area is encouraged by warmth and sweat and usually the warts are multiple, quite large, soft, and fleshy, although those on the penis may be flat. Anal warts are commonest in male homosexuals, although they occur in other people as well. In women, warts tend to occur around the vagina, and certain strains of wart virus, when they affect the cervix, seem to be associated with the development of abnormal cells and possibly cancer. However, this has not yet been proved. Large fleshy warts may ulcerate or bleed and if they become infected they may produce an unpleasant discharge.

TESTS

Occasionally a wart on the foot may be difficult to differentiate from a corn or local hardening of the skin (callosity). In such a case, the doctor may take a scalpel and gently scrape away at the overlying layers. This is painless because there are no nerve endings in these layers of skin. In a wart, tiny blood vessels came quite close to the surface and these will be seen as tiny red or black points. Such points are not visible in a callosity.

TRADITIONAL TREATMENT

Most doctors recommend that unless warts are particularly unsightly or uncomfortable they should be left alone. The exceptions to this are anal and genital warts, which are very contagious, and plantar warts, which can become very painful. The main reason for leaving warts untreated is that eventually they will resolve of their own accord without scarring whereas treatment can occasionally leave a scar that is more troublesome than the wart itself. The aim of all forms of treatment is to kill the wart virus, either directly or by changing the properties of the skin in which it is living, making its continued existence there difficult.

Occlusion
In some situations, an airtight plaster put over warts and changed weekly for six to eight weeks may destroy them by softening the

underlying skin to such an extent that the virus can no longer live there. This is particularly useful when there is only a small group of warts situated on delicate skin, such as that around the nails or on the toes, which may react poorly to chemical treatment.

Salicylic Acid

This is available as a paint and is particularly suitable for treating multiple warts on the hands, head, and neck. One of its actions is to soften the wart, making it less conspicuous. When treating a plantar wart, the patient must first rub it with pumice stone or an emery board to remove the top surface before applying the paint. The wart is then covered with an airtight plaster. As the treatment starts to work, the wart turns white and the area becomes slightly tender.

Formaline

This method of treatment is suitable only for plantar warts. The patient smears Vaseline around the wart, to protect the surrounding skin, and then soaks the wart in a saucer of formaline solution for fifteen minutes every day. Treatment needs to be continued for at least a month and before each soak the hard surface tissue must be scraped or rubbed away. Three dilutions of formaline are available. It is usual to start with the weakest and progress to a stronger solution if the treatment does not seem to be working.

Podophyllin

This is available as a paint or an ointment. Used two to three times a week, it may be effective for plantar warts when other treatments have failed and is the treatment of choice for anal or genital warts. It is also useful for warts around the nails or on the toes, but should not be used on the face or neck. The surrounding skin must be protected with Vaseline and the podophyllin must be washed off after about six hours because otherwise there is a risk of burning. Treatment is usually effective within a few weeks. Like formaline, podophyllin comes in different dilutions and increasing strengths can be used if patients fail to respond. Because a small amount of podophyllin may be absorbed into the bloodstream and because it may cause fetal abnormalities, it should not be used by pregnant women.

Cryotherapy
Carbon dioxide snow or liquid nitrogen can be used to freeze warts, but they are not suitable for treating large clusters. They may, however, be used for warts around the nails and for the toes and, if all else fails, for plantar warts. The treatment has about a 70 percent success rate, but very occasionally it may leave a painful scar.

Curettage and Cautery
This is done under local anesthetic. The wart is scooped out of the skin and the area is cauterized to stop bleeding and to kill any of the wart virus that may remain. It cannot be used on warts around the nails because it may damage the nail bed and result in nail deformities. It may be useful for genital and anal warts if these keep recurring or if there is no response to podophyllin. Like cryotherapy, it may very occasionally leave a painful scar.

Other Treatments
These include the use of preparations containing silver nitrate. Lasers may also be used to burn out warts.

RECENT ADVANCES

Interferons are proteins that occur naturally in the body and that are involved in the process of immunity, especially against viruses. In recent years it has become possible to make synthetic interferons and one of these (Interferon A) has been used in a trial to treat genital warts. Injected into the warts three times a week for three weeks, it was found to produce good results. Up to 60 percent of patients developed flulike symptoms during treatment, but these seemed to be the only side effects. Unfortunately, interferons are extremely expensive and so for the time being it seems likely that they will only be used for treating genital and anal warts that have not responded to any other form of treatment.

COMPLEMENTARY TREATMENT

Aromatherapy
Lemon and tea tree are among the oils that may help to combat warts.

Herbalism

Various herbal remedies may be effective against warts. Patients may be advised to rub the wart each day with the sap from a fresh dandelion stalk, a slice of garlic, or the juice of a sour apple, a fresh pineapple, or fresh green figs. Calendula juice, celandine juice, and thuja (arborvitae) tincture may also be helpful.

Homeopathy

Calc. carb. may be prescribed if the patient has large numbers of warts, especially on the sides of the fingers, the hands, and arms. Thuja is useful if there are crops of warts on the backs of the hands and dulcamara if they are on the back of the fingers. Fleshy warts may be treated with causticum or natrum mur. and flat, hard warts with antimony crud.

Hypnotherapy

Because "mind over matter" may sometimes be effective in getting rid of warts, hypnotherapy may be useful if all else has failed.

TRADITIONAL DRUGS AND THEIR TRADE NAMES

SOME OF THE DRUGS mentioned in the text may be better known to patients by their trade names. A selection of these is given below.

Those drugs and groups of drugs about which specific information is given in the text will also be found in the main index.

ACNE

Benzoyl peroxide	Acnegel, Benoxyl, Benzagel, Desquam X, Nericur, Panoxyl
Sulphur	Night cast, Sebulex
Tretinoin	Retin-A
Tetracycline	Achromycin, Sumycin
oxytetracycline	Terramycin, Urobiotic
Trimethoprim-sulfamethoxazole	Bactrim, Septra
Minocycline	Minocin
Doxycycline	Vibramycin, Doryx, Vibra-Tabs
Erythromycin	Erthrocin, Ilosone, EES, ERYC, Ery Ped, PCE, E-Mycin
Isotretinoin	Accutane

ANXIETY AND PHOBIAS

Diazepam	Valium
Chlordiazepoxide	Librium
Oxazepam	Serax

Temazepam	Restoril
Lorazepam	Ativan
Chlorpromazine	Thorazine
Trifluoperazine	Stelazine

ARTHRITIS

Ibuprofen	Advil, Nuprin, Mediprin, Motrin, Rufen
Indomethacin	Indocin
Naproxen	Naprosyn
Aspirin	Aspergum, Ecotrin, Bayer Aspirin, Bufferin, Anacin, Excedrin, Zorprin
Sodium aurothiomalate	Myochrisine
Auranofin	Ridaura
Penicillamine	Cuprimine, Depen
Azathioprine	Imuran
Methotrexate	Methotrexate

Steroids include:

betamethasone	Celestone
cortisone	Cortisone
dexamethasone	Decadron
hydrocortisone	Hydrocortisone
methylprednisolone	Medrol
prednisolone	Prednisolone
prednisone	Prednisone
triamcinolone	Aristocort
Piroxicam	Feldene
Allopurinol	Zyloprim
Probenecid	Benemid

ASTHMA

Sodium cromolyn	Intal
Theophylline	Quibron, Uniphyl, Primatene, Theo-Dur, Elixophylin
Aminophylline	Somophyllin
Isoetharine	Bronkosol, Bronkometer
Albuterol	Proventil
Terbutaline	Bricanyl, Brethine

Steroids—see Arthritis
Methotrexate   Methotrexate

BACK PAIN
Indomethacin   Indocin
Flurbiprofen   Assaid

BED-WETTING
Imipramine   Tofranil
Propantheline   Pro-Banthine
Desmopressin   DDAVP

BREAST LUMPS
Danazol   Danocrine
Bromocriptine   Parlodel
Tamoxifen   Nolvadex

BRONCHITIS
Digoxin   Lanoxin

CONSTIPATION
Bran   Bran
Bulking agents include:
psyllium husk   Fiberall, Effer-Syllium
methycellulose   Citrucel
Lactulose   Dulphalac, Cephulac, Chronulac
Docusate sodium   Colace, Peri-Colace
Senna   Senokot
Magnesium sulphate   Epsom salts

DEPRESSION
Imipramine   Tofranil
Amitriptyline   Elavil, Endep, and in Limbitrol and
                                      Triavil
Nortriptyline   Pamelor
Doxepin   Sinequan, Adapin
Trazodone   Desyrel

Monoamine oxidase inhibitors include:

phenelzine	Nardil
isocarboxazid	Marplan
tranylcypromine	Parnate
L-tryptophan	L-tryptophan
Lithium carbonate	Eskalith, Lithane, Lithobid
Carbamazepine	Tegretol
Fluoxetine	Prozac

DIABETES

Glyburide	Micronase, Diabeta Orinase
Chlorpropamide	Diabinese
Tolazamide	Tolinase
Cyclosporin	Sandimmun
Glipizide	Glucotrol

DIVERTICULAR DISEASE

Belladonna	Donnatal, Kinesed
Dicyclomine hydrochloride	Bentyl
Hyoscine	Scopolamine
Propantheline bromide	Pro-Banthine

EPILEPSY

Sodium valproate	Depakene
Ethosuximide	Zarontin
Phenytoin	Dilantin
Carbamazepine	Tegretol
Primidone	Mysoline
Phenobarbital	Phenobarbital

GALLBLADDER DISEASE

Chenodeoxycholic acid	Chenix, Chenodiol
Ursodeoxycholic acid	Ursodiol, Actigall

HAIR LOSS

Minoxidil	Rogaine

HERPES SIMPLEX

Povidone iodine	Betadine
Acyclovir	Zovirax
Vidarabine	Vira-A

HIGH BLOOD PRESSURE

Digoxin	Lanoxin
Bendroflumethazide	Naturetin
Chlorothiazide	Diuril
Hydrochlorothiazide	Hydrodiuril
Furosemide	Lasix
Bumetanide	Bumex
Amiloride	Midamor
Triamterene	Dyrenium
Propranolol	Propranolol
Nadolol	Corgard
Metoprolol	Lopressor
Teruzosin	Hytrin
Atenolol	Tenormin
Hydralazine	Apresoline
Minoxidil	Loniten
Prazosin	Minipres
Labetalol	Trandate, Normodyne
Nifedipine	Adalat, Procardia
Verapamil	Isoptin, Calan, Verelan
Captopril	Capoten; with hydrochlorthiazide, Capozide
Enalapril	Vasotec
Methyldopa	Aldomet
Clonidine	Catapres
Doxazosin	Cardura

IMPOTENCE

Guanethidine	Ismelin
Metaraminol	Aramine

INCONTINENCE

Propantheline	Pro-Banthine
Imipramine	Tofranil
Bethanechol	Urecholine

INFERTILITY

Clomiphene citrate	Clomid
Tamoxifen	Nolvadex
Bromocriptine	Parlodel

INSOMNIA

Flurazepam	Dalmane
Temazepam	Restoril
Triazolam	Halcion
Chloral hydrate	Noctec
Dichloralphenazone	Welldorm
Chlormethiazole	Heminevrin
Promethazine	Phenergan
Imipramine	Tofranil
Trimipramine	Surmontil

IRRITABLE BOWEL SYNDROME

Mebeverine	Colofac, Colven
Propantheline	Pro-Banthine
Psyllium husk	Metamucil, Regulan, Effer-sylium, Fiberall
Methylcellulose	Citrucel

ISCHEMIC HEART DISEASE

Nitroglycerin	Nitrolingual spray, Nitrostat, Nitro-Bio, Nitrogard
Isosorbide dinitrate	Isordil, Sorbitrate
Propranolol	Inderal
Nifedipine	Adalat, Procardia
Verapamil	Isoptin, Calan, Verelan
Diltiazem	Cardizem
Labetalol	Trandate, Normodyne

Digoxin	Lanoxin
Clofibrate	Atromid-S
Gemfibrozil	Lopid

MENOPAUSE

Hormone replacement	Premarin, Protera
Estrogen cream	Ortho Dienoestrol, Premarin
Clonidine	Catapres

MENSTRUAL PROBLEMS

Flurbiprofen	Ansaid
Mefenamic acid	Ponstel
Naproxen	Naprosyn
Ibuprofen	Advil, Mediprin, Motrin, Nuprin, Rufen
Piroxicam	Feldene
Norethindrone	Norlutin
Tranexamic acid	Cyklokapron
Clomiphene	Clomid
Danazol	Danocrine

MIGRAINE

Propranolol	Inderal
Metoprolol	Lopressor
Nadolol	Corgard
Timolol	Blocadren
Methysergide maleate	Sansert
Cyproheptadine	Periactin
Naproxen	Naprosyn
Clonidine	Catapres
Metoclopramide	Reglan
Ergotamine	Cafergot

MOUTH ULCERS

Carbamide peroxide	Gly-Oxide
Benzocaine	Anbesol, Chloraseptic, Oragel
Salicylates	Bonjela, Pyralvex, Teejel

Chlorhexidine   Peridex
Steroids   Orabase

NOSEBLEEDS
Tranexamic acid   Cyklokapron

OSTEOPOROSIS
Hormone replacement—see Menopause
Etidronate disodium   Didronel
Calcitonin   Calcimar

PEPTIC ULCER
Cimetidine   Tagamet
Ranitidine   Zantac
Famotidine   Pepcid
Nizatidine   Axid
Bismuth subsalicylate   Pepto-Bismol
Sucralfate   Carafate
Misoprostol   Cytotec

PREMENSTRUAL SYNDROME
Progesterone   Progesterone
Spironolactone   Aldactone
Bromocriptine   Parlodel

PROSTATE PROBLEMS
Prazosin   Minipres
Flutamide   Eulexin
Terazosin   Mytrin

PSORIASIS
Salicylic acid   Sebulex
Tar   Balnetar, Estar, Sebutone, Pentrax, Zetar
Anthralin   Anthra-Derm, Drithocreme
Methotrexate   Methotrexate
Etretinate   Tegison

RHINITIS

Astemizole	Hismanal
Terfenadine	Seldane
Oxymetazoline	Afrin
Cromolyn sodium	Intal
Beclomethasone	Beconase, Vancenase

RINGWORM

Griseofulvin	Fulvicin, Grifulvin, Grisactin, Gris-PEG
Clotrimazole	Lotrimin, Mycelex
Econazole	Spectazole
Miconazole	Monistat
Sulconazole	Exelderm
Salicylic acid	Fungi-Nail

SCHIZOPHRENIA

Chlorpromazine	Thorazine
Thioridazine	Melleril
Trifluoperazine	Stelazine
Haloperidol	Haldol
Procyclidine	Kemadrin
Trihexiphenidyl	Artane
Orphenadrine	Norflex
Fluphenazine	Prolixin
Benz-tropine	Cogentin

SHINGLES

Acyclovir	Zovirax
Prednisolone	Prednisolone
Vidaribine	Vira-A

THRUSH

Nystatin	Mycostatin
Clotrimazole	Lotrimin, Mycelex
Ketoconazole	Nizoral
Econazole	Spectuzole
Miconazole	Monistat

THYROID DISEASES

Thyroxine	Synthroid, Levothroid
Tri-iodothyronine	Cytomel, Euthroid
Propylthiouracil	Propylthiouracil

URINARY TRACT INFECTIONS

Potassium citrate	Urocit-K, Citrolith, Polycitra

VAGINAL DISCHARGE

Metronidazole	Flagyl, Protostat
Tetracycline—see Acne	
Trimethoprim-sulfamethoxazole	Septra
Erythromycin	Erythrocin, EES, ERYC, Ery Ped, PCE, E-Mycin, Ilosone, Ilotycin

VARICOSE VEINS

Stanozolol	Winstrol

VERTIGO AND TINNITUS

Scopolamine	Transderm-Scop
Cyclizine	Marezine
Dimenhydrinate	Dramamine
Prochlorperazine	Compazine
Promethazine	Phenergan
Thiethylperazine	Torecan, Norzine
Meckzine	Antivert, Bonine

WARTS

Formaldehyde (formaline)	Lazenformaldehyde
Podophyllin	Pod-Ben-25, Verrex

APPENDIX B

PRONUNCIATION GUIDE

VOWELS

a	as in cap, mad, hat	oh	as in spoke, boat, low
ā	as in tape, date, male	u	as in but, stud, shut
ah	as in far, mark, jar	ū	as in put, wood, look
e	as in met, kept, wed	yoo	as in due, new, mute
ee	as in meet, weak, seem	aw	as in saw, naughty,
er	as in term, learn, perm		taught
i	as in with, miss, list	oi	as in coin, annoy, void
ī	as in might, line, wide	oo	as in do, boot, fruit
o	as in soft, lost, dot	ow	as in how, stout, loud

There are some words in which, when one is speaking normally, one glosses over a vowel and this I have shown as "eh"—for example, the word *normally* would be shown as nawm-eh-lee rather than nawm-a-lee and *ballerina* as bal-eh-ree-neh.

CONSONANTS

g	as in grand, grant, girl	s	as in soft, speak, less
j	as in jelly, just, giant	z	as in raising, was, exercise

The syllable on which emphasis is put is shown in capital letters.

adenoma—a-den-OH-mah
adenomyosis—a-den-oh-mī-OH-sis
alkalosis—al-kah-LOH-sis
alopecia—a-loh-PEE-sheh

amenorrhea—ay-men-oh-REE-ah
ampulla—am-PŪL-ah
anagen—AN-a-jen
androgens—AN-droh-jens
angiogram—AN-jee-oh-gram
ankylosing—AN-kil-oh-sing
aorta—ay-OR-tah
aortography—ay-or-TOG-raf-ee
apnea—AP-nee-ah
arthritides—ar-THRIT-id-eez
arthrodesis—ar-throh-DEE-sis

biguanide—bī-GWAN-īd
bronhchi—BRON-kee
bronchioles—BRON-kee-ohls
bulimia—bul-IM-ee-ah

catagen—KAT-a-jen
cheilosis—kee-LOH-sis
chemonucleolysis—KEE-moh-nyoo-klee-O-li-sis
chenodeoxycholic—KEE-noh-dee-oks-ee-KOH-lik
chlamydia—kla-MID-ee-ah
cholangiogram—koh-LAN-jee-oh-gram
cholangitis—koh-lan-JĪ-tis
cholecystitis—KOH-lee-sis-TĪ-tis
cholecystokinin—KOH-lee-sis-toh-KĪ-nin
choledocholithiasis—koh-lee-DOH-koh-li-THĪ-ah-sis
cholesteatoma—koh-LES-tee-ah-TOH-meh
chymopapain—kī-moh-pa-PAYN
cilia—SI-lee-ah
cirrhosis—si-ROH-sis
coarctation—koh-ark-TAY-shun
colporrhaphy—kol-PO-ra-fee
coronary—KO-ron-air-ree
cruris—KRAW-ris
curettage—KYAW-re-tazh
cystocele—SIS-toh-seel

defecation—de-feh-KAY-shun
déjà vu—DAY-zhah voo
diuretic—DĪ-yaw-re-tik
dysmenorrhea—dis-men-oh-REE-ah
dysplasia—dis-PLAY-zee-ah
dysuria—dis-YAW-ree-ah

eicosapentenoic—ī-KOH-sah-pen-tah-en-OH-ik
emphysema—em-fi-ZEE-mah
endometrium—en-doh-MEE-tree-um
enuresis—en-YAW-ree-sis
eosinophils—ee-oh-SIN-oh-filz
epidermis—e-pi-DER-mis
epididymitis—e-pi-di-dim-Ī-tis
erythrodermic—e-ri-throh-DER-mik
exogenous—eks-O-jeh-nus
exophthalmos—EKS-off-thal-mos

fecal—FEE-kal
fibroadenosis—FĪ-broh-a-de-NOH-sis
fluorescein—FLAW-re-seen

gingivitis—JIN-ji-VĪ-tis
glucagon—GLOO-ka-gon
glucosidase—gloo-koh-SĪ-dayz
goiter—GOI-ter
gynecology—gī-neh-KO-leh-jee

hematoma—hee-mah-TOH-mah
hematuria—hee-mah-TYAW-ree-eh
hemorrhoids—HEM-ah-roids
herpes—HER-peez
hypertrophy—hī-PER-tro-fee
hypoglycemia—hī-poh-glī-SEE-mee-ah

idiopathic—i-dee-oh-PA-thik
ileus—Ī-lee-us
intertriginous—in-ter-TRĪ-geh-nus

ischemic—is-KEE-mik
interstitial—in-ter-STI-shal

keratolytics—ke-ra-toh-LI-tiks
ketoacidosis—kee-toh-a-si-DOH-sis

libido—li-BEE-doh
lipodermatosclerosis—li-poh-der-mah-toh-skleh-ROH-sis
luteinizing—LOO-ti-nī-zing

maceration—MA-ser-ray-shun
malleus—MA-lee-us
meibomian—mī-BOH-mee-ehn
melena—ma-LEE-nah
menorrhagia—me-noh-RAY-jee-ah
methyl—me-THĪL
myometrium—mī-oh-MEE-tree-um
myxoedema—miks-ah-DEE-mah

nephropathy—ne-FRO-pa-thee
neuropathy—nyaw-RO-pa-thee
nystagmus—ni-STAG-mus

esophagus—ee-SO-fa-gus
onycholysis—on-ee-KO-li-sis
ophthalmoscope—off-THAL-mo-skohp
orchidectomy—or-ki-DEK-to-mee
otitis—oh-TĪ-tis

paronychia—pa-roh-NI-kee-ah
pedis—PEE-dis
percutaneous—per-kyoo-TAY-nee-us
petit mal—PE-tee mal
pheochromocytoma—fee-oh-KROH-moh-sī-TOH-mah
phlebography—fle-BO-graf-ee
phlegm—flem
photocoagulation—foh-toh-koh-ag-yoo-LAY-shun
phylloides—fī-LOI-deez

physiology—fi-zee-O-lo-jee
placebo—pla-SEE-boh
procidentia—pro-si-DEN-sheh
psoralens—SO-ra-lenz
psoriasis—so-RĪ-ah-sis
psoriatic—so-ree-A-tik
pulmonary—PUL-mehn-ree
pyelogram—PĪ-ah-loh-gram

rectocele—REK-toh-seel
Reiter's—RĪ-terz
renal   REE-nal
retinopathy—re-ti-NO-pa-thee
rhinitis—rī-NĪ-tis

salicylic—sal-li-SI-lik
saphena—sa-FEE-nah
scintigraphy—sin-TI-gra-fee
sebaceous—seh-BAY-shus
seborrheic—se-bah-RAY-ik
sebum—SEE-behm
septicemia—sep-ti-SEE-mee-ah
sphenoidal—sfee-NOI-dahl
sphincterotomy—sfink-ter-O-to-mee
sphygmomanometer—sfig-moh-ma-NO-mi-ter
spondylolisthesis—spon-di-loh-lis-THEE-sis
spondylosis—spon-di-LOH-sis
stapes—STAY-peez
sulphanylurea—sul-fa-nīl-yaw-REE-ah
suppurative—SUP-yaw-ray-tiv
systolic—sis-TO-lik

telogen—TEE-loh-jen
terbutylether—ter-byoo-tīl-EETH-er
testosterone—tes-TOS-ter-ohn
thyroxine—thī-ROKS-in
tinea—TI-nee-ah
tinnitus—TI-ni-tus

trachea—tra-KEE-ah
transhepatic—tranz-he-PA-tik
transurethral—tranz-yaw-REE-thral
trichomonas—trī-koh-MOH-nas
triiodothyronine—trī-ī-O-doh-THĪ-roh-neen
tumescence—tyoo-ME-sens
tympanic—tim-PA-nik

unguium—UN-gwee-ūm
urethra—yaw-REE-thrah
urethrocele—yaw-REE-throh-seel
uric—YAW-rik
ursodeoxycholic—ER-soh-dee-oks-ee-KOH-lik
uterine—YOO-ter-īn

varicella—va-ri-SE-lah
vasodilator—vay-zoh-dī-LAY-teh
ventricular—ven-TRI-kyoo-lah
vertigo—ver-TĪ-goh
vesicoureteric—VEE-si-koh-yaw-ri-TE-rik
videocystourethrography—vi-dee-oh-sis-toh-yaw-ree-THRO-gra-fee

HOW TO FIND A QUALIFIED COMPLEMENTARY PRACTITIONER

THE FOLLOWING ORGANIZATIONS hold registers of qualified practitioners. Not every practitioner is on every register covering his therapy (for example, some will appear only on that held by the school at which they qualified). So, if one organization is unable to give you the name of a practitioner near your home, try another.

ACUPUNCTURE

American Acupuncture Association, 4262 Kissena Boulevard, Flushing, NY 11355. 718/886-4431

American Association of Acupuncture and Oriental Medicine, 1414 16th Street, NW, Suite 501, Washington, DC 20036. 202/232-1404

ALEXANDER TECHNIQUE

The American Center for the Alexander Technique, Inc., 142 West End Avenue, New York, NY 10023 *and* 931 Elizabeth Street, San Francisco, CA 94114

AROMATHERAPY

Body Essentials, 108 Central Avenue, Westfield, NJ 07090. 201/322-5099

Bonne Sante Health Products, 642 62nd Street, Brooklyn, NY 11220. 718/492-3887

Margot Latimer, P.O. Box 65, Pineville, PA 18946. 215/598-3802

Julia Meadows, 323 E. Matilija 112, Ojai, CA 93023. 805/640-1300

Just Good Scents Co Ltd., 20b Collingwood Court, Edmonton, Alberta T5T OH5, Canada. 416/897-7120

LNJ Trading, 844 North Star Mall, San Antonio, TX 78216. 512/341-1709

Swedish Health Care Center, 178 Milcreek Road, Livingston, MT 59047. 406/333-4216

The S.E.E.D. Institute, 3170 Kirwin Avenue, No. 605, Mississauga, Ontario L5A 3R1, Canada. 416/897-7120

For information about essential oils, training courses, and qualified practitioners in your area, contact the following:

Margot Latimer, P.O. Box 65, Pineville, PA 18946. 215/598-3802

Julia Meadows, 323 E. Matilija 112, Ojai, CA 93023. 805/640-1300

The International Society of Professional Aromatherapists (ISPA), 41 Leicester Road, Hinckley, Leics LE 10 1LW, England. 0455-637987

BACH FLOWER REMEDIES

Dr. Edward Bach Healing Society, 644 Merrick Road, Lynbrook, NY 11563. 516/593-2206

Bach Center Seminars, 457 Rockaway Avenue, Valley Stream, NY 11580

CHIROPRACTIC

American Chiropractic Association, 1701 Clarendon Boulevard, Arlington, VA 22209. 202/276-8800

American Chiropractic Association, 2200 Grande Avenue, Des Moines, IA 50312

International Chiropractors Association, 741 Brady Street, Davenport, IA 52808

HEALING

The best way to find a healer is probably by word of mouth—people are always ready to recommend someone who has helped them, so ask around.

Consciousness Research and Training Project, 315 East 68th Street, Box 90, New York, NY 10021

HERBALISM

The American Botanical Council, P.O. Box 201660, Austin, TX 78720

The Herb Research Foundation, 1007 Pearl Street, Suite 200, Boulder, CO 80302

HOMEOPATHY

American Institute of Homeopathy, 1500 Massachusetts Avenue, NW, Suite 41, Washington, DC 20005. 202/223-6182

International Foundation for Homeopathy, 2366 Eastlake Avenue, East, #301, Seattle, WA 98102. 206/324-8230

HYPNOTHERAPY

The American Society of Clinical Hypnosis, 2250 East Devon Avenue, Suite 336, Des Plaines, IL 60018. 312/297-3317

Associate Trainers in Clinical Hypnosis, 567 Split Rock Road, Syosset, NY 11791

Milton H. Erickson Foundation, 3606 N. 24th Street, Phoenix, AZ 85016

International Society of Hypnosis, 111 N. 49th Street, Box 144, Philadelphia, PA 19139

NATUROPATHY

American Association of Naturopathic Physicians, P.O. Box 2579, Kirland, WA 98083-2579. 206/827-6035

NUTRITION THERAPY

American Holistic Medical Association, 2002 Eastlake Avenue, East, Seattle, WA 98102. 206/322-6842

American Holistic Nurses Association, 205 St. Louis Street, Springfield, MO 65806

Association for Holistic Health, P.O. Box 9532, San Diego, CA 92109

Omega Institute, P.O. Box 571, Lebanon Springs, NY 12114

OSTEOPATHY

American Academy of Osteopathy, P.O. Box 750, Newark, OH 43055. 614/349-8701

American Osteopathic Association, 142 E. Ontario Street, Chicago, IL 60611. 312/280-5800

North American Academy of Manipulative Therapy, 12238 113th Avenue, Suite 106, Youngtown, AZ 85363

RADIONICS

American Society of Dowsers, Danville, VT 05828

REFLEXOLOGY

International Institute of Reflexology, P.O. Box 12642, St. Petersburg, FL 33733

Reflexology Center, 1307 Avenue J, Brooklyn, NY 11230

GLOSSARY

Achilles tendon: the tendon lying at the back of the ankle joint

Acute: short-term, often having a sudden onset

Adenoidectomy: removal of the adenoids

Adenoids: lymphatic tissue lying at the back of the nose

Allergen: a substance capable of causing an allergic reaction

Allergy: overreaction to a substance that is normally harmless (such as grass pollen)

Amenorrhea: absence of the monthly periods

Amino acid: one of the "building blocks" out of which protein is made and into which protein food is broken down by the digestive system

Anemia: a condition in which the number of red blood cells (which are responsible for carrying oxygen) is reduced

Anterior: at the front

Antibiotic: a drug that will kill bacteria; antibiotics have no action on viruses and therefore are not given to patients with viral infections

Antibody: a substance produced by the cells involved in the immune system to neutralize foreign invaders such as viruses

Anticoagulant: a drug that prevents the blood from clotting abnormally; sometimes known as a "blood-thinning" drug

Antihistamine: a drug that prevents histamine from being released from the cells that produce it

Antispasmodic: a drug that prevents spasm in the muscle layers of the intestines and airways and in other muscle that is not under voluntary control

Anus: the end of the digestive system, consisting of a ring of muscle that relaxes to allow the bowels to be opened

Arrhythmia: an abnormality of the heart's rhythm

Arterial: concerning the arteries (the blood vessels that take blood from the heart to the rest of the body)

Arteriography: an X-ray of arteries into which a radioopaque substance has been injected

471

Articulating surfaces: the surfaces of two bones that move against each other at a joint

Aspirate: (verb) to draw off or suck out; (noun) that which is drawn off or sucked out

Asymptomatic: having no symptoms

Atheroma: a fatty substance that is laid down in plaques along the inside of arteries

Atrophy: wasting

Auditory: concerning the hearing

Aura: symptoms occurring before an attack of epilepsy or migraine by which the patient knows that an attack is imminent

Autoimmune disease: a disease in which the patient's immune system attacks his own body

Bacteria: tiny organisms that invade the body and can cause disease; germs

Benign: not malignant, relatively harmless

Biliary: concerning the bile and the organs that produce and transport it

Biliary tract: the bile ducts and gallbladder

Biopsy: the removal of a small piece of tissue in order to examine it under a microscope

Bipolar depression: depression that alternates with mania; manic depressive psychosis

Bone marrow: the central part of a bone in which the blood cells are manufactured

Bronchi: the larger airways of the lungs

Bronchioles: the smaller airways of the lungs

Bronchodilator: a drug that relaxes the muscles in the walls of the airways, allowing them to dilate

Buccal: concerning the cheek or mouth

Calcified: having calcium laid down in it

Carbohydrate: sugars and starches

Carcinogen: a substance capable of causing cancer

Carcinoma: one form of cancer

Cardiac: concerning the heart

Cardiovascular: concerning the heart and blood vessels

Cartilage: gristle; a firm substance of great strength and rigidity that is found on the articulating surfaces of bones and elsewhere

Cataract: an opacity in the lens of the eye that can cause blindness

Catheter: a tube

Caucasian: white races

Cautery: literally burning, but used to mean anything that will have the same effect of sterilizing the area and sealing off any bleeding vessels

Cerebrovascular: concerning the blood vessels of the brain

Cervix: neck (usually the neck of the uterus); **cervical:** concerning the neck

Chemotherapy: literally treatment with chemicals, but usually applied to the drugs used in the treatment of cancer and related diseases

Chromosomes: the microscopic bodies within the nucleus of each cell that carry the hereditary factors; it is the chromosomes that are responsible for children inheriting the attributes of their parents, and it is abnormalities in the chromosomes that cause diseases such as Down's syndrome

Chronic: long term

Compression fracture: a fracture of an osteoporotic vertebra caused by the weight of the body pressing down on the thinned bone

Congenital: something that is present at or before birth

Conjunctivitis: inflammation of the conjunctiva, the membrane that covers the eyeball

Contractile: having the ability to contract

Convulsion: a seizure

Coronary: to do with the heart

Cranial nerves: nerves that arise directly from the brain and run to the head and parts of the neck and chest

Curettage: scraping material (e.g., pus) out of a cavity

Cyst: a sac containing liquid or semisolid material

Cystitis: inflammation of the bladder

Cystoscopy: examination of the inside of the bladder with a small telescope, done under anesthetic

Cytotoxic: cell killing; usually applied to drugs used to kill cancer cells

Deep vein thrombosis: clotting of blood in the deep system of veins in the leg

Defecation: moving of the bowels

Dehydrated: lacking in fluid; dry

Delusion: a false unshakable belief

Dermatologist: a specialist in skin diseases

Desensitization: treatment with a series of injections to try to reduce a patient's allergic state; starting with a very low concentration, increasingly larger doses of the allergen are given until the patient can tolerate large doses without reacting

Detrusor: the muscle in the wall of the bladder

Dialysis: a mechanism that acts as an artificial kidney

Diaphragm: the sheet of muscle that divides the chest from the abdomen

Diffuse: widespread

Dilatation (or dilation): stretching

Dilate: to stretch

Diuretic: a drug that makes the kidneys pass more water

Double-blind trial: a trial of a drug or other form of treatment in which neither the patients nor the doctors know until the end who has been given the real treatment and who has received a placebo

Duct: a canal or tube

Duodenum: the first part of the small intestine

Dysmenorrhea: painful periods

Dysplasia: an abnormality of cells not necessarily signifying malignancy

Dysuria: pain when passing water

Electrode: a conductor of electricity

Emollient: a substance that softens and moisturizes the skin

Emulsify: to mix an oily substance in water, producing a uniform fluid

Encephalitis: inflammation of the brain

Endometrium: the lining of the womb

Endoscope: a flexible telescope used for inspecting the inside of the stomach and duodenum

Enzyme: a substance that speeds a chemical reaction within the body while remaining unchanged itself

Esophagus: the gullet

Estrogen: one of the female hormones secreted by the ovaries

Eustachian tube: the canal that links the middle ear and the throat

Expectorant: a medication that loosens phlegm on the chest, enabling it to be coughed up more easily

Exudate: fluid that oozes out through tiny blood vessels

Feces: the waste matter expelled from the bowels; **fecal:** concerning the feces

Feedback mechanism: a mechanism controlling the secretion of certain body chemicals and hormones. A lack of substance A causes gland B to secrete substance B; this stimulates gland A to secrete substance A. Once the level of substance A rises, this stops the secretion of substance B until the level drops again

Fetus: an unborn child; **fetal:** concerning the fetus

Fissure: a split

Fistula: an abnormal hole between two body cavities, for example, between the bowel and the bladder

Flaccid: limp, flabby

Follicle: a small sac; **hair follicle:** the sac from which the hair grows

Fracture: a broken bone

Frequency: the need to pass water frequently

Gait: the way in which one walks

Gangrene: death of part of the body tissues, often due to an inadequate blood supply

Gastric: concerning the stomach

Gastrointestinal: concerning the stomach and intestines

Genetically: concerning heredity and inherited characteristics

Genital: concerning the genitalia

Genitalia: literally all the reproductive organs but, in a woman, usually used to mean the external genitalia—the vulva and vagina

Goiter: a swelling of the thyroid gland

Gynecology: the science of diseases of women; **gynecologist:** a specialist in women's diseases

Hallucination: a false perception—seeing, hearing, tasting, smelling, or feeling something that is not there

Hematuria: blood in the urine

Hemorrhage: bleeding

Hepatitis: inflammation of the liver

Histamine: a chemical manufactured by the body that is involved in allergic reactions and also in the normal function of the nervous system

Hormone: a substance secreted by an endocrine gland (e.g., thyroid, ovaries) directly into the bloodstream that has an effect on the function of other organs

Hormonelike: acting in a similar way to a hormone but not produced by an endocrine gland

Hyperthyroid: overactivity of the thyroid gland

Hypertrophy: overgrowth

Hyperventilation: overbreathing

Hypoallergenic: having a low capacity for causing allergic reactions

Hypothermia: a condition in which the body temperature drops below normal

Hypothyroid: underactivity of the thyroid gland

Hysterectomy: surgical removal of the womb, with or without the ovaries

Idiopathic: having an unknown origin

Immune system: the system that protects the body against invasion by bacteria and viruses and, probably, cancer, and that is made up of the lymphatic system and the white blood cells together with the substances that they produce (see also Antibody)

Immunosuppressant: a substance that suppresses the activity of the immune system

Incision: a cut

Interstitial: within the tissues

Intertriginous areas: skin folds

Intervertebral: between the vertebrae

Intraabdominal: within the abdomen

Intraepithelial: within or into the skin

Intramural: within the walls

Intramuscular: within or into the muscles

Intrauterine: within the uterus (womb)

Intravenous: within or into the veins

Jaundice: yellowing of the skin caused by bile in the blood

Keratin: a hard dead substance that forms the basis of hair and nails and that is found in the top layer of skin cells

Keratolytic: a substance that smooths the skin surface by encouraging the shedding of superficial scales

Ketoacidosis: a condition occurring in diabetics who have an excess of sugar in the blood; this is broken down into acidic compounds called ketones, which may cause vomiting, abdominal pain, kidney failure, coma and, if untreated, death

Labyrinthitis: inflammation of the inner ear

Laryngeal: concerning the larynx

Larynx: the voice box

Laser: an extremely concentrated beam of light capable of cutting or burning tissue (see also Cautery)

Lateral: at the sides

Ligament: a strong fibrous band that supports an organ or holds bones together

Lipodermatosclerosis: a fan-shaped flare of blood vessels over the ankle bone, associated with abnormal firmness and darkening of the skin, resulting from incompetent valves in the veins and pooling of blood

Lobule: a small, round section of an organ

Low-grade: subacute; usually used to describe an infection that is causing a minimum of symptoms

Lymphatic system: a system of vessels through which flows lymph, a colorless fluid containing white blood cells that are involved in the process of immunity

Lymph glands: patches of tissue that act as sieves, catching invaders (such as bacteria, viruses, and cancer cells) in the lymphatic system in an attempt to prevent further spread

Maceration: waterlogging of skin, which looks white and soggy

Maintenance therapy: treatment to keep a patient with a chronic disease in good health and to prevent a relapse into the disease state

Malignant: harmful; something that without treatment is likely to have a fatal outcome

Mastectomy: surgical removal of a breast

Mastoid: the section of the skull behind the ear that contains pockets of air and that communicates with the middle ear

Membrane: a thin layer of tissue, often acting as a lining to a body cavity

Meningitis: inflammation of the meninges, the membranes that cover the brain and spinal cord

Menorrhagia: excessively heavy, frequent, or prolonged periods

Menstrual: concerning the periods

Menstruation: the monthly periods

Micturition: passing water

Mucosa: see Mucous membrane

Mucous membrane: a thin layer of tissue containing glands that secrete mucus

Multinodular: having many nodules

Murmur: an abnormal heart sound or sound heard over a large artery

Musculoskeletal: concerning the muscles and bones

Myelogram: an X-ray in which a radioopaque substance is injected into the spinal canal to outline the spinal cord and show up any abnormalities of the intervertebral discs

Myringotomy: a cut made in the eardrum to release fluid behind it

Nail bed: that part of the end of the finger from which the nail grows

Neoplasia: literally new growth, usually applied to cancer

Neurological: having to do with the nerves and nervous system

Neuropathy: a disease affecting the nervous system

Neurosis: a mental condition in which the patient still retains touch with reality (c.f. Psychosis)

Neurotransmitter: a chemical that carries messages across the gap between two nerve cells and is essential to the normal functioning of the nervous system

Nocturnal: by night

Nodule: a swelling

Nucleus: the central part of each cell, containing all the equipment needed for the function of that cell, together with the chromosomes

Ophthalmoscope: an instrument for looking at the back of the eyes

Optic disc: the point at which the optic nerve enters the eyeball, seen at the back of the eye as a round, pale area

Ossicles: the tiny bones in the middle ear that transmit vibrations to the inner ear

Otoscope: an instrument for looking into the ears
Ovulation: the production of an egg by the ovary

Pacemaker: a device that, by means of an electrical stimulus, can keep the heart rhythm regular in a diseased or damaged heart
Pancreas: an organ in the upper part of the abdomen that secretes digestive juices into the intestines and insulin into the bloodstream
Pancreatitis: inflammation of the pancreas
Paranoid: having a fear of persecution
Partial thyroidectomy: removal of part (usually one half) of the thyroid
Pedunculated: on a stalk
Pelvic cavity: that part of the abdomen lying within the pelvis
Pelvis: the hip bones; **pelvic:** concerning the pelvis
Percutaneous: through the skin
Perineum: the area between the legs
Peritonitis: inflammation of the peritoneum, the membrane that lines the abdominal cavity and covers its contents
Pessary: something inserted into and retained within the vagina
Phlebitis: inflammation of the veins
Phlebography: an X-ray taken of veins into which a radioopaque venography substance has been injected
Phlegm: mucus, catarrh, sputum
Physiology: the way in which the body works
Pigment: a colored substance
Pinna: the ear flap
Placebo: a substance that has no medical action (e.g., a sugar pill)
Placenta: the structure joined to a growing fetus through its umbilical cord and by which it receives its blood supply; the afterbirth
Plain X-ray: an X-ray taken without any contrast medium being used (i.e., no radioopaque substance is given beforehand)
Polyp: a tumor (usually benign) attached to the body by a stalk
Posterior: at the rear
Postpartum: after birth
Precursor: that which goes before; something from which another substance is derived
Prodromal: before the main illness
Progestogen: a substance having similar properties to progesterone
Progesterone: one of the hormones secreted by the ovaries

Prognosis: forecast of the likely outcome of a disease

Prolapse: dropping down

Prophylactic: preventive

Psychogenic: arising from the mental state

Psychomotor: the effect of the nervous system or the mind on movement

Psychosis: a mental condition in which the patient loses touch with reality

Purulent: involving pus

Pyloroplasty: cutting of the pylorus (the ring of muscle at the outlet of the stomach) to allow food to flow more freely into the duodenum

Radioopaque: opaque to X-rays, showing up as white on an X-ray

Rectum: lowest part of the colon

Referred pain: irritation of a nerve, which causes pain lower down the nerve as well as at the actual site of irritation

Remission: a state in which the symptoms and signs of a disease disappear, although they may return later

Renal: concerning the kidneys

Renal colic: pain caused by a kidney stone

Reproductive organs: the vagina, uterus, tubes, and ovaries in a woman; the penis, testes, and the vas (tube) linking them in a man

Resection: cutting out

Respiratory: concerning the lungs and breathing

Retina: the light-sensitive cells at the back of the eye

Retinopathy: disease affecting the retina

Retrograde: backward

Retropubic: behind the pubic bone, which forms the anterior part of the hip bones

Saline: a salt solution, used as the basis for most intravenous drips

Sciatica: pain running from the back down the leg

Sclerosing: hardening

Sebaceous cyst: a cyst arising in the skin and containing a thick oily substance

Second line: not first choice (usually in reference to drugs); backup where other treatments have failed

Septicemia: infection of the bloodstream, blood poisoning

Serum: the fluid part remaining after blood has clotted

Sign: see Symptom

Sphincter: a ring of muscle that keeps an orifice (such as the anus) shut but that can relax to allow it to open

Sphincterotomy: cutting through a sphincter

Spinal cord: a continuation of the tissue of the brain, contained within the vertebral column and giving rise to the nerves that supply the body below the head

Spleen: an organ situated in the upper left side of the abdomen that can bleed profusely if ruptured, threatening life; it can safely be removed since it is not essential to the normal workings of the body

Staphylococci: a common type of bacteria

Stenosis: narrowing

Stools: the waste product eliminated from the bowels

Streptococci: a common type of bacteria

Stress fracture: a broken bone caused by continued stress being put on it, often occurring in the foot.

Stress incontinence: a condition in which anything that raises the intraabdominal pressure (such as coughing) will cause a leakage of urine

Subacute: less dramatic than acute but usually not as long term as chronic

Submucosal (or submucous): below the lining (mucosa) of an organ

Subserosal (or subserous): below the outer covering (serosa) of an organ

Suppository: something inserted into and retained within the rectum

Suppurative: pus-forming

Suspension: a liquid in which something is evenly mixed although not dissolved

Symptom: what the patient feels; often used in a wider sense to include what the doctor sees (which, strictly speaking, is a sign); thus, pain in the eye is a symptom but redness of the eye is a sign

Syndrome: a condition in which certain well-defined symptoms and signs appear together, although not all cases are necessarily due to the same cause—or the cause may be unknown

Synovectomy: removal of the synovial membrane within a joint

Systemic: generalized (e.g., systemic treatment is distributed to all the tissues by the bloodstream, a systemic illness affects the whole body)

Tendon: a fibrous band that attaches a muscle to a bone

Testes: the organs that produce sperm and are contained within the scrotum

Thoracic: concerning the chest

Thyrotoxicosis: overactivity of the thyroid gland

Tinnitus: ringing in the ears

Tolerance: when applied to drugs, means a state in which a higher dose is needed in order to achieve the same effect

Topical: applied to the skin

Torsion: twisting

Tourniquet: a very tight band that cuts off the blood supply to part of the body

Trachea: the windpipe

Transhepatic: through the liver

Transurethral: through the urethra

Transvesical: through the bladder

Trauma: injury

Tumor: a swelling, not necessarily malignant

Ulna: one of the bones of the forearm; **ulnar:** to the side of the ulna (the side of the little finger)

Ultrasound: the use of an instrument that sends an ultrasound beam through the body tissues and analyzes the beam they reflect back; in some cases it can be used instead of X-ray

Umbilicus: the navel

Unipolar depression: depression in which the patient never has episodes of mania

Urgency: a condition of having to pass water as soon as one feels the need or risk incontinence

Urinary tract: the kidneys, ureters, bladder, and urethra

Uterine: concerning the womb

Uterus: the womb

Vagina: the female front passage, leading to the uterus

Vagotomy: cutting of the vagus nerve to reduce acid secretion in the stomach

Varices: dilated veins (plural of varix)

Vasectomy: cutting of the vas or tube that leads from the testes to the penis, to prevent sperm from getting through

Vertebra: one of the individual bones making up the spine or backbone

Vertigo: dizziness

Vesicoureteric reflux: a condition in which urine can flow backward from the bladder up the ureter due to a faulty valve mechanism

Virus: a tiny organism, smaller than a bacterium, that causes disease by getting into the body cells; it is not affected by antibiotics

Vulva: the area surrounding the vagina

Whitlow: inflammation around a fingernail

INDEX OF COMPLEMENTARY REMEDIES

GENERAL INDEX